PRACTICAL PRINCIPLES OF CYTOPATHOLOGY

To Alexander, David, and Jacqueline
Love, Dad

PRACTICAL PRINCIPLES of CYTOPATHOLOGY

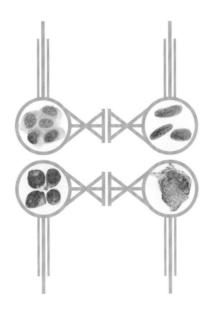

Richard M. DeMay, MD
Professor of Clinical Pathology
Director of Cytopathology
University of Chicago

ASCP Press
American Society of Clinical Pathologists
Chicago

Publishing Team
Jeffrey Carlson (design/production)
Michael Methe (digital imaging/production)
Philip Rogers (editorial)
Joshua Weikersheimer (publisher)

Author's Acknowledgments
Thanks to the outstanding staff of the section of cytopathology, Sandra Reina,
Traci Jennings, Patsy Lin, Sean Macleish, Jodi Ozan, Ann Marie Maslan, and
Joan Hives; to my current fellow, Sam Gupta; to my valued colleagues, including
(but certainly not limited to) Jim Vardiman, John Anastasi (also for figure 13.1),
Cyril Abrahams, Barb Doss, John Hart, Wendy Recant, and Tony Montag
(the font of pathology knowledge); most especially to my friend and associate,
Ward Reeves, whose hard work and good humor made it possible for me to
write this book; to Joshua Weikersheimer, simply the best, and finally, to
Mary King, a continuing source of inspiration.

Notice
Trade names for equipment and supplies described herein are included as
suggestions only. In no way does their inclusion constitute an endorsement or
preference by the American Society of Clinical Pathologists. The ASCP did not
test the equipment, supplies, or procedures and therefore urges all readers to
read and follow all manufacturers' instructions and package insert warnings
concerning the proper and safe use of products.

Library of Congress Cataloging-in-Publication Data
DeMay, Richard M.
Practical principles of cytopathology / Richard M. DeMay.
p. cm.
Includes index.
ISBN 0-89189-437-3
1. Pathology, Cellular. 2. Cytodiagnosis. I. Title.
[DNLM: 1. Pathology. 2. Cytodiagnosis. QZ 4 D373p 1999]
RB43.D453 1999
616.07—dc21
DNLM/DLC   98-32155
for Library of Congress   CIP

03 02 01 00 99   5 4 3 2 1

Printed in the United States.

Table of Contents

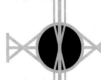

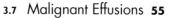

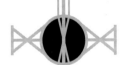

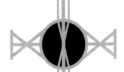

Preface

vade mecum *n*: **1**: a portable, practical reference **2**: go with me

Evade, invade, pervade—ever on the go with a prefix to steer us. This book is for those with limited time and immediate information needs. Going against the trend for ever larger information sources in print, this book follows instead the trend from desktop to palmtop.

A *vade mecum* is supposed to be concise and *at hand*: in *Practical Principles of Cytopathology* readers can expect *handy* information. The surgical pathologist needing quick cytomorphologic consult will find it here—and in a form easily carried to a colleague's office. The resident with only a few months' time to master the essentials can fall asleep (when exhaustion strikes) without fear of injury when this book falls!

The Art & Science of Cytopathology is encyclopedic: it comprises synoptic atlases, thousands of references, etc. *Practical Principles of Cytopathology* dispenses with atlases and references, offering instead what the diagnostician needs *at hand*, without urging more going to yet another set of pages. Nonetheless, because cytopathology is a visual art and science, we've built in over 1200 images, each of them *at hand* within a page of the information you are seeking.

Rabbi Hillel was once challenged to teach the whole Torah while his challenger stood on one foot. He replied, "That which is hurtful to you do not do to others. That is the whole of the Torah, now *go study*." We've striven to make *Practical Principles of Cytopathology* a wealth of information for the hand (we can't stop to stand on one foot), but when further study is needed, *The Art & Science of Cytopathology* stands ready.

Mac DeMay
Author

Joshua Weikersheimer
Publisher, ASCP Press

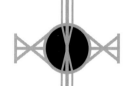

The Pap Smear

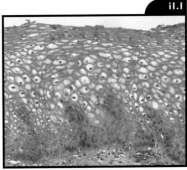
Normal histology

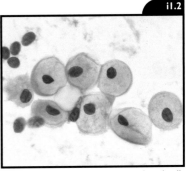
Parabasal cells

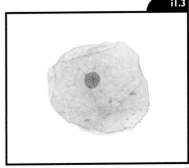
Intermediate cell

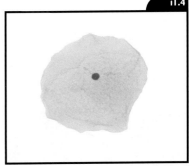
Superficial cell

Pap smears are the most effective cancer prevention tests ever invented. Before Pap smear screening was introduced into clinical practice, carcinoma of the cervix was a leading cause of cancer-related deaths in women. Today, cervical cancer mortality has been reduced by as much as 99% among women who are screened regularly. Unfortunately, despite its outstanding success, the Pap smear is not perfect. Problems occur at every level, from failure of women to get regular Pap tests in the first place, to sampling and interpretation errors, and finally, to inadequate clinical follow-up. Still, no other test, indeed no other public health measure of any kind, has been as effective as the Pap smear in eradicating cancer.

1.1 Squamous Epithelium

1.1.1 Normal Cytology

The normal maturation of the human vaginal mucosa proceeds from basal to parabasal to intermediate to superficial cells (the Icons). The names for these cells correspond to their histologic location in a fully mature, nonkeratinized, stratified squamous epithelium |i1.1|.

Basal cells are small undifferentiated cells that resemble small histiocytes. Basal cells are seldom identified in the Pap smear, except in severe atrophy, in which case they usually are associated with the next most mature cell type, parabasal cells.

Parabasal cells are the first cells to acquire squamous features, ie, dense cytoplasm and distinct cell boundaries (the two hallmarks of squamous differentiation) |i1.2|. The cytoplasm is moderately abundant. The nucleus of a parabasal cell is round to oval, with smooth nuclear membranes and fine chromatin. The nuclear area averages 50 μm^2.

Intermediate cells are the next cell type |i1.3|. The nucleus of the intermediate cell is a key reference for nuclear size and chromatin quality (staining and texture). The normal intermediate nucleus averages 35 μm^2 (about the size of an RBC), and, by definition, its chromatin is normochromatic and has a fine texture. Any squamous nucleus that is significantly larger and more hyperchromatic than an intermediate cell nucleus is probably dysplastic. Intermediate cells range in overall size from slightly larger than parabasal cells to the size of superficial cells. The cytoplasm of mature intermediate cells is abundant, thin, and transparent.

Superficial cells are the final cell type in a normal nonkeratinizing squamous mucosa |i1.4|. Superficial cells are

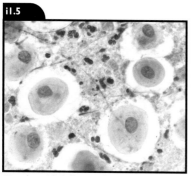

i1.5

Atrophy with inflammation

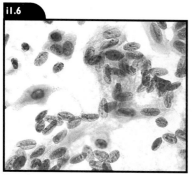

i1.6

Atrophy—transitional metaplasia

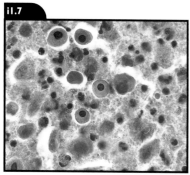

i1.7

Atrophy—pseudokeratinization

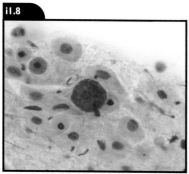

i1.8

Atrophy—blue blob

almost identical in appearance to the most mature intermediate cells, except that their nuclei are pyknotic (India ink dot–like). Also, the cytoplasm tends to stain pink, while intermediate cell cytoplasm tends to stain blue, but the color reaction is not reliable in distinguishing the two cell types.

1.1.2 Hormonal Cytology

To evaluate maturation of the vaginal mucosa, cells are obtained from the midvagina by gentle scrape to sample recently exfoliated cells. (Note: An ordinary Pap smear is obtained by vigorous scrape.) For the examination, 300 single, not clustered, cells are evaluated, and the results are written as a ratio of parabasal to intermediate to superficial cells, eg, 0:80:20, which is known as the maturation index, or MI. In this example, the Pap smear was dominated by 80% intermediate cells, with 20% superficial cells and no parabasal cells. For the MI to be valid, there should be no evidence of inflammation or dysplasia, and representatives from only two cell layers should be present. The presence of three cell layers usually indicates inflammation. A complete clinical history, including age, menstrual history, drugs or hormones, radiation or chemotherapy, and so forth, must be provided by the clinician. The report should state whether the MI is or is not compatible with the patient's age and history; the numbers are of secondary importance.

A Pap smear that is dominated by basal/parabasal cells indicates that the mucosa is atrophic |i1.5|. Atrophy is common in the late postmenopausal period, the postpartum period, and during childhood. Syncytial sheets of basal and parabasal cells are characteristic of atrophy. Spindle parabasal cells also are common (transitional metaplasia) |i1.6|. Atrophy can be associated with nuclear enlargement into the range seen in dysplasia, accompanied by mild hyperchromasia. Air drying is common in atrophic smears and contributes to nuclear enlargement. However, the nuclear membranes are uniform, and the chromatin is bland, often smudgy (see atypia of atrophy, p 17). Atrophy commonly is associated with evidence of inflammation ("atrophy with inflammation"), such as evidence of cellular degeneration, including numerous naked nuclei, nuclear pyknosis, pseudokeratinization |i1.7|, abundant inflammation, and a granular basophilic background ("benign diathesis") in which "blue blobs" (mummified parabasal cells) may be identified |i1.8|.

Under the influence of progesterone, the vaginal epithelium matures to the intermediate cell level; intermediate cell predominant maturation is characteristic of the luteal phase (second half) of the menstrual cycle and pregnancy |i1.9|. Under the influence of estrogen, complete maturation of the mucosa to the superficial cell layer can occur; the Pap smear is dominated by superficial cells. This is characteristic of the follicular phase (first half) of the menstrual cycle, peaking at midcycle |i1.10|.

A newborn girl's vaginal mucosa matures to the level of intermediate cells under the (transplacental) influence of her mother's hormones. Within a few weeks after birth, the baby's vaginal mucosa atrophies and remains atrophic until around the time of puberty. Obese women may maintain a mature epithelium into their postmenopausal years because androstenedione, from the adrenal glands, is converted in the peripheral fat into estrone, an estrogen. Similarly, postmenopausal women with cirrhosis can maintain a mature smear pattern due to relative excess of estrogen caused by decreased hepatic catabolism of this hormone. Inflammation can cause nonhormonal maturation of the epithelium (pseudomaturation). Many other things, including drugs such as digitalis, vitamins, radiation, and chemotherapy, can affect the maturation of the vaginal mucosa.

Barr bodies (inactivated X chromosomes) can be evaluated along with the maturation pattern |i1.11|. For example, normal maturation and a normal complement of Barr bodies is normal. But normal maturation also can be seen in testicular feminization syndrome in which the patients, who are XY, do not have Barr bodies. Abnormal maturation can be seen in the presence of Barr bodies, eg, ovarian failure or Down syndrome (trisomy 21), as well as in the absence of Barr bodies, eg, in Turner (XO) syndrome.

1.2 Benign Proliferative Reactions

Benign proliferative reactions include squamous metaplasia and keratosis. Squamous metaplasia ranges from immature to mature; keratosis includes hyperkeratosis and parakeratosis. These proliferative reactions, particularly squamous metaplasia, are the milieu in which precursor lesions of cervical carcinoma may arise, but they are not in and of themselves premalignant.

1.2.1 Squamous Metaplasia

Squamous metaplasia begins with the reserve cell, which has the unique ability to differentiate into either a glandular or a squamous cell. The earliest change, known as reserve cell hyperplasia (RCH), is proliferation of undifferentiated reserve cells underneath the endocervical glandular epithelium. Although commonly seen in tissue, RCH is rarely recognized in the Pap smear |i1.12|.

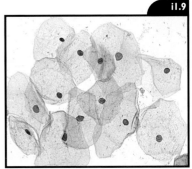
i1.9

Intermediate predominant MI

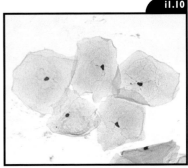
i1.10

Superficial predominant MI

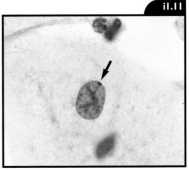
i1.11

Barr body (oil)

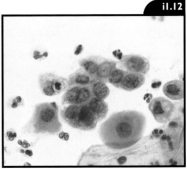
i1.12

Reserve cell hyperplasia

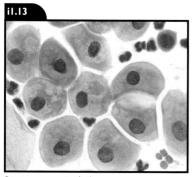
Squamous metaplasia

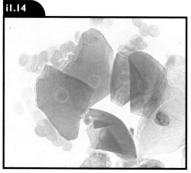
Hyperkeratosis

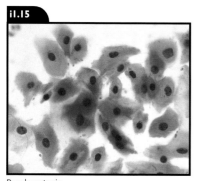
Parakeratosis

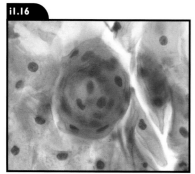
Parakeratosis

Next, the cells start to acquire squamous features, which is the beginning of true squamous metaplasia. In contrast with RCH, this immature form of squamous metaplasia is commonly recognized in Pap smears. Immature squamous metaplastic cells are parabasal cell–sized, with rounded cell borders that are very sharply defined: the cells look as if they were cut out of cardboard |i1.13|. They tend to form loosely aggregated, flat sheets in a characteristic cobblestone pattern. The nuclei are the size of those of parabasal cells (50 μm^2), which is slightly larger than the intermediate nucleus (35 μm^2), but otherwise similar. The cytoplasm is thick and dense and typically stains cyanophilic. Immature metaplasia differentiates to mature squamous metaplasia characterized by intermediate-sized cells that eventually become indistinguishable from native squamous cells.

1.2.2 Keratosis

Keratosis, including hyperkeratosis and parakeratosis, occurs in response to severe stress or irritation, such as a pessary or uterine prolapse. In this condition, the normally nonkeratinizing epithelium "hyperdifferentiates" into a skin-like epithelium by adding two additional cell layers at the surface, namely a granular cell layer, characterized by superficial cells with dark keratohyaline granules in the cytoplasm, and a stratum corneum, characterized by anucleate squames. Anucleate squames are diagnostic of hyperkeratosis |i1.14|. Another surface keratotic reaction, parakeratosis, is characterized by the presence of miniature superficial cells in the Pap smear, which can be seen as single cells |i1.15|, layered strips, or pearls |i1.16|. Although these keratotic conditions are benign, they could mask an underlying squamous abnormality, possibly including cancer.

1.3 Dysplasia and Carcinoma In Situ

The terminology for cervical carcinoma precursor lesions has changed several times through the years. The traditional nomenclature, dysplasia and carcinoma in situ (CIS), has the advantage of being readily understood by many practitioners and being descriptive of the lesions. Cervical intraepithelial neoplasia (CIN) was introduced to emphasize the spectrum of abnormalities that these lesions represent and to help standardize treatment. The latest entry, from the Bethesda System, divides precursor lesions into two groups: low- and high-grade squamous intraepithelial lesions (LSIL and HSIL, respectively). Equivalent terms are mild dysplasia, CIN 1, and LSIL; moderate dysplasia, CIN 2,

t1.1 Comparative Terminology for Cervical Carcinoma Precursor Lesions

Traditional Nomenclature	CIN	The Bethesda System
(Condyloma)	(Condyloma)	LSIL
Mild dysplasia	1	LSIL
Moderate dysplasia	2	HSIL
Severe dysplasia	3	HSIL
Carcinoma in situ	3	HSIL

CIN, cervical intraepithelial neoplasia; LSIL, low-grade squamous intraepithelial lesion; HSIL, high-grade squamous intraepithelial lesion.

and HSIL; severe dysplasia, CIN 3, and HSIL; and CIS, CIN 3, and HSIL |t1.1|. Human papillomavirus (HPV) changes and condyloma are considered LSIL in the Bethesda System |i1.17|. Note that with each succeeding new terminology, there was an amalgamation of the high-end diagnostic categories. Consequently, the traditional nomenclature, dysplasia and CIS, can always be translated into the other terminology, but the reverse is not true.

Carcinoma in situ is defined histologically as a noninvasive abnormal reaction of the squamous epithelium in which, through the full thickness of the epithelium, no squamous differentiation takes place |i1.18|, |f1.1|, |t1.2|. Dysplasia refers to all similar abnormal reactions, but in which some squamous differentiation occurs toward the surface |i1.19|. In dysplasia and CIS, the full thickness of the epithelium is abnormal; the key difference is the presence or absence of any squamous differentiation. The Pap smear samples cells from the mucosal surface. Therefore, in CIS, undifferentiated, abnormal cells are obtained. In dysplasia, abnormal cells also are obtained, but in contrast with CIS, they show varying degrees of squamous differentiation.

Dysplasia also can be graded (mild, moderate, severe), depending on how much squamous differentiation occurs. Normally, undifferentiated basal cells are confined to a single layer at the bottom of the epithelium. In dysplasia, the undifferentiated cells proliferate and ascend above the basal layer. In mild dysplasia, the undifferentiated basaloid cells are confined to the bottom one third of the epithelium, and considerable maturation can occur toward the surface. In moderate dysplasia, undifferentiated basaloid cells occupy at least one third, but no more than two thirds, of the thickness of the epithelium. In severe dysplasia, at least two thirds of the epithelium is replaced with basaloid cells, but some squamous differentiation occurs near the surface. In CIS, the entire thickness of the epithelium is replaced by undifferentiated basaloid cells; there is no squamous differentiation. To reiterate a key point: in all grades of dysplasia, as well as in CIS, the entire thickness of the epithelium is composed of abnormal cells; if this were not true, the Pap smear could not detect precursor lesions less severe than CIS.

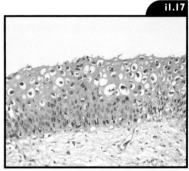

Flat condyloma (LSIL), tissue

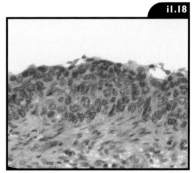

Carcinoma in situ, tissue

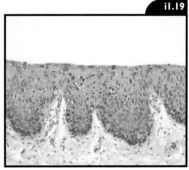

Dysplasia, tissue

f1.1 Precursor Lesions of Cervical Carcinoma

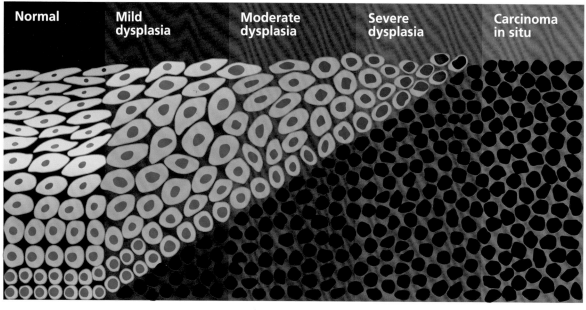

	L SIL	H SIL		
	CIN I	CIN II	CIN III	
Normal	Mild dysplasia	Moderate dysplasia	Severe dysplasia	Carcinoma in situ

t1.2 Mean and Peak Ages for Occurrence of Intraepithelial Lesions

Disease	Mean Age, y	Peak Age, y
Condyloma	28.2	19
Mild dysplasia	29.0	22
Moderate dysplasia	28.3	22
Severe dysplasia	30.3	23
Carcinoma in situ	36.0	30
Squamous cell carcinoma	52.8	39

t1.3 Diagnosing Dysplasia

First: Is the cell dysplastic?
    Look at the nucleus, compare with intermediate cell nucleus
    In essence, "if it's big and it's dark, it's dysplasia"
        Intermediate cell nucleus = 35 μm^2
        Dysplasia = 120-200+ μm^2 (>3 times the size of the intermediate nucleus)

Second: How dysplastic is it?
    Evaluate nuclear/cytoplasmic ratio:
        Higher nuclear/cytoplasmic ratio indicates more advanced dysplasia
        Carcinoma in situ exfoliates hyperchromatic crowded groups

The first step in diagnosing dysplasia in the Pap smear is to evaluate the nucleus |t1.3|. Cervical dysplasia is characterized by nuclear enlargement and hyperchromasia. Compare the nucleus in question with the nucleus of an intermediate cell. In essence: *If it's big and it's dark, it's dysplasia*. Of interest is that the largest nuclei occur in mild dysplasia, with nuclear enlargement four to six times the area of an intermediate cell nucleus (ie, from 120-200+ μm^2) |i1.20|. As the degree of dysplasia advances, cytologic abnormalities also tend to increase, including number of abnormal cells, nuclear membrane irregularities, and abnormalities of the chromatin (coarsening, clumping). Also, the nuclear/cytoplasmic ratios increase, although the overall size of the cell and the nucleus diminish.

After determining that a cell is dysplastic, the next step is to grade the dysplasia |t1.3|. The nuclear/cytoplasmic ratio is a measure of cell maturity and, therefore, a key feature to evaluate when grading dysplasia. As the severity of the dysplasia increases, so does the nuclear/cytoplasmic ratio. In mild dysplasia, relatively well-differentiated cells are obtained from the mucosal surface. Although these mildly dysplastic cells have the largest nuclei, they also have the most abundant cytoplasm and, hence, low nuclear/ cytoplasmic ratios. In severe dysplasia, small, poorly differentiated cells with irregular "raisinoid" nuclei, scant cytoplasm, and high nuclear/cytoplasmic ratios are obtained |i1.21|. The highest nuclear/cytoplasmic ratios are seen in CIS, but instead of squamous cytoplasm with distinct cell borders, there are "hyperchromatic crowded groups" of abnormal cells, ie, three-dimensional aggregates, with undifferentiated cytoplasm, ill-defined ("syncytial") cell borders, and loss of nuclear polarity (chaotic architecture) |i1.22|.

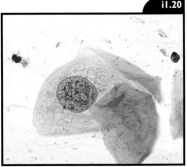
i1.20

Mild dysplasia (LSIL)

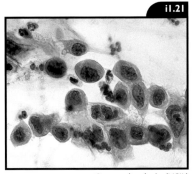
i1.21

Severe dysplasia (HSIL)

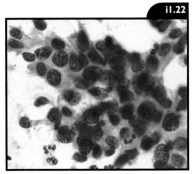
i1.22

Carcinoma in situ (HSIL)

1.3.1 Morphologic Types of Dysplasia

There are two basic morphologic types of squamous dysplasia, metaplastic and keratinizing, which arise in or mimic the

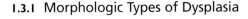

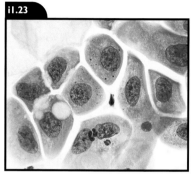

Metaplastic dysplasia (HSIL)

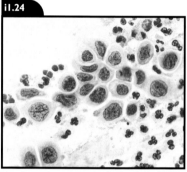

Very immature metaplastic dysplasia (HSIL)

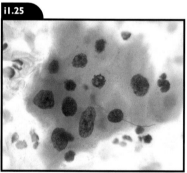

Keratinizing dysplasia (LSIL)

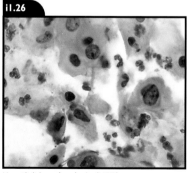

Keratinizing dysplasia (HSIL)

corresponding benign proliferative reactions of metaplasia and keratosis, respectively. Although there may be some differences in prognosis, the principal reason for this subdivision is to recognize various cytologic patterns of dysplasia to facilitate diagnosis.

Metaplastic Dysplasia

Metaplastic dysplasia simply looks like ordinary squamous metaplasia, except that the cells have "dysplastic" (ie, big, dark) nuclei |i1.23|. And, like ordinary metaplasia, metaplastic dysplasia can be further divided into immature and mature types. Immature metaplastic dysplasia resembles immature squamous metaplasia (parabasal-sized cells with big dark nuclei), while mature metaplastic dysplasia resembles mature metaplasia (intermediate-sized cells with big dark nuclei). Although either form of metaplastic dysplasia can range from mild to severe in degree, the immature form of metaplastic dysplasia (or simply, metaplastic dysplasia) is more often high grade than the mature form (also known as large cell, nonkeratinizing dysplasia), which tends to be low grade (ie, mild). Low-grade metaplastic dysplasias can be difficult to distinguish from benign reactive changes, while high-grade metaplastic dysplasias may be overlooked because the cells may be small ("no-see-ums," difficult to spot while screening) or cytologically bland (difficult to interpret; irregular raisinoid nuclear membranes are an important diagnostic clue) |i1.24|. In some cases, high-grade dysplastic cells resemble histiocytes.

Keratinizing Dysplasia

Keratinizing dysplasia usually arises in a background of abnormal keratinization, including hyperkeratosis, parakeratosis, and atypical parakeratosis (also known as pleomorphic parakeratosis). Low-grade keratinizing dysplasia resembles superficial cells with dysplastic (big, dark) nuclei |i1.25|. As the grade of the dysplasia increases, the cells become more pleomorphic, including spindle- and bizarre-shaped cells; "pleomorphic dysplasia" is a synonym |i1.26|. Low-grade keratinizing dysplasia is closely associated with flat condyloma; the keratinized dysplastic cells could be considered "dyskeratocytes," which are, in essence, koilocytes without halos. High-grade keratinizing dysplasia can be difficult to distinguish from invasive keratinizing squamous cell carcinoma in some cases.

1.4 Microinvasive Carcinoma

Microinvasive carcinoma represents a gray area between noninvasive CIS and fully invasive squamous cell carcinoma. Although microinvasive carcinoma is an invasive cancer, it can be

t1.4 Differential Diagnosis: CIS, MicroCA , SCC

	Nucleus		Cytoplasm	Background
	Prominent Nucleoli	Irregular Chromatin Distribution*	Squamous Differentiation	Diathesis
CIS	–	–	–	–
MicroCA	+	+	±	±
SCC	++	++	++	++

CIS, carcinoma in situ; MicroCA, microinvasive carcinoma; SCC, squamous cell carcinoma.
–, absent; ±, may be present; +, present; ++, conspicuous.
* To judge chromatin texture, think of ice cream. Fine, even chromatin, such as in normal intermediate cell nuclei, is smooth and uniform, like chocolate ice cream (smooth chromatin texture). Coarse, evenly distributed chromatin, as may be seen in dysplasia/carcinoma in situ, is like chocolate chip ice cream (uniform chromatin chips, evenly dispersed). Coarse, irregularly distributed chromatin, as seen in invasive carcinoma, is like chocolate chunk ice cream (irregular chromatin chunks, randomly dispersed).

cured with conservative therapy (eg, cone biopsy with adequate margins). The usual cutoff for depth of microinvasion is 3 mm, measured from the basement membrane at the point of invasion (which could be from a deep-lying gland) |i1.27|.

The key cytologic parameters to evaluate relate to the nucleus, cytoplasm, and background; the deeper the invasion, the more the cytology resembles frankly invasive cancer |t1.4|. Look carefully at CIS-like syncytial aggregates |i1.28|. Do many of the nuclei have prominent nucleoli? (First clue to invasion, but non-specific.) Is the chromatin irregularly distributed? (May be subtle at first, but this is the first truly malignant feature of the nucleus.) As invasion progresses, the cells reacquire squamous cytoplasm (dense; well-defined borders), and a tumor diathesis begins to appear in the background of the slide. A tumor diathesis is characterized by a granular background composed of fresh and old blood, fibrin, and necrotic debris. When a diathesis is present, invasive squamous cell carcinoma must be excluded. However, certain benign conditions can be associated with a granular background mimicking a tumor diathesis, eg, severe inflammation (especially due to *Trichomonas* infection), severe atrophy, and pyometra. In practice, microinvasive carcinoma is a histologic, not a cytologic, diagnosis.

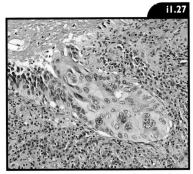

i1.27

Microinvasive carcinoma, tissue

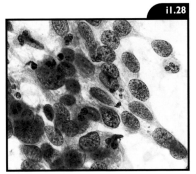

i1.28

Microinvasive carcinoma

1.5 Squamous Cell Carcinoma

In essence, the cytologic features of fully invasive squamous cell carcinoma (SCC) represent a progression of the developments that began in microinvasive carcinoma, ie, prominent nucleoli, abnormal chromatin, squamous cytoplasm, and a tumor diathesis |t1.4|. The cytologic appearance of the tumor depends

t1.5 Characteristic Features of Squamous Cell Carcinomas

	Small Cell	Nonkeratinizing	Keratinizing
Arrangements			
Single cells	+	+	++
Hyperchromatic crowded groups	+	++	+
Cells			
Size	Small	Medium	Large
Variance	Uniform	Relatively uniform	Pleomorphic
Shape	Oval	Round/polygonal	Spindle or bizarre
Cytoplasm			
Density	Delicate	Moderate	Dense
Stain	Basophilic	Cyanophilic	Orange
Nucleus			
Chromatin	Coarse	Moderately coarse	Pyknotic
Macronucleolus	+	++	±
Background			
Diathesis	+	+	±

±, may be present; +, present; ++, conspicuous.

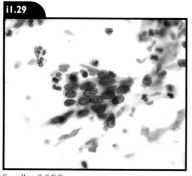

Small cell SCC

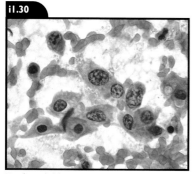

Nonkeratinizing SCC

on the degree of differentiation. Squamous cell carcinoma can be divided into three grades: poorly differentiated (also known as small cell squamous carcinoma), moderately differentiated (also known as nonkeratinizing squamous cell carcinoma), and well-differentiated squamous cell carcinoma (also known as keratinizing squamous cell carcinoma) |t1.5|. There is probably no significant difference in prognosis between keratinizing and nonkeratinizing squamous cell carcinomas; however, small cell (poorly differentiated) carcinomas are more aggressive. Also note that not all poorly differentiated squamous carcinomas are composed of small cells.

Small cell (poorly differentiated) squamous carcinoma is composed of small uniform cells that have only subtle features of squamous differentiation |i1.29|. The malignant squamous cells are present in hyperchromatic crowded groups and singly. They have high nuclear/cytoplasmic ratios and hyperchromatic ovoid nuclei with coarse chromatin; nucleoli may be conspicuous. The cytoplasm is scant, basophilic, and delicate. A tumor diathesis is usually present. These cancers may progress rapidly.

Nonkeratinizing squamous cell carcinoma is characterized by a relatively uniform population of medium-sized malignant cells, present in loose clusters, hyperchromatic crowded groups, and singly |i1.30|. The cells have moderate nuclear/cytoplasmic ratios and definite squamous cytoplasm (ie, dense, with distinct cell boundaries) that typically stains cyanophilic. The nuclei tend to be round and have moderately coarse, irregular chromatin and prominent nucleoli. A tumor diathesis is usually present.

Keratinizing squamous cell carcinoma is characterized by a dispersed population of spindle- to bizarre-shaped cells |i1.31|; aggregates are less common than in nonkeratinizing squamous cell carcinoma. The cytoplasm is heavily keratinized and, most characteristically, orangeophilic (but not all cells stain orange). The nuclei are markedly pleomorphic. The chromatin tends to be dense and pyknotic or coarsely granular and irregularly distributed |i1.32|. Nucleoli are less conspicuous than in nonkeratinizing squamous cell carcinoma (they may be hidden in the condensed chromatin). Although occasional dyskeratotic cells can be seen in nonkeratinizing squamous cell carcinoma, pearls are pathognomonic of keratinization. A tumor diathesis may be lacking because of the characteristic exophytic growth pattern of keratinizing squamous cell carcinoma.

The differential diagnosis of small cell squamous carcinoma includes small cell neuroendocrine carcinoma |i1.33|. Compared with small cell neuroendocrine carcinoma, squamous cell carcinoma has less nuclear molding, but coarser chromatin, more prominent nucleoli, and denser cytoplasm, and crush artifact is minimal. The differential diagnosis of nonkeratinizing squamous cell carcinoma includes adenocarcinoma |i1.34|. Compared with adenocarcinoma, squamous cell carcinoma tends to have denser chromatin, less prominent nucleoli, and denser cytoplasm but lacks acinar formation, cytoplasmic secretory vacuoles, and evidence of mucin production. Keratinizing squamous cell carcinoma may be difficult to distinguish from high-grade keratinizing dysplasia; the presence of numerous abnormal cells, very heavy keratinization, markedly abnormal nuclei, and a diathesis favor invasive carcinoma.

I.6 Cervical Cancer: Further Considerations

Cervical cancer, particularly squamous cell carcinoma, is caused, at least in part, by a virus (HPV), the same virus that causes condyloma. Epidemiologic evidence suggests that a woman is most susceptible to this infectious agent at a young age and that the development of cancer requires long continued exposure. Thus, early age of first intercourse, promiscuity, and intercourse with high-risk males are important risk factors. High-risk males are promiscuous, have penile condylomas (which may be invisible to the naked eye), or have had other partners with cervical neoplasia. Smoking is considered a cofactor in the development of cervical carcinoma; products of cigarette smoke have been found in cervical mucus. Several other cofactors also have been identified, including immunocompetency (related to transplants, AIDS, etc), trauma, pregnancy, hormones (eg, diethylstilbes-

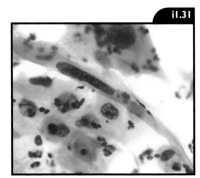

Keratinizing SCC

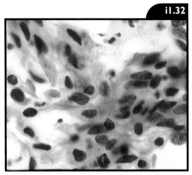

Keratinizing SCC

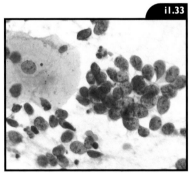

Small cell neuroendocrine carcinoma

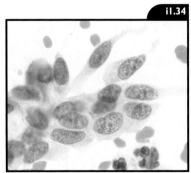

Adenocarcinoma (endocervical)

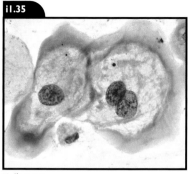

Koilocytes

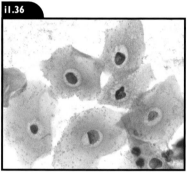

"Trich" halos

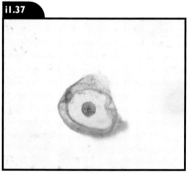

Glycogenated cell

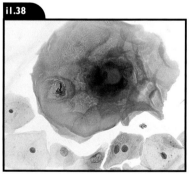

Macrocyte

trol, birth control pills), venereal infections, vitamin deficiencies (A, B, C), and genetic susceptibility.

1.6.1 HPV, Condyloma, and Cervical Cancer

HPV, a member of the papovavirus family, is thought to be a necessary but not sufficient condition for the development of cervical carcinoma. Many studies now support the role of HPV in the development of squamous cell carcinoma, and the molecular biology of viral carcinogenesis is being worked out. The key event seems to be integration of the viral DNA into the host genome, which usurps the host's genetic machinery, causing aneuploidy and uncontrolled cellular proliferation. However, the mere presence of virus is insufficient for the development of cancer. In fact, the virus very commonly infects the female genital tract, yet relatively few women develop cancer. There are dozens of viral types, and low-risk (eg, 6, 11) and high-risk (eg, 16, 18) types have been identified. However, currently, it is not clinically important to know *if* virus is present, let alone its type. Moreover, aneuploidy can be found in low-grade lesions with little tendency to progress. What is clinically important is the lesions the viruses produce. Any virus associated with a high-grade lesion has the proven ability to induce cellular anaplasia. Thus, morphology is still the most important indicator of outcome, even though the prognosis for *individual* patients cannot be predicted.

Koilocytes are diagnostic of HPV infection and condyloma, which is considered an LSIL in the Bethesda System |i1.35|. Of course, the mere presence of koilocytes does not exclude a more advanced lesion, including cancer. By definition, koilocytes have a large cytoplasmic vacuole surrounding the nucleus, and the nucleus is abnormal (big and dark, ie, dysplastic) |t1.6|. The cytoplasm peripheral to the vacuole is condensed.

Important differential diagnostic possibilities include inflammatory ("Trich") halos |i1.36|, which are smaller and less sharply defined, surrounding inflamed nondysplastic nuclei, and glycogenated cells, which contain yellow-staining glycogen and normal nuclei |i1.37|. Bona fide koilocytes are usually found in a background of dysplasia, often keratinizing type (dyskerato-

t1.6 Characteristics of Koilocytes

Cytoplasmic vacuoles
   Sharp, dense periphery
Nuclear dysplasia
   Big, dark
Background
   Dyskeratocytes

cytes). Other minor (nondiagnostic) criteria also are identified frequently, including macrocytes |i1.38|, polka-dot cells |i1.39|, kite cells |i1.40|, two-tone cells, cracked cells, balloon cells, and hyaline cytoplasmic inclusions, as well as binucleation, spindle nuclei, chromatin smudging, and karyorrhexis. The presence of these minor criteria should alert the cytologist to search carefully for diagnostic findings.

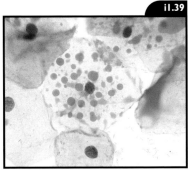

Polka-dot cell

1.7 Atypical Squamous Cells of Undetermined Significance

Atypical squamous cells of undetermined significance, or ASCUS, is a potpourri of abnormalities that includes cells that fall qualitatively or quantitatively short of being diagnostic of a squamous intraepithelial lesion or are of uncertain nature. Also included in the ASCUS category are squamous atypia and atypical squamous metaplasia—entities that are actually of fairly well-defined clinical significance. Squamous atypia and atypical squamous metaplasia are minimally dysplastic lesions, which could be thought of as "CIN 1/2." They occur in mature and immature squamous cells, respectively. Unfortunately, in practice, ASCUS has become a wastebasket diagnosis used almost indiscriminately for "funny-looking" cells, and some cytology laboratories have practically abandoned this nebulous category.

Squamous atypia resembles intermediate or superficial cells with nuclear enlargement falling short of dysplasia (ie, two to three times vs four to six times the area of an intermediate cell nucleus) |i1.41|. The nuclei have smooth or only slightly irregular nuclear membranes, and the chromatin varies from almost normal appearing to distinctly hyperchromatic. In essence, the cytoplasm is normal, but the nucleus is sick ("dyskaryosis"). The differential diagnosis is marked inflammation vs LSIL. Mild dysplasia tends not only to have bigger nuclei, but the cytoplasm also appears thick and dense ("immature").

Atypical squamous metaplasia resembles typical parabasal-like squamous metaplasia but has abnormal nuclei similar to those described for squamous atypia |i1.42|. In practice, atypical squamous metaplasia is a difficult diagnosis: it can be very hard to distinguish atypical squamous metaplasia from either benign metaplasia or HSIL (metaplastic dysplasia).

The theoretical importance of a diagnosis of squamous atypia or atypical squamous metaplasia is that it identifies a patient at high risk for developing squamous intraepithelial lesions; the practical importance is that many women (>25%) already have a squamous lesion, often (>10%) high-grade.

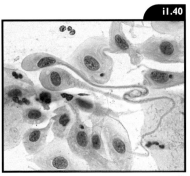

Kite cells

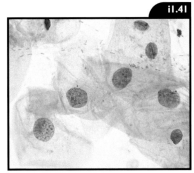

Squamous atypia

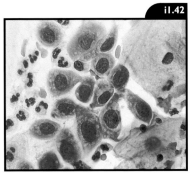

Atypical squamous metaplasia

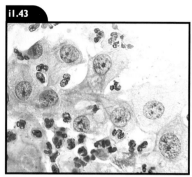

Inflammatory change

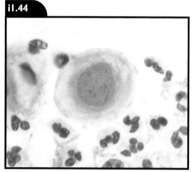

Inflamed red chromatin

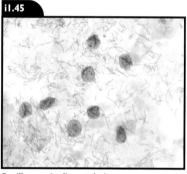

Bacillus vaginalis, cytolysis

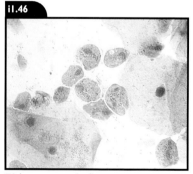

Trichomonas vaginalis

1.8 **Benign Cellular Changes**

Distinguishing inflammatory change (inflammatory "atypia") from dysplasia is one of the most common everyday problems in cytology. The essential difference between inflammatory atypia and dysplasia is the nucleus: remember, if it's big and it's dark, it's dysplasia. In contrast, although inflammatory change can cause slight nuclear enlargement and hyperchromasia, they are usually less marked than what is seen in dysplasia (usually less than twice the area of an intermediate cell nucleus). The chromatin typically appears fine, pale, and uniform |i1.43|. A peculiar feature is the tendency of the inflamed chromatin to "shine red" |i1.44|, while dysplastic chromatin tends to stain dark blue. The presence of nucleoli, which can be single or multiple, suggests inflammatory change (nucleoli are unusual in exfoliated dysplastic cells). Inflamed nuclei often are degenerated (pyknotic, karyorrhectic). A common feature of inflammatory change is the formation of perinuclear halos. These are often—but not always—related to *Trichomonas* infection; the designation "Trich halos" is apt because they may trick the unwary into a diagnosis of condyloma by mimicking koilocytes |i1.36|. In contrast with koilocytes, inflammatory halos are smaller and the nuclei do not appear dysplastic (big, dark), although they frequently appear inflamed. Inflamed cells with cytoplasmic pseudokeratinization (eosinophilia, orangeophilia) and mild nuclear enlargement and hyperchromasia can mimic low-grade keratinizing dysplasia. Again, this change is particularly common in—but not limited to—*Trichomonas* infection. Some other features that can be seen in inflammation are nuclear and cytoplasmic degeneration, including vacuolization; cytoplasmic polychromasia; and a dirty, inflammatory background that can mimic a tumor diathesis.

Some important points to keep in mind: inflammatory change usually mimics low-grade, not high-grade, dysplasia; inflammatory change and dysplasia frequently coexist; and patients with "only" inflammatory change, particularly when persistent, are at increased risk of having dysplasia.

1.8.1 Specific Infections

Bacillus vaginalis, Döderlein bacillus, is actually a mixed bag of rod-shaped organisms that comprise the normal vaginal flora |i1.45|. These organisms, also known as lactobacilli, attack intermediate cells for their glycogen, causing cytolysis, and maintain normal vaginal acid pH by producing lactic acid as a byproduct of glycolysis.

Trichomonas vaginalis is a pear-shaped organism that ranges in size from a parabasal nucleus to a parabasal cell |i1.46|. To be diagnostic, the elliptical nucleus must be identified; red cytoplasmic granules often are present, but the flagella are essentially never identified in Pap smears. The clinical effects of *Trichomonas* range from asymptomatic infestation to severe inflammation.

Leptothrix is a group of long thin organisms (*Lactobacillus, Actinomyces*). When present, they are usually associated with *Trichomonas* (however, the reverse is not true, ie, *Trichomonas* is commonly present without *Leptothrix*).

Candida |i1.47| is recognized as branching pseudohyphae (sticks) and spores (stones). *Candida* is associated with neutrophil lysis, slight hyperkeratosis, and mild nuclear enlargement with slight hyperchromasia that can closely mimic squamous atypia (ASCUS). The presence of these features is a clue to look for *Candida* organisms, which may be sparse. Culture is required to speciate the organism.

Gardnerella vaginalis can be normal flora or can be associated with bacterial vaginosis. *Gardnerella* agglomerates onto random squamous cells, forming a purple, velvety coat; these coated cells provide an important clue to the diagnosis ("clue cells") |i1.48|. When the normal vaginal flora is replaced with mixed coccobacilli, this is reported in the Bethesda System as "bacteria morphologically consistent with shift in vaginal flora." The background is usually clean (ie, free of inflammation), although there is frequently a touch of parakeratosis. Note that clue cells are not necessary to diagnose a shift in flora. The descriptive diagnosis of shift in vaginal flora must be correlated clinically. If the patient is symptomatic, then this finding is compatible with bacterial vaginosis; if not, the finding may be normal for this patient.

Actinomyces is seen in the Pap smear as aggregates of long filamentous organisms, which tend to stain reddish, and are accompanied by fuzzy masses of bacteria living in symbiosis ("dust bunnies") |i1.49|. *Actinomyces* is associated with the use of an intrauterine device (IUD).

Herpes simplex can be asymptomatic or cause painful ulcerating blisters in adults |i1.50|. However, in neonates, herpes can cause life-threatening disease; therefore, the diagnosis of genital herpes is very important in pregnant patients, especially near term. The diagnostic cells are multinucleated, the nuclei mold one another, and the nuclear material marginates, resulting in thick-appearing nuclear membranes and—a key feature—ground-glass chromatin. Intranuclear viral inclusions may be present, particularly in secondary infection.

Chlamydia is an important cause of nongonococcal urethritis or cervicitis and pelvic inflammatory disease. Although certain types of cytoplasmic vacuoles have been associated with chlamydial infection, the Pap smear usually is considered an unreliable method for its diagnosis.

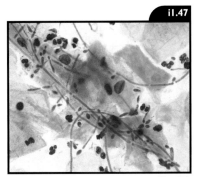

Candida

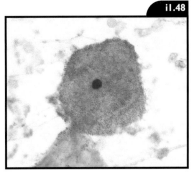

Clue cell

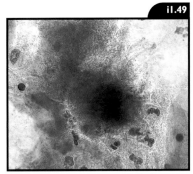

Actinomyces

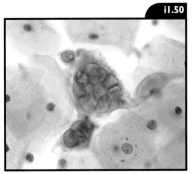

Herpes

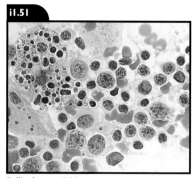

Follicular cervicitis

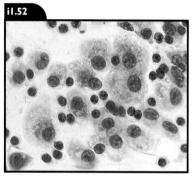

Histiocytes

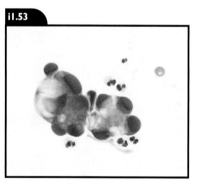

IUD changes

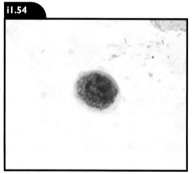

IUD changes (oil)

1.8.2 Other Inflammatory Reactions

Follicular cervicitis looks like an imprint of a reactive lymph node: there is a range of maturation of the lymphocytes with a predominance of small mature lymphocytes, accompanied by immature (follicular center) lymphocytes and tingible body macrophages |i1.51|. Follicular cervicitis is associated with *Chlamydia* infection. Although women of any age can be affected, follicular cervicitis is more commonly observed in Pap smears from older women who have thin, atrophic, overlying epithelium. The differential diagnosis includes malignant lymphoma that, unlike follicular cervicitis, causes gross abnormality of the cervix and is extremely rare in this site.

Histiocytes are a common observation in Pap smears, especially during exodus (days 6-10) |i1.52|. However, histiocytes also are commonly observed during the postpartum period and in postmenopausal women (see risk factors for endometrial carcinoma, p 21). Multinucleated giant cell histiocytes also are common in postmenopausal patients, as well as after radiation therapy or surgery.

IUD-associated changes include cytologic atypia affecting glandular cells and squamous metaplastic cells. Patients with IUDs can shed endometrial cells at any time of the menstrual cycle. Also, patients with IUDs may shed reactive, hypervacuolated glandular or metaplastic cells, with prominent nucleoli, in a clean background, mimicking metastatic adenocarcinoma |i1.53|. Single endometrial cells with high nuclear/cytoplasmic ratios and undulating nuclear membranes can mimic CIN 3 |i1.54|. Important clues to the differential diagnosis of IUD changes with CIN 3 include the following: IUD cells are sparse and exclusively single, do not form hyperchromatic crowded groups, are not associated with dysplasia, and there is a history of IUD use. Psammoma bodies may be present. Patients with IUDs may harbor *Actinomyces* and, very rarely, amebae.

Repair/regeneration is a common reaction to injury |i1.55|. The cells of repair/regeneration can resemble endocervical, squamous, or metaplastic cells or can be indeterminate. Repair is characterized by flat cohesive sheets of well-ordered cells; single reparative cells usually are absent and, when present, are found in the vicinity of the sheets. The nuclei tend to line up in orderly rows ("nuclear streaming"). Although prominent nucleoli, or macronucleoli, typically are present, the chromatin is fine and pale. Mitotic figures may be seen but are not abnormal. An inflammatory reaction often is present in the background, and it is common to observe neutrophils in the cytoplasm of the reparative cells. The major differential diagnosis is with carcinoma, which is characterized by poorly cohesive, disorderly cells with a conspicuous component of atypical single cells. The malignant chromatin is abnormal, often hyperchromatic and irregularly distributed. Nucleoli are not too helpful in this differential diagnosis; similarly, the presence of mitoses does not differentiate repair from cancer unless the mitotic figures are abnormal. Good intercellular cohesion, orderliness, and fine pale chromatin are three of the most helpful features favoring repair.

Atypical repair is characterized by significant nuclear atypia, including crowding, pleomorphism, irregular membranes, abnormal chromatin, and nucleolar pleomorphism, which goes beyond that seen in typical repair |i1.56|. A few single atypical cells may be present but are not numerous, and a tumor diathesis is lacking. Atypical repair is associated with a high risk of squamous (or glandular) lesions; in fact, some cases may represent repair occurring *in* a dysplastic epithelium.

Atypia of atrophy is a common and sometimes difficult diagnostic problem in the Pap smear |i1.57|. Parabasal cells in atrophy are normally variable in appearance and have high nuclear/cytoplasmic ratios; when coupled with nuclear enlargement and hyperchromasia, atypia of atrophy can mimic significant dysplasia. The chromatin in atypia of atrophy, although it may be somewhat hyperchromatic, usually appears degenerated, or "smudgy," rather than crisp and distinct as in dysplasia. Of course, significant nuclear enlargement and hyperchromasia, irregular nuclear membranes, irregular chromatin, and marked pleomorphism (eg, "snakes," "tadpoles") are findings suggestive of dysplasia or cancer. A helpful point to bear in mind is that most squamous dysplasia occurs before menopause (as a rule, dysplasia is not a disease of older women). Also, dysplasia usually occurs in an estrogenic, not an atrophic, environment. Note well, however, that CIS and invasive carcinomas can occur in older women or in an atrophic background. In cases of doubt, an estrogen test may be helpful: merely atypical cells will mature into recognizably benign cells, while neoplastic cells will remain abnormal, although they too may mature somewhat. Another course is simply to refer patients for colposcopy.

Radiation effect is characterized, in essence, by the presence of "macrocytes," ie, cytomegalic cells with enlarged or multiple nuclei and voluminous cytoplasm but relatively normal nuclear/cytoplasmic ratios |i1.58|. The nuclei range from pale to hyperchromatic (but smudgy) and may be vacuolated. The cytoplasm often stains pink and blue (polychromasia or two-tone staining) and also may be vacuolated; the cytoplasmic vacuoles sometimes contain leukocytes. Radiation change is frequently accompanied by repair/regeneration. Radiation effect may regress after therapy or persist for life. Certain chemotherapeutic agents can produce changes similar to those seen with radiation therapy. Macrocytes also can occur in condyloma and vitamin deficiency (folate, B_{12}).

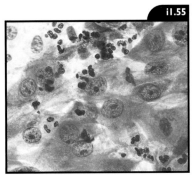
Repair/regeneration

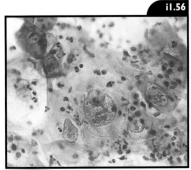
Atypical (radiated) repair

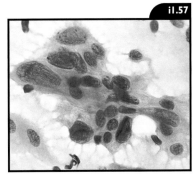
Atypia of atrophy

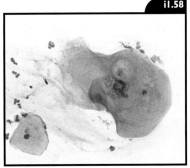
Radiation effect

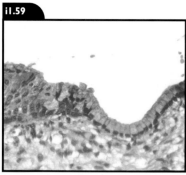

Squamocolumnar junction

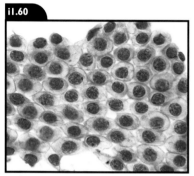

Endocervical cells

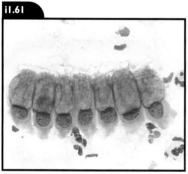

Endocervical cells

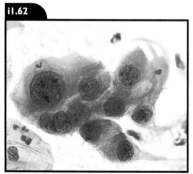

Reactive endocervical cells

Postradiation dysplasia is a serious lesion that sometimes develops after radiation therapy, usually for squamous cell carcinoma. It is probably more closely related to ionizing radiation than to HPV. Patients who develop this lesion are at high risk of recurrence of their cancer, particularly if the postradiation dysplasia occurs within 3 years of therapy. Morphologically, postradiation dysplasia resembles ordinary dysplasia, often the keratinizing type, and is diagnosed by the usual criteria. In practice, mild postradiation dysplasia may be difficult to distinguish from ordinary radiation effect.

1.9 Glandular Epithelium

1.9.1 Endocervical Cells in Health and Disease

The endocervix is normally lined by a single layer of glandular cells |i1.59|. The cervical "glands" are actually mucosal folds that form crypts mimicking glands in histology, but are not true tubuloacinar glands.

Endocervical cells in the Pap smear form cohesive flat sheets or strips of uniform cells. In sheets, the cells line up in orderly ranks and files. Where apposing cells touch, the cytoplasmic membranes appear thick, resulting in the highly characteristic "honeycomb" pattern |i1.60|. Strips of endocervical cells, viewed from the side, form orderly "picket fence" or "palisade" arrangements |i1.61|. Individual endocervical cells are columnar, with nucleocytoplasmic polarity, uniform nuclei, smooth nuclear membranes, and inconspicuous nucleoli. The cytoplasm appears slightly dense or vacuolated. Occasional cells may be ciliated (see tubal metaplasia, p 19).

Reactive endocervical cells are common. Significant nuclear enlargement, hyperchromasia, and prominent nucleoli all can be observed in benign reactive endocervical cells |i1.62|. However, reactive nuclei tend to remain round with smooth or only slightly irregular nuclear membranes and have fine chromatin (although it may be dark). The reactive cells remain fairly orderly, forming flat sheets or strips without significant crowding, stratification, or overlapping. The cytoplasm is abundant with distinct cell borders (honeycomb), maintaining relatively normal nuclear/cytoplasmic ratios. The differential diagnosis includes endocervical glandular neoplasia, which is characterized by abnormalities of architecture (eg, marked crowding, microacinar formation) and nuclei (nuclear elongation, hyperchromasia, coarse chromatin, mitotic figures, high nuclear/cytoplasmic ratios). In contrast, reactive cells tend to "lie flat" and have adequate cytoplasm.

t1.7 Atypical Endocervical Cells

	Favors Reactive	Favors Neoplastic
Architecture	Cells lie flat, minimal crowding Honeycomb Picket fence	Hyperchromatic crowded groups, feathery edges Microacini Stratification
Nuclei (nuclear enlargement, per se, not too helpful)	Rounded Smooth membrane More uniform	Elongated Irregular membrane More pleomorphic
Chromatin	Finer	Coarser, darker
Nucleoli	Can be prominent	In situ: usually none Invasive: usually present
Cytoplasm	More Distinct borders	Less (high nuclear/cytoplasmic ratio) Indistinct borders
Background	Clean/inflammatory	In situ: clean Invasive: diathesis
Other	Cilia	Mitoses

Tubal metaplasia has become a common observation in the Pap smear, probably due to the increased use of the endocervical brush |i1.63|. Tubal metaplastic cells can form hyperchromatic crowded groups, stratified strips, and rosettes, mimicking endocervical glandular neoplasia. However, marked crowding, feathery edges, and mitoses are uncommon in tubal metaplasia. The nuclei of tubal metaplasia tend to be round to oval and have fine, even chromatin. The nuclei of endocervical neoplasia tend to be elongated and have coarse, dark chromatin. Terminal bars and cilia are the most important clues to the diagnosis of tubal metaplasia. Unfortunately, cilia can degenerate, making the differential diagnosis more difficult.

Microglandular hyperplasia is characterized by reactive endocervical cells (a nonspecific finding) and pseudoparakeratosis |i1.64|. Pseudoparakeratosis refers to degenerated endocervical cells, with nuclear pyknosis and cytoplasmic orangeophilia (although staining is variable), mimicking parakeratosis. The cells tend to line up in rows in mucus. The differential diagnosis is parakeratosis. Pseudoparakeratotic cells show nucleocytoplasmic polarity and may be associated with better preserved cells clearly recognizable as endocervical. True parakeratotic cells resemble miniature superficial cells and may be associated with other signs of keratinization.

Endocervical glandular neoplasia is characterized by abnormalities of the glandular architecture and nuclei |t1.7|. An abundance of endocervical cells may be the first clue to the diagnosis of a glandular lesion. Architectural abnormalities, including

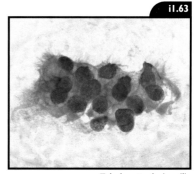
i1.63

Tubal metaplasia, cilia

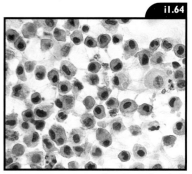
i1.64

Pseudoparakeratosis

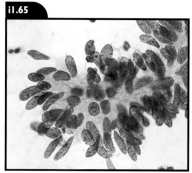

il.65

Adenocarcinoma in situ

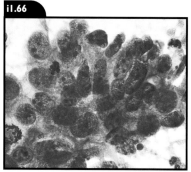

il.66

Endocervical adenocarcinoma

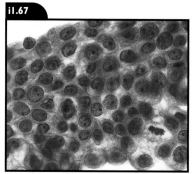

il.67

Adenoma malignum

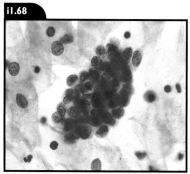

il.68

Endometrial cells

marked nuclear crowding (such as hyperchromatic crowded groups with "feathery edges") and abnormal glandular arrangements (particularly microacinar structures or rosettes), are key findings |il.65|. Nuclear abnormalities include high nuclear/cytoplasmic ratios, nuclear elongation, and coarse, dark chromatin. Mitotic figures in endocervical cells are a highly suspicious finding. The cells are tall columnar, with decreased cytoplasm and indistinct cell borders; the honeycomb pattern is lost. In situ adenocarcinoma, like in situ squamous carcinoma, usually lacks prominent nucleoli. However, a poorly differentiated variant, with vesicular chromatin and prominent nucleoli, can occur that is cytologically similar to invasive adenocarcinoma. Invasive adenocarcinoma is characterized by the presence of single cells, irregular chromatin, prominent nucleoli, and a tumor diathesis |il.66|. Of important note, however, is that invasion cannot be excluded by cytology. A variety of subtypes of endocervical adenocarcinoma are recognized, including endometrioid (identical in appearance to endometrial adenocarcinoma), intestinal (identical to colon cancer), adenoma malignum (minimal deviation tumor, similar in appearance to endocervical repair) |il.67|, clear cell, and serous. Endocervical adenocarcinoma can also undergo squamous differentiation. Endocervical glandular neoplasia frequently coexists with squamous lesions (and it sometimes can be difficult to distinguish squamous CIS from glandular neoplasia).

1.9.2 Endometrial Cells in Health and Disease

(Note: The following discussion refers primarily to *spontaneously exfoliated* endometrial cells rather than to those directly obtained by endometrial aspiration or biopsy.)

Endometrial glandular cells or stromal cells, or both, can be identified in the Pap smear. Endometrial cells are normally present only during the first half of the menstrual cycle; their presence during the second half of the menstrual cycle, and particularly in the postmenopausal period, is considered abnormal shedding—a risk factor for endometrial hyperplasia or neoplasia |t1.8|.

Endometrial glandular cells typically form small clusters (hyperchromatic crowded groups) of degenerated small cells with high nuclear/cytoplasmic ratios and ill-defined cell borders |il.68|. Single cells are uncommon. The nucleus is normally small (about the size of an intermediate cell nucleus), round, and single; nucleoli are small and inconspicuous. The cytoplasm is scant and basophilic, occasionally vacuolated. Ciliated endometrial cells are associated with tubal metaplasia of the endometrium. Two key features to distinguish endometrial cells from endocervical cells are the way the endometrial cells are "packed together" and their

t1.8 Endometrial Cell Pathology

Abnormal shedding
    Second half of cycle or anytime after menopause
    Risk factor for endometrial hyperplasia or neoplasia
    Particularly glandular cells, also stromal cells
Atypical endometrial cells
    Nuclear enlargement (> intermediate cell nucleus)
    Nucleoli present, conspicuous
Notes:
    Shedding of abnormal endometrial cells is always abnormal,
       regardless of relationship to menstrual cycle
    No criteria to distinguish reactive from neoplastic atypia

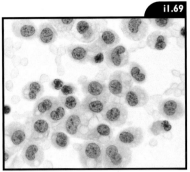

Superficial stromal cells

scant cytoplasm. Endocervical cells usually form looser clusters of larger cells with more abundant cytoplasm.

    Endometrial stromal cells are divided into two types: superficial and deep. Superficial stromal cells are identical in appearance to small histiocytes but typically form loose aggregates ("sticky histiocytes") |i1.69|. Deep stromal cells range from round to spindle shaped, with small oval nuclei and scant cytoplasm |i1.70|.

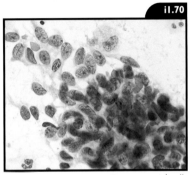

Deep stromal cells

    The most characteristic appearance of endometrial cells is "double-contoured" endometrial cell balls with paler staining glandular cells surrounding darker staining central aggregates of stroma |i1.71|. These cell balls are particularly associated with the phase of the menstrual cycle known as exodus (days 6-10, when stromal histiocytes are most abundant).

    Endometrial adenocarcinoma occurs in two clinically distinct settings. The first, or classic, type of endometrial adenocarcinoma typically occurs in perimenopausal women who tend to be obese, hypertensive, and diabetic. These cancers arise in a background of endometrial hyperplasia, tend to be well differentiated, and have a favorable prognosis. The second type typically occurs in elderly women who are thin and lack the classic risk factors for endometrial carcinoma. Their cancers arise in an atrophic background and tend to be poorly differentiated and aggressive.

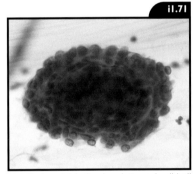

Endometrial gland and stromal cell ball

    Risk factors for endometrial carcinoma observable in the Pap smear include abnormal shedding of endometrial cells (particularly glandular cells, but also stromal, as defined previously); presence of numerous histiocytes (increased histiocytic activity), especially lipophages or siderophages; necrosis and old blood; and increased maturation (postmenopausal). Abnormally shed endometrial cells can be normal or abnormal in appearance. (Note: Shedding of abnormal-appearing endometrial cells is always abnormal, regardless of the relationship to the menstrual cycle.) Nuclear enlargement (greater than an intermediate cell nucleus) and the presence of nucleoli are two key features of abnormal endometrial cells |i1.72|. Nuclear size, hyperchromasia, and nucleoli increase with the grade of the

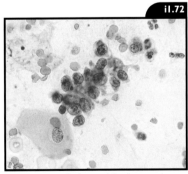

Endometrial adenocarcinoma

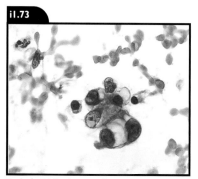

Endometrial adenocarcinoma

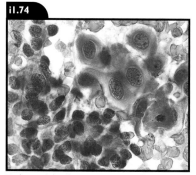

Endometrial AdCA, squamous differentiation

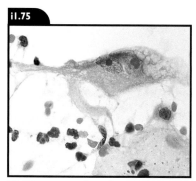

MMMT—sarcomatous element

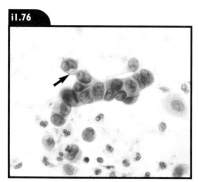

Metastatic breast CA—ICL

tumor |i1.73|. The cytoplasm is typically scant, cyanophilic, and vacuolated. The diathesis in endometrial carcinoma is characteristically basophilic and finely granular (watery), compared with the coarsely granular diathesis associated with invasive squamous or endocervical carcinoma. Compared with endocervical adenocarcinoma, endometrial carcinoma sheds fewer, smaller, more rounded cells with scant cytoplasm and smaller nuclei. Variants of endometrial adenocarcinoma include adenocarcinoma with squamous differentiation |i1.74|, secretory carcinoma, clear cell carcinoma, mucinous carcinoma, and papillary serous carcinoma. "Atypical Endometrial Cells of Undetermined Significance" is used in the Bethesda System lexicon for cases suggestive but not diagnostic of endometrial carcinoma. There are no criteria to help distinguish reactive from neoplastic atypical endometrial cells as there are for atypical endocervical cells.

1.10 Rare Tumors

1.10.1 Sarcoma

Sarcomas are usually fairly easy to recognize as malignant, but they may be difficult to classify. Most cases shed spindle-shaped malignant cells with conspicuous nuclear abnormalities and glassy or fibrillar cytoplasm. Endometrial stromal sarcoma, leiomyosarcoma, and rhabdomyosarcoma, among others, may occur.

1.10.2 Mixed Mesodermal (Müllerian) Tumor

Mixed mesodermal (müllerian) tumor, or MMMT, also known as carcinosarcoma, is the combination of adenocarcinoma and sarcoma |i1.75|. The sarcomatous elements can be homologous to the uterus (eg, stromal sarcoma, leiomyosarcoma) or heterologous (eg, rhabdomyosarcoma, chondrosarcoma), although the sarcomatous elements are thought to derive from epithelium by metaplasia.

1.10.3 Metastatic Malignancy

Most patients with metastatic tumor have a known history of cancer; the Pap smear is rarely the first place metastasis from a nongenital primary tumor is diagnosed. The cells are usually clearly malignant appearing, with features of adenocarcinoma. The most characteristic property, however, is that the background is usually clean (ie, no tumor diathesis); a "floater" may be considered in the differential diagnosis. Metastatic ovarian carcinoma is the most frequent source, followed by gastrointestinal tract, breast |i1.76|, and lung. Other types of tumors, including melanoma |i1.77|, can also metastasize to the cervix.

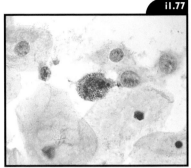
Metastatic melanoma

1.11 Pregnancy-Associated Changes

Pregnancy cannot be diagnosed by the Pap smear, but certain types of cells are associated with pregnancy. During pregnancy, intermediate predominant maturation is normal; characteristically, the intermediate cells are heavily glycogenated and form elongated, boat-like shapes—the so-called navicular cells |i1.78|. Other types of cells, including decidual cells, Arias-Stella reaction, and trophoblasts, may be identified, rarely, in the Pap smear during pregnancy.

Decidual cells are about the size of parabasal cells and have large nuclei that may mimic moderate dysplasia; however, the chromatin usually appears bland to reactive, and nucleoli may be present.

Arias-Stella reaction (hypersecretion with polyploidy) can occur in the endocervical cells, causing nuclear enlargement, pleomorphism, and hyperchromasia |i1.79|.

Trophoblastic cells, either giant cell syncytiotrophoblasts or mononucleated cytotrophoblasts, can also be seen, rarely.

Cockleburrs, which are radiate crystalline arrays formerly thought to be hematoidin crystals, are found in a small number of pregnant (and sometimes nonpregnant) patients |i1.80|. They range up to 100 μm in diameter, have club-shaped spokes that stain reddish to golden brown, and are typically surrounded by histiocytes. Their presence is not associated with any adverse effect on maternal or fetal prognosis.

Cervical neoplasia, ranging from low-grade dysplasia to invasive carcinoma, can and does occur during pregnancy. Cervical neoplasia is diagnosed by the usual criteria. Pregnancy represents an ideal opportunity for Pap smear screening, since most women seek health care at this time. Although there is a high regression rate of dysplasia during the postpartum period, many cases recur.

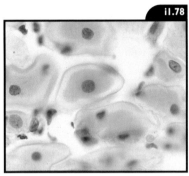
Navicular cells

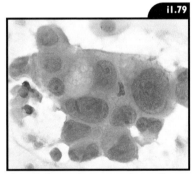
Arias-Stella reaction—progesterone therapy

1.12 Miscellaneous Findings

Glandular cells in patients with hysterectomies are not all that rare. Possible explanations include wrong history (no hysterectomy or supracervical hysterectomy), well-ordered atrophic parabasal

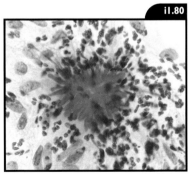
Cockleburr

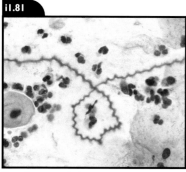

Curschmann spiral

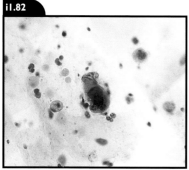

Seminal vesicle

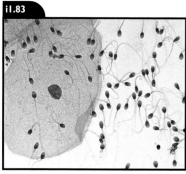

Sperm

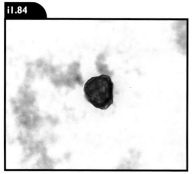

Psammoma body

cells or goblet-like cells, fallopian tube cells, and vaginal adenosis. Well-differentiated adenocarcinoma must be excluded.

Curschmann spirals, identical to those occurring more commonly in respiratory specimens, occasionally can be seen in the Pap smear |i1.81|. These spirals probably form owing to an intrinsic property of the mucus itself and have no special diagnostic significance.

Seminal vesicle cells can be seen—rarely—in the Pap smear, particularly in those of women whose sexual partners are older men |i1.82|. These cells are columnar and can have big "ugly" nuclei mimicking adenocarcinoma. Two important clues to the diagnosis are golden brown cytoplasmic lipochrome pigment and the presence of sperm |i1.83| in the vicinity. The chromatin tends to be smudgy, and the abnormal cells are usually sparse.

Psammoma bodies are a rare observation in Pap smears that can be associated with a wide variety of conditions, ranging from benign (eg, IUD or birth control pill use and genital tract infections) to malignant (eg, papillary serous carcinoma) |i1.84|.

1.13 Summary and Conclusions

The Pap smear is an excellent tool for the prevention of cancer. It is primarily effective in preventing cervical squamous cell carcinoma; it has little proven effect in preventing cervical adenocarcinoma (which is increasingly common) and is completely ineffective in preventing other kinds of cancer. The Pap smear works primarily by detecting precursor lesions of squamous carcinoma, which can then be destroyed (by laser, cryotherapy, or excision) before becoming invasive cancer. The practical problem is that millions and millions of women have these precursor lesions, but only a small minority will progress to cancer if left untreated. Unfortunately, there is currently no way to predict which individual lesions will ultimately progress. Thus, the cost of treating all lesions vs the risk of not treating is an important clinical dilemma.

Moreover, the Pap smear is not perfect. Although it can detect as many as 80% to 90% of squamous precursor lesions, this immediately implies that the Pap smear fails to detect at least 10% of cases. *It is simply not possible to detect all significant cervical abnormalities with the Pap smear.* Problems include sampling and diagnostic errors. Sampling error refers to failure of abnormal cells to be transferred from the patient to the glass slide ("no cells, no diagnosis"). Diagnostic errors include problems with screening (failure to find abnormal cells) and problems with interpretation (failure to properly categorize cells).

In analyzing errors that are made, certain cytologic factors stand out as contributing to false-negative diagnoses. These include the presence of few abnormal cells (particularly <100), small cells (difficult to find), bland cells (difficult to interpret) |i1.85|, and hyperchromatic crowded (HCGs) groups (diagnostically difficult: usually benign, but occasionally malignant) |i1.86|, |i1.87|, |i1.88|. Certain types of tumors are more difficult to detect or diagnose in the Pap smear (eg, adenocarcinomas, adenosquamous carcinomas, lymphoma, or sarcomas, and minimal deviation tumors such as adenoma malignum or verrucous carcinoma). Also, when the smear is obscured by excess exudate or blood, or the cells are poorly preserved, the Pap smear is less effective. Inadequate patient information also contributes to false diagnoses.

Although it is commonly assumed that most diagnostic errors occur because screeners examine too many cases, because they are incompetent, or because they are poorly supervised, the simple truth is that most diagnostic errors occur because cytologists are human and humans make mistakes. Any system that depends on perfect human performance all of the time is doomed to fail at least some of the time, even if the punishment for error is severe. But errors must be kept in perspective. It is thought that only a small percentage, probably less than 3%, of cases of cervical cancer can be traced to misread Pap smears. The vast majority, between 60% and 90% of cases, are related to inadequate screening of the population at risk. In other words, the most important source of error, by far, is failure of women to be screened adequately in the first place.

There are steps that can be taken to help improve cancer prevention. Patients should be informed of the fallibility of the Pap test, the need to be screened regularly, and availability of ancillary diagnostic techniques. Women should have at least three consecutive, satisfactory negative smears before being reassured. High-risk patients should be followed up more closely. High risk includes early onset of sexual activity (teenage), multiple sexual partners, sexually transmitted diseases, and history of abnormal Pap smears. Patients should be informed of steps they can take to reduce their risk of developing cervical cancer, including practicing "safe sex" (eg, abstinence or monogamy—both partners, use of condoms) and not smoking. All abnormal Pap smear results should be carefully followed up, and all suspicious clinical symptoms should be investigated and suspicious lesions biopsied, regardless of the Pap smear results.

In conclusion, the Pap smear can reduce cervical cancer mortality in a *population* of patients who are screened regularly. Unfortunately, it cannot guarantee the prevention of cancer in any *individual* patient, even if screened regularly, much less so if not.

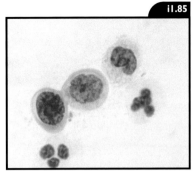

i1.85

Few, small, bland CIN 3 cells (oil)

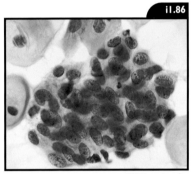

i1.86

HCG—atrophy

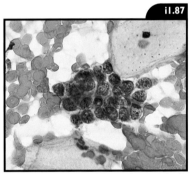

i1.87

HCG—endometrial cells

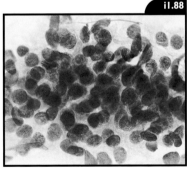

i1.88

HCG—carcinoma in situ

The Respiratory Tract

Respiratory cytology consists of three basic types of exfoliative specimens: sputum, bronchial cytology (including washings and brushings), and bronchoalveolar lavage (BAL). In general, large central tumors are more readily detected by exfoliative methods than small peripheral ones. Squamous and small cell carcinomas are more accurately diagnosed than adenocarcinomas. Poorly differentiated cancers are more readily detected than well-differentiated ones; benign tumors may not shed any diagnostic cells. Most diagnostic problems relate to sampling (false negatives) and inflammation (false positives).

2.1 Diagnostic Respiratory Cytology

2.1.1 Sputum

Sputum is composed predominantly of mucus but also contains cells and other elements. Significant spontaneous sputum production indicates pulmonary disease is present. Most smokers, as well as many patients with bronchogenic carcinoma, have a cough and can produce sputum. Sputum production also can be induced. Unfortunately, sputum screening has not been able to prevent lung cancer in the way that Pap smear screening has prevented cervical cancer.

Sputum is the most readily accessible pulmonary cytology specimen, but it cannot be used to localize lesions. To look for cancer in (spontaneous) sputum specimens, it is best to examine morning pooled secretion. At least three specimens should be submitted to diagnose cancer; a single specimen is unreliable in tumor detection. Fresh specimens are preferred. Although sputum can be preserved in alcohol, it is not recommended because alcohol can shrink the cells, making them more difficult to interpret; it can fail to penetrate mucus, leaving embedded cells poorly fixed; and it can make smearing difficult because it coagulates mucus. Specimens can be prepared by the Saccomanno (blender) technique or by the "pick and smear" technique. The major advantage of the Saccomanno technique is that it concentrates cells, thereby increasing diagnostic yield. Disadvantages include fragmentation of fungal organisms, disruption of glands, dispersion of cells of small cell carcinoma, and creation of potentially infectious aerosols. Postbronchoscopy sputum has the highest sensitivity of any exfoliative respiratory cytology specimen.

2.1.2 Bronchial Cytology

Patients with abnormal sputum cytology should undergo bronchoscopy. Bronchial cytology, including bronchial brushings and washings, is better suited for diagnosis of peripheral lung lesions than sputum cytology. Bronchoscopy also is useful in diagnosing patients with central lesions and negative sputum cytology who are not candidates for surgery.

2.1.3 Bronchoalveolar Lavage

BAL often is used to diagnose opportunistic infections in immunocompromised hosts (eg, patients with AIDS or transplants). BAL also can be helpful in diagnosis of interstitial lung disease, granulomatous disease including sarcoid, hypersensitivity pneumonia, drug-induced pulmonary toxicity, asbestosis, pulmonary hemorrhage, and cancer (particularly when peripherally located).

In a BAL specimen, it is important to look for fungus, *Pneumocystis*, viral changes, hemosiderin-laden macrophages, and malignant cells; some of the specimen also should be cultured. BAL can help separate inflammatory processes in which lymphocytes predominate (eg, sarcoid, hypersensitivity pneumonia including drug reaction, berylliosis) from those in which neutrophils or macrophages predominate (eg, pneumonia, idiopathic pulmonary fibrosis, cytotoxic drug reaction, Langerhans histiocytosis). Hemosiderin-laden macrophages suggest pulmonary hemorrhage but also can be seen in infection and cancer.

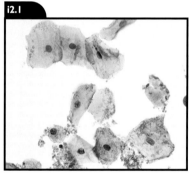

Squamous cells

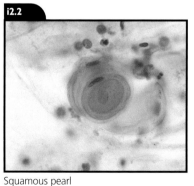

Squamous pearl

2.2 The Cells

Cells obtained in bronchial washings and brushings usually are better preserved than those in sputum. Cells from squamous cell carcinoma in sputum usually are more keratinized (differentiated) than those found in bronchial washing or brushing specimens of the same tumor. All cell types of bronchogenic carcinoma tend to appear less mature in bronchial brush specimens. Although single tumor cells are an important feature of malignancy, occasionally they are not present in bronchial brushing specimens of malignant tumors.

2.2.1 Squamous Cells

Most squamous cells come from the mouth, as contaminants. Their cytologic appearance is identical to that of those in the Pap smear |**i2.1**|. There is a predominance of superficial cells. Anucleate squames and intermediate cells also may be present. Benign pearls |**i2.2**| and occasionally spindle squamous cells may be seen. Reactive or degenerative changes are common: squamous cells originating in the mouth often show cytologic atypia that can cause diagnostic problems.

2.2.2 Glandular Cells

The tracheobronchial tree is lined by a pseudostratified glandular epithelium composed predominantly of ciliated columnar and mucous goblet cells, normally in a ratio of at least 5:1. Other cell types include Clara cells, reserve cells, and Kulchitsky cells. Lymphoid follicles are present in the walls of the bronchi (bronchial associated lymphoid tissue, BALT).

Ciliated Columnar Cells

The most characteristic cytologic feature of ciliated columnar cells is, of course, the presence of cilia on the apical surface, anchored into a terminal bar |**i2.3**|. At the other end, the cells often have a cytoplasmic tail by which they were attached to the basement membrane. The cytoplasm is usually basophilic and homogeneous, with basally oriented, round to oval nuclei. The chromatin ranges from fine to mildly coarse and dark. Small nucleoli may be present. Occasionally, as a nonspecific reaction to injury, the ciliary tufts become detached from the cells (ciliocytophthoria).

Mucous Goblet Cells

Goblet cells degenerate rapidly in sputum but commonly are seen in bronchial cytology. Goblet cells have abundant, vacuolated cytoplasm, filled with mucin |**i2.4**|. The nuclei are uniform and basally located. Mucous goblet cells are more numerous in asthma, chronic bronchitis, bronchiectasis, and allergic conditions. When goblet cells are *abundant,* consider mucinous bronchioloalveolar carcinoma (BAC).

Benign Reactive Atypia, Bronchial Irritation Cells

Reactive atypia can include nuclear enlargement and pleomorphism with abnormally coarse dark chromatin and prominent nucleoli |**i2.5**|. Multinucleation is common |**i2.6**|. Reactive changes are seen more frequently in bronchial than in sputum cytology. In contrast with cancer, benign cells usually have good intercellular cohesion with fewer single cells. There is a range of atypia in benign conditions, whereas in malignant neoplasms there is usually a discrete population of abnormal cells. When a cell is ciliated, it is almost certainly benign, but cilia can degenerate rapidly, eliminating a valuable diagnostic clue.

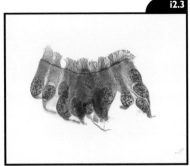

Ciliated bronchial cells

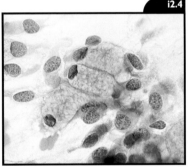

Goblet cells

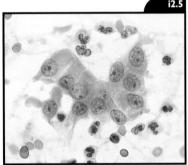

Reactive bronchial cells

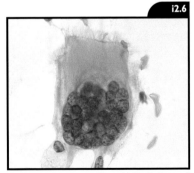

Bronchial irritation cell

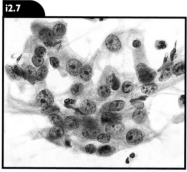

Bronchial repair

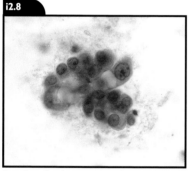

Reactive alveolar pneumocytes

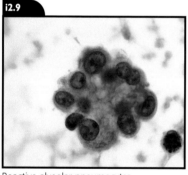

Reactive alveolar pneumocytes

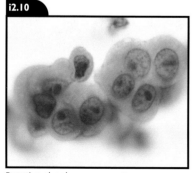

Reactive alveolar pneumocytes

Reparative/Regenerative Bronchial Cells

Repair/regeneration in bronchial cells is similar to that seen in the Pap smear |i2.7|. Cytologic atypia can range from mild to severe, mimicking cancer. Repair is characterized by cohesive, orderly, flat sheets of cells with adequate cytoplasm; single cells are absent or rare. Although the nuclei can be enlarged and pleomorphic with large or irregular nucleoli, the nuclei are not significantly crowded or disorderly, and the nuclear/cytoplasmic ratios remain within normal limits. The chromatin is usually fine, but the nuclei can degenerate, undergoing karyopyknosis, karyorrhexis, or karyolysis. Cancer is characterized by crowded disorderly groups and single atypical cells with hyperchromatic coarse chromatin. Mitotic figures are not too helpful in the differential diagnosis with cancer, unless they are abnormal.

2.2.3 Pneumocytes

Alveoli are lined by two kinds of pneumocytes, type I and type II.

Type I alveolar pneumocytes are flat cells (squamous or membranous) and cover most (> 90%) of the alveolar surface. They usually are not specifically recognized in cytologic specimens.

Type II, or granular, alveolar pneumocytes are columnar cells that normally are found scattered in the alveoli, and they secrete surfactant. They usually are recognized only when they are hyperplastic (reactive).

Reactive (type II) pneumocytes can occur in many conditions, notably pulmonary infarcts and viral pneumonia |i2.8|, |i2.9|, |i2.10|. Markedly reactive pneumocytes can closely mimic adenocarcinoma. Reactive cells occur singly and in clusters; highly atypical reactive cells are usually sparse. The cytoplasm ranges from finely to coarsely vacuolated but usually lacks inclusions. Reactive cells can have increased nuclear/cytoplasmic ratios, angular nuclear membranes, chromatin clumping or clearing, and macronucleoli, and they can be multinucleated.

The primary differential diagnosis is with adenocarcinoma, particularly BAC. Briefly, BAC is characterized by the presence of numerous well-preserved tumor cells, while reactive cells are usually fewer and may be degenerated. Benign groups tend to have scalloped (flower-like) borders and less depth of focus. Cilia, if present, point to a benign diagnosis. Be cautious diagnosing BAC in the presence of a known cause of reactive changes, eg, pneumonia or pulmonary embolism.

2.2.4 Alveolar Macrophages

Alveolar macrophages are bone marrow–derived histiocytes that are found free in the alveolar space. The presence of alveolar macrophages is a necessary but not sufficient condition for adequacy of a sputum specimen. Macrophages indicate that at least some of the "deep lung" (ie, most peripheral, alveolar part) has been sampled. Ciliated respiratory cells (so-called bronchial cells) are insufficient evidence of a deep lung sample in sputum. In BAL specimens, alveolar macrophages should not simply be present but abundant.

Alveolar macrophages are morphologically identical to other histiocytes. They vary in size; have round to oval or bean-shaped nuclei; and may be mononucleated, binucleated, or multinucleated. Multinucleated alveolar macrophages (giant cell histiocytes) |i2.11| are found in increased numbers in granulomatous diseases, such as sarcoid and tuberculosis, but are not specific for granulomas. The chromatin characteristically has a "salt and pepper" texture but is variable. One or more nucleoli may be present. The cytoplasm is foamy and stains variably. Characteristically, the cells are phagocytic and often contain various particles, such as carbon. These cells often are named for the particles found in them.

Carbon histiocytes are common in smokers and urban dwellers and numerous in anthracosis. They also are known as "dust cells" and contain black carbon pigment.

Siderophages |i2.12| occur in reaction to bleeding. These macrophages contain the blood pigment, hemosiderin (hence, "hemosiderin-laden macrophages"). The presence of siderophages usually indicates "old" bleeding, which may be associated with benign conditions, such as infarcts, heart failure ("heart failure cells"), and hemosiderosis, or with malignant conditions.

Lipophages |i2.13| have lacy bubbly cytoplasm owing to their lipid content. The source of the lipid can be exogenous (eg, oily nose drops) or endogenous (related to tissue destruction). Lipophages can be seen in conditions such as lipid pneumonia, fat embolism, and acute pancreatitis. In children, lipid-laden macrophages may be associated with aspiration pneumonia. However, when lipophages are present, particularly in adults, malignant conditions must be considered.

2.2.5 Acellular Material

Curschmann spirals |i2.14| usually are found in conditions associated with excess mucus production, eg, asthma and smoking. Curschmann spirals were formerly thought to represent inspissated mucus casts of small bronchioles; however, rarely, they are found in other specimens, eg, in the Pap smear or body cavity fluids. Therefore, their formation is probably due to an intrinsic property of mucus itself.

Curschmann spirals have a darkly staining center with a lighter staining periphery and usually spiral like a corkscrew.

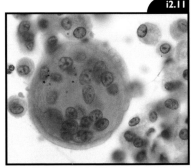
i2.11
Alveolar macrophages

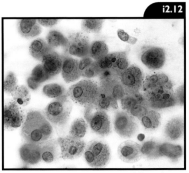
i2.12
Siderophages

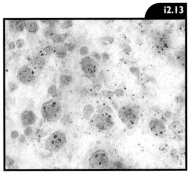
i2.13
Lipophages (oil red O)

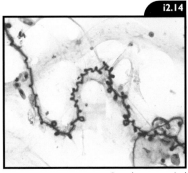
i2.14
Curschmann spiral

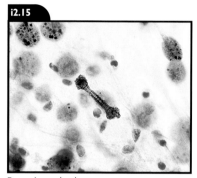

Ferruginous body

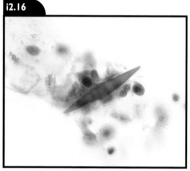

Charcot-Leyden crystals

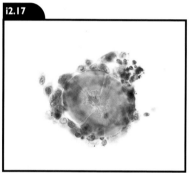

Corpus amylaceum

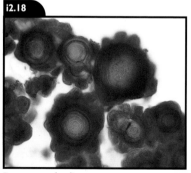

Psammoma bodies

Curschmann spirals may be associated with eosinophils, in patients with asthma, or with neutrophils, in patients exposed to air pollution or who smoke.

Ferruginous bodies |i2.15| form when iron salts precipitate onto tiny rounded or fibrous inhaled dusts. The fiber is often asbestos (asbestos bodies) but can be other particles, eg, fiberglass, carbon, or other minerals. Ferruginous bodies are typically golden brown and beaded and have bulbous tips. They are frequently engulfed by macrophages.

Charcot-Leyden crystals |i2.16| are bipyramidal or needle-like red crystals composed of condensed granules derived from eosinophils. Eosinophils also are usually present near the crystals. Charcot-Leyden crystals are particularly associated with asthma but also can be seen in other allergic conditions.

Other Acellular Material

Alveolar proteinosis, due to an enzymatic disorder of macrophages, results in coarsely granular, periodic acid–Schiff (PAS)–positive debris.

Corpora amylacea |i2.17| are concentrically laminated, noncalcified, alveolar casts associated with preceding pulmonary edema.

Psammoma bodies |i2.18| are concentrically laminated, calcified bodies associated with BAC but can also be seen in benign disease (eg, tuberculosis or microlithiasis).

Amyloid is dense, acellular, waxy material that has a characteristic "apple green" birefringence under polarized light after Congo red staining.

2.2.6 Contaminants

Starch from glove powder typically has a cracked center and a Maltese cross polarization.

Pollen appears as colorful bodies with cell walls and spikes.

Food particles are common in sputum and may be a source of diagnostic error. Meat is recognized by cross striations. Vegetable cells have translucent refractile cell walls (cellulose).

2.3 Benign Proliferation

In response to a wide variety of chronic irritations or inflammations, ranging from air pollution to infections to cancer, the bronchial epithelium can undergo a series of transformations, including reserve cell hyperplasia, squamous metaplasia, and bronchial hyperplasia. Squamous epithelium is more mechanically resistant but less specialized than the respiratory epithelium. Although not premalignant, squamous metaplasia is the milieu in which cancer may arise.

2.3.1 Reserve Cell Hyperplasia

Reserve cell hyperplasia is most commonly observed in bronchial brush specimens. Reserve cell hyperplasia exfoliates as tightly cohesive groups of small uniform cells, often lined on one surface by small, ciliated, columnar cells |i2.19|. Individual reserve cells resemble lymphocytes or histiocytes. They have small, dark, round nuclei with a thin rim of basophilic cytoplasm and high nuclear/cytoplasmic ratios. The nuclei resemble those of ordinary ciliated cells but may show some nuclear molding. Nucleoli are usually absent, unless the cells are irritated. The background is clean. The main differential diagnosis is small cell carcinoma, which has more nuclear pleomorphism, more nuclear molding, crush artifact, and a tumor diathesis.

2.3.2 Squamous Metaplasia

Squamous metaplasia is essentially normal and ranges from focal to extensive. It is frequently associated with reserve cell hyperplasia.

Squamous metaplasia can be morphologically similar to that seen in the Pap smear, with rounded parabasal-sized cells. However, when immature, it has smaller cells (similar in diameter to bronchial cells) with more angulated or polygonal outlines |i2.20|. As in the Pap smear, the cells often appear in loose "cobblestone" sheets. Metaplastic cytoplasm is particularly dense with distinct cell borders and usually stains cyanophilic (blue-green). The nuclei are round with granular chromatin; nucleoli are present when the cells are irritated ("repairish") |i2.21|. Other degenerative and regenerative changes include cytoplasmic eosinophilia or orangeophilia and nuclear karyorrhexis or pyknosis.

Degenerated metaplastic cells with angular outlines, orange cytoplasm, and pyknotic nuclei may be difficult to distinguish from parakeratosis. Atypical squamous metaplasia, often associated with necrotizing pneumonia (classically due to *Aspergillus*), is a possible cause of false-positive diagnoses.

2.3.3 Parakeratosis and Atypical Parakeratosis

The cytology of bronchial parakeratosis |i2.22| and atypical parakeratosis is similar to that of the Pap smear. Parakeratosis and atypical parakeratosis usually result from severe irritation, eg, from a tracheostomy tube. However, atypical parakeratosis

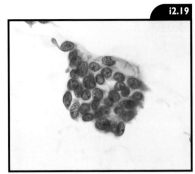

i2.19

Reserve cell hyperplasia

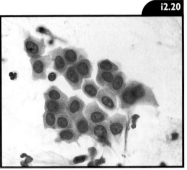

i2.20

Squamous metaplasia

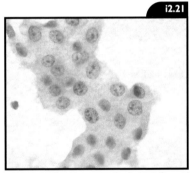

i2.21

Squamous metaplasia, inflamed

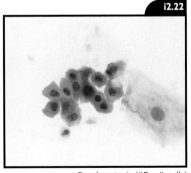

i2.22

Parakeratosis ("Pap" cells)

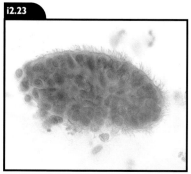

Creola body

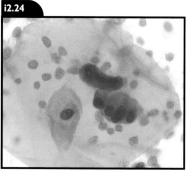

Radiation effect—squamous cells

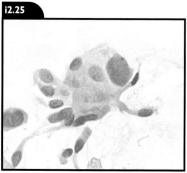

Radiation effect—gland cells

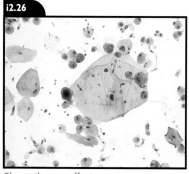

Chemotherapy effect

also can occur with squamous cell dysplasia or carcinoma. Moreover, atypical parakeratosis, also known as pleomorphic parakeratosis, can mimic keratinizing squamous cell carcinoma, except that the parakeratotic cells are small. Look carefully for clear-cut (large) malignant tumor cells to diagnose cancer.

2.3.4 Bronchial Hyperplasia and Creola Bodies

Bronchial hyperplasia results in papillary-like mucosal folds. The most characteristic finding is creola bodies, which are compact three-dimensional groups of reactive bronchial cells that can mimic adenocarcinoma. An important clue to the benign diagnosis is the presence of cilia, which usually are found along the surface |i2.23|.

2.4 Therapeutic Agents

Radiation and chemotherapy can induce severe cytologic atypia, which can mimic cancer. Clinical history is essential in diagnosis.

2.4.1 Radiation

As in the Pap smear, radiation induces changes that are characterized by cytomegaly of squamous |i2.24| or glandular |i2.25| cells (ie, macrocytes). Irradiated malignant cells show characteristic malignant features, plus radiation effect. Radiation-induced changes may subside with time or persist for life.

Radiation effect on squamous cells causes enlargement of cytoplasm and nucleus in concert, so that the nuclear/cytoplasmic ratio remains within normal limits. Multinucleation is common. The nuclei may be hyperchromatic or hypochromatic and sometimes are vacuolated. Prominent nucleoli or macronucleoli may be seen. The cytoplasm is thick and dense, but frequently vacuolated, and stains polychromatically (ie, two-tone stain). In addition, squamous metaplasia, which may be atypical, can be present.

Radiation effect on glandular cells causes many of the changes described for bronchial irritation cells, including multinucleation and reactive nuclear changes; cytomegaly also occurs. Occasionally, disorganized groups of atypical cells with large dark nuclei, coarse chromatin, and prominent nucleoli in a "dirty" background of necrosis, WBCs, and debris may be seen. These findings could suggest malignancy. Clues to a benign diagnosis include cilia or terminal bars, maintained nuclear/cytoplasmic ratios, and smudgy degenerated chromatin.

2.4.2 Chemotherapy

Chemotherapy often causes cytologic changes similar to those of radiation, ie, cytomegaly |i2.26|, that may particularly affect glandular cells. The cells are enlarged and pleomorphic and may have large nuclei with dark chromatin and prominent nucleoli. Mitotic figures can be seen. In addition, there may be an increase in the number of goblet cells and the amount of mucin. Histiocytes and inflammatory cells typically are seen in the background. In chemotherapy effect, the atypical cells tend to be few, degenerated, and single, and they maintain their columnar shape. Cilia, if present, indicate the cells are benign.

2.5 Granulomatous Inflammation

Granulomatous inflammation can be seen in a wide variety of conditions, including tuberculosis, fungus, or other infections; rheumatoid arthritis; sarcoid; and as a reaction to cancer (particularly with squamous differentiation). Granulomas are nodular collections of epithelioid histiocytes |i2.27|; giant cells are not required for diagnosis |i2.28|. In bronchial cytology, epithelioid histiocytes usually are found in loose syncytial aggregates. In sputum, epithelioid histiocytes usually are about the size of bronchial cells and stain red to orange when degenerated ("carrot cells"). They also can be rounded and resemble ordinary histiocytes. The nuclei usually are elongated and often have folded nuclear membranes, fine pale chromatin, and tiny nucleoli. When well preserved, as in bronchial brush specimens, the cytoplasm is more abundant, eccentrically located around the nucleus, and often has a fibrillar quality, with poorly defined cell borders. In foreign body granulomas, phagocytosis is prominent.

2.5.1 Tuberculosis

The typical features of tuberculosis are epithelioid histiocytes, giant cells (particularly Langhans type with peripheral nuclei), lymphocytes, and a caseous (necrotic) background. The combination of both Langhans giant cells and epithelioid histiocytes is characteristic but not pathognomonic. Acute inflammation can be seen early in the course of the disease. Identification of beaded, red, acid-fast bacilli or positive culture clinches the diagnosis. Reactive atypia of bronchial or squamous metaplastic

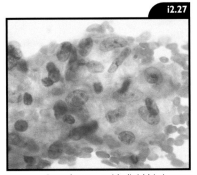

i2.27

Granuloma—epithelioid histiocytes

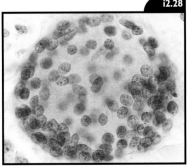

i2.28

Granuloma—giant cell histiocyte

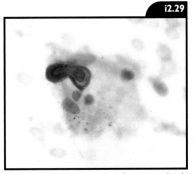

i2.29

Schaumann body

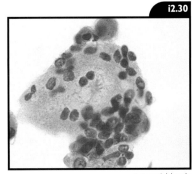

i2.30

Asteroid body

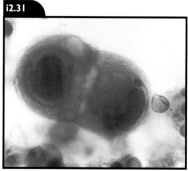

Cytomegalovirus (P)

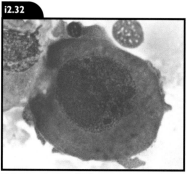

Cytomegalovirus (DQ)

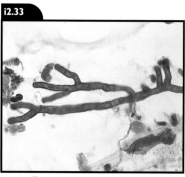

Aspergillus

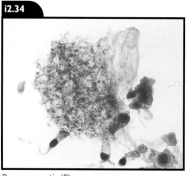

Pneumocystis (P)

cells or alveolar pneumocytes in a necrotic background could result in a false-positive diagnosis.

2.5.2 Sarcoid

Sarcoidosis, or simply sarcoid, is a chronic granulomatous disease of unknown etiology. Noncaseating (hard) granulomas are characteristic but not pathognomonic. Schaumann or asteroid bodies are suggestive of sarcoid but also are not specific. Schaumann bodies |i2.29| are concentrically laminated calcifications found in the cytoplasm of giant cells. Asteroid bodies |i2.30| are intracytoplasmic, radiate, crystalline arrays.

2.5.3 Rheumatoid Granuloma of Lung

Rheumatoid granulomas can exfoliate epithelioid histiocytes with bizarre shapes. These cells may have hyperchromatic, degenerated, smudged nuclei and variably colored cytoplasm ranging from blue to red to orange. The background shows marked inflammation and necrotic debris. Occasional degenerated multinucleated giant cells may be seen.

Bizarre cells with dark nuclei and pseudokeratinized cytoplasm in a necrotic background can mimic keratinizing squamous cell carcinoma. Atypical squamous metaplasia can further confuse the picture. Clinical history can be helpful in diagnosis.

2.6 Specific Infections

Respiratory cytology is increasingly used to diagnose infections, particularly in immunocompromised patients (see also the Appendix).

2.6.1 Viral Pneumonia

Specific viral changes, such as those due to cytomegalovirus |i2.31|, |i2.32| or herpes, may be identified in cytologic specimens. Viral infection can cause reactive changes in bronchial cells, which in the absence of cilia, may be virtually indistinguishable from BAC. However, atypical cells usually are sparse in infection, while in BAC, atypical cells are usually numerous. Be cautious in diagnosis of BAC in a patient with an acute illness or fever.

2.6.2 Other Infections

If *Candida* or bacterial colonies are found, suspect contamination or overgrowth. *Actinomyces* is a common saprophyte in the tonsils. Respiratory cytology is generally not too helpful in specific identification of bacteria.

Fungi, eg, *Aspergillus* |**i2.33**|, *Pneumocystis* |**i2.34**|, |**i2.35**|, and other organisms, are more commonly diagnosed in immuno-suppressed patients but also can be seen in apparently immuno-competent hosts.

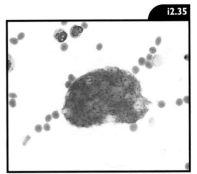

Pneumocystis (DQ)

2.7 Pulmonary Embolism/Infarct

A solitary pulmonary embolism can mimic a neoplasm, clinically and radiologically. Some cases exfoliate markedly reac-tive (ie, atypical) cells that may be confused with malignancy. Three-dimensional clusters of pleomorphic cells with enlarged nuclei, irregular chromatin clearing, and macronucleoli can mimic adenocarcinoma (see p 30). Sheets of cells with orangeophilic cytoplasm and enlarged hyperchromatic nuclei can mimic squa-mous cell carcinoma. Blood, inflammation, and siderophages may be seen in the background. Squamous metaplasia is common. Clues to the benign nature of the changes may include sparsity of atypical cells, few or no single atypical cells, variability within groups (ie, typical and atypical cells together), shallow depth of focus, tight cell grouping, presence of cilia, and smudgy chromatin. Benign atypia is transient. (See reactive pneumocytes, p 30.)

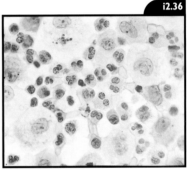

Eosinophilic pneumonia (P)

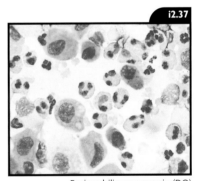

Eosinophilic pneumonia (DQ)

2.8 Miscellaneous Benign Diseases

Asthma: Creola bodies, Curschmann spirals, Charcot-Leyden crystals, and eosinophils are characteristic of asthma. Bacteria may be decreased.

Silicosis: Silica is weakly birefringent, silvery particles. Brightly birefringent silicates also can cause disease.

Löffler's Pneumonia: This is also known as eosinophilic pneumonia |**i2.36**|, |**i2.37**|. It may be associated with worm infes-tation, notably ascariasis, with allergy, including drug reactions, and with connective diseases such as systemic lupus erythematosus.

Giant Cell Interstitial Pneumonia: Pneumoconiosis often is due to industrial exposure to hard metals. It is characterized by multinucleated giant cell histiocytes that may contain phagocy-tosed cells or debris.

Storage Diseases: Gaucher disease is a lysosomal storage disease with accumulation of glucocerebroside in phagocytes. Gaucher cells are characterized by their abundant cytoplasm with a "rumpled tissue" appearance |**i2.38**|.

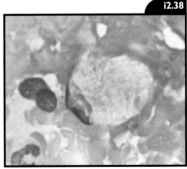

Gaucher cell (DQ)

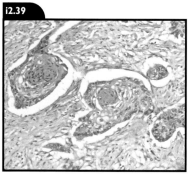

Keratinizing SCC, tissue

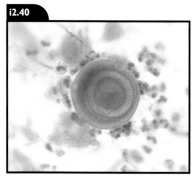

Keratinizing SCC—pearl

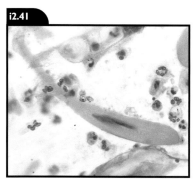

Keratinizing SCC—bizarre cell

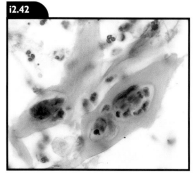

Keratinizing SCC—orangeophilia

2.9 Malignant Diseases

2.9.1 General Cytodiagnostic Principles

As a general rule, cancer cells are larger and more pleomorphic than normal or reactive cells and have increased nuclear/cytoplasmic ratios. Abnormal, coarse, dark, and, especially, irregularly distributed chromatin are key diagnostic features of malignant cells. Mitotic figures, particularly when atypical, are suspicious. Conversely, ciliated cells are virtually always benign.

Lung cancer can occur as pure lesions, eg, pure squamous cell carcinoma. However, most lung cancers are actually mixtures of cell types; even a single cell can show evidence of glandular, squamous, and neuroendocrine differentiation. Mixtures of squamous cell carcinoma and adenocarcinoma are particularly commonly observed in cytologic specimens. In practice, a diagnosis of small cell carcinoma or non–small cell carcinoma in primary lung cancer is usually sufficient to initiate therapy.

2.9.2 Squamous Cell Carcinoma

Squamous cell carcinoma tends to arise centrally and usually can be diagnosed by sputum or bronchial cytology. Sputum usually contains more differentiated keratinized cells with denser cytoplasm, more pyknotic nuclei, and fewer nucleoli compared with bronchial cytology that selects less differentiated, nonkeratinized cells with more open chromatin and more prominent nucleoli. Bronchial brush specimens may contain large tissue fragments of malignant cells.

Keratinizing (Well-Differentiated) Squamous Cell Carcinoma

Keratinizing squamous cell carcinoma is characterized by malignant cells with heavy keratinization and marked pleomorphism |i2.39|. Pearls are pathognomonic of keratinization |i2.40|. The heavier the keratinization, the more single cells are present. Cytologic features of keratinization usually are more apparent in sputum than bronchial cytology.

Bizarre cell shapes (eg, snakes, tadpoles) |i2.41| and "pumpkin" cells (large, round, bright orange) are characteristic findings. Single cells are numerous. The cytoplasm is dense, waxy, or "hard," with sharply defined cell borders. Cytoplasm varies from scant to abundant; therefore, nuclear/cytoplasmic ratios range from high to low. Cyanophilic tumor cells often predominate in bronchial brush specimens and eosinophilic or orange cells in sputum |i2.42|. Features of keratinization include refractile, concentric, cytoplasmic rings; Herxheimer spirals (twisted ropy aggregates of filaments); and pearls (pathognomonic).

The nuclei also are pleomorphic. The chromatin varies from coarse and dark, with clearing and clumping (especially bronchial cytology), to pyknotic or ink dot–like (especially sputum). Further nuclear degeneration, including karyorrhexis and karyolysis (with nuclear "ghosts"), is common. Multinucleation with nuclear molding may occur. Prominent nucleoli can be seen, particularly in brush specimens, but nucleoli often are inconspicuous to invisible, particularly in sputum. Mitotic figures are rare.

Keratinizing squamous cell carcinoma can undergo extensive necrosis, producing a central cavity (cavitary carcinoma), that results in an abundance of necrotic material; markedly pleomorphic, degenerated, keratinized tumor cells; and marked inflammation. The differential diagnosis includes necrotic granulomas (eg, fungal infection or tuberculosis).

Various nonneoplastic reactive processes and factors (eg, infections, infarction, and tracheostomy tubes) can cause inflammatory atypia, repair/regeneration, or atypical parakeratosis that can mimic squamous cell carcinoma (as previously discussed). Very well-differentiated squamous cell carcinoma may suggest low-grade dysplasia rather than cancer in cytologic specimens. Such highly differentiated carcinomas are more commonly metastatic (particularly from the head and neck region) than primary.

Nonkeratinizing (Moderately to Poorly Differentiated) Squamous Cell Carcinoma

The cells of nonkeratinizing squamous cell carcinoma |i2.43| are characteristically more cohesive and uniform than those of keratinizing squamous cell carcinoma. They tend to form disorderly sheets, particularly in brush specimens. However, single cells also are present, particularly in bronchial washings and sputum specimens.

The malignant cells are fairly uniform |i2.44|, |i2.45|, |i2.46|, although from case to case they range from relatively small (can resemble small cell carcinoma) to relatively large (can resemble adenocarcinoma). Bizarre cells are absent.

The cytoplasm is dense, often cyanophilic, and has distinct cell boundaries. Refractile rings of keratinization may be seen in the cytoplasm. Nuclear/cytoplasmic ratios are increased. Although occasional dyskeratotic cells may be present, marked keratinization, diffuse orangeophilia, and pearls are not seen.

The nuclei are enlarged and hyperchromatic. The chromatin is coarse and irregular but somewhat more open than that of keratinizing squamous cell carcinoma. Pyknotic nuclei are unusual. Nucleoli are usually more prominent than in keratinizing squamous cell carcinoma but less so than in adenocarcinoma.

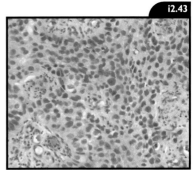

i2.43

Nonkeratinizing SCC, tissue

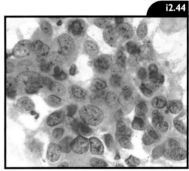

i2.44

Nonkeratinizing SCC

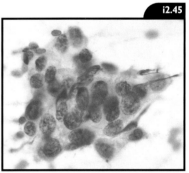

i2.45

Nonkeratinizing SCC

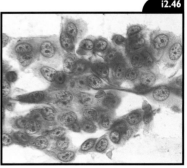

i2.46

Nonkeratinizing SCC

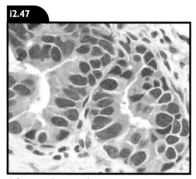

Adenocarcinoma, tissue

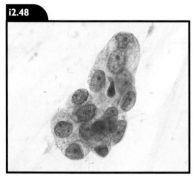

Adenocarcinoma—cell ball

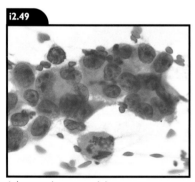

Adenocarcinoma—acini

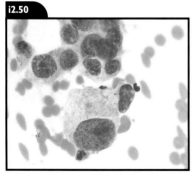

Adenocarcinoma—nucleocytoplasmic polarity

Repair/regeneration, with its pleomorphic nuclei and prominent nucleoli, can mimic nonkeratinizing squamous cell carcinoma but usually has other cytologic features that help point to a benign diagnosis (eg, cohesive orderly sheets, little nuclear crowding, and fine pale chromatin). Distinguishing poorly differentiated adenocarcinoma from poorly differentiated squamous cell carcinoma also can be difficult (and remember, many tumors are mixed). Dense cytoplasm with distinct cell boundaries is a squamous feature, while nucleocytoplasmic polarity, delicate vacuolated cytoplasm, and mucin secretion are glandular features. An occasional keratinized (dyskeratotic) cell is a squamous feature. However, coagulative necrosis of adenocarcinoma cells can result in "pseudokeratosis" that mimics squamous differentiation. Another common problem is distinguishing poorly differentiated squamous cell carcinoma, composed of small cells, from small cell (neuroendocrine) carcinoma. Distinct dense cytoplasm, minimal nuclear molding, conspicuous nucleoli, and lack of crush artifact favor squamous cell carcinoma. (For more discussion, see "Small Cell Carcinoma," p 43.)

Squamous Dysplasia and Carcinoma In Situ

Dysplasia of the respiratory mucosa usually arises in the milieu of squamous metaplasia. Dysplasia also is known as atypical squamous metaplasia, which gives a good clue to its morphology. Low-grade dysplasia resembles ordinary metaplasia but has slightly abnormal nuclei. Nuclear atypia, including enlargement and hyperchromasia, increased nuclear/cytoplasmic ratios, and chromatin abnormalities, increases with grade. High-grade dysplasia/carcinoma in situ is composed of small round to pleomorphic cells with high nuclear/cytoplasmic ratios, irregular nuclear membranes, and chromatin abnormalities, found singly or in loose clusters; syncytia are not required to diagnose carcinoma in situ in the bronchus. Nucleoli, often basophilic, may be seen. The cytoplasm may be keratinized. The presence of frankly malignant appearing cells (ie, bizarre shapes, heavy keratinization, irregular chromatin, prominent nucleoli), high cellularity, and a tumor diathesis favor invasive squamous cell carcinoma. If the lesion exfoliating malignant cells is radiologically visible, it is invasive (an incidental abnormality, such as a granuloma, could coexist).

2.9.3 Adenocarcinoma

Adenocarcinoma usually arises in the lung periphery. Adenocarcinomas usually are detected more readily by bronchial cytology than by sputum cytology. The incidence of adenocarcinoma has been increasing, particularly among women, and it has become the most commonly diagnosed primary lung cancer. Adenocarcinoma is associated with smoking but less strongly than squamous or small cell carcinoma. Adenocarcinoma of the lung can be divided into two major types: bronchogenic carcinoma (the usual type) and bronchioloalveolar carcinoma.

Bronchogenic Adenocarcinoma

The cells of bronchogenic adenocarcinoma |i2.47| occur in characteristic papillae, cell balls |i2.48|, or acini (rosette-like structures) |i2.49|, as well as singly. Crowded sheets of disorderly cells with ill-defined cell borders also can be seen, particularly in brush specimens. Syncytial aggregates, with little evidence of glandular differentiation, are seen in poorly differentiated adenocarcinoma. Nucleocytoplasmic polarity is a characteristic feature of adenocarcinoma, even when poorly differentiated |i2.50|.

The cytoplasm ranges from homogeneous to foamy, although large vacuoles suggest metastasis or reactive/degenerative conditions. The cytoplasm usually stains faintly basophilic. Secretory vacuoles containing mucin indicate glandular differentiation.

The nuclei are enlarged, sometimes multiple, with high nuclear/cytoplasmic ratios. The nuclear membranes are often irregular, and the chromatin varies from fine to coarse. Classically, a single cherry red macronucleolus is seen in the center of a relatively pale nucleus, but the chromatin quality and size and number of nucleoli are variable.

Occasionally, adenocarcinoma undergoes coagulative necrosis: the cells become pseudokeratinized (stain eosinophilic or orangeophilic), and the nuclei become dark and pyknotic, mimicking keratinizing squamous cell carcinoma. On the other hand, squamous cell carcinoma can develop nonspecific, degenerative vacuoles that can mimic secretory vacuoles of adenocarcinoma. (For further discussion of differential diagnoses of adenocarcinoma, see the following sections.)

Bronchioloalveolar Carcinoma

BAC is a group of tumors that can arise from different cell types, including ciliated terminal bronchiolar cells, Clara cells, or type II alveolar pneumocytes. BAC grows along the preexisting bronchioloalveolar framework of the lung, without invasion |i2.51|. The pattern of growth can be a single mass, multiple nodules, or massive/diffuse. The classic chest x-ray resembles nonresolving pneumonia. Mucin production can be abundant, producing copious amounts of mucoid sputum (bronchorrhea).

The cytology of BAC is similar to the usual type of adenocarcinoma, although BAC is more often well-differentiated. Although there are poorly differentiated BACs, they are essentially indistinguishable from ordinary adenocarcinoma by cytology. Abundant clusters of strikingly uniform cells provide a clue to the cytodiagnosis of BAC. The tumor cells may be present in flat

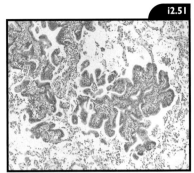

i2.51

BAC, tissue

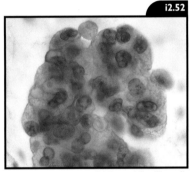

i2.52

BAC—goblet-like cells

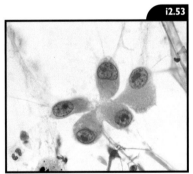

i2.53

BAC—mesothelial-like cells

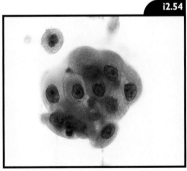

i2.54

BAC—alveolar-like cells

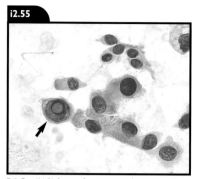

BAC—INCI (arrow), compare benign cells

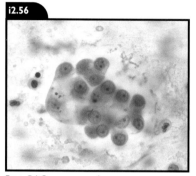

Faux BAC—pneumonia

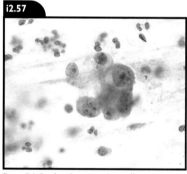

Faux BAC—benign reactive cells

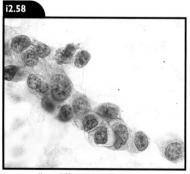

Large cell undifferentiated carcinoma

sheets or cell balls with great depth of focus (especially sputum). Cell balls often have flowery or hobnail outlines, and the cells do not mold one another. Papillary growth is a particularly characteristic feature of BAC. Acini and single cells also may be seen, although single cells may be sparse in sputum.

In cytologic specimens, two basic types of tumor cells can be recognized: mucinous and nonmucinous (or serous). Mucinous tumor cells are large and columnar and resemble goblet cells |i2.52|, but they frequently have prominent nucleoli. Nonmucinous tumor cells are smaller and cuboidal and reminiscent of mesothelial cells |i2.53|. Nonmucinous tumor cells also can closely resemble reactive alveolar pneumocytes or macrophages |i2.54|. Benign macrophages also may be present in large numbers.

The cytoplasm varies from scant to abundant and finely granular to clear, depending on cell type. Mucous vacuolization, similar to goblet cells, is characteristic of mucinous tumors. The tumor cells may have microvilli that can mimic cilia or terminal bars, but true cilia are not present.

The nuclei are round, and the chromatin is usually pale and fine but can be moderately hyperchromatic. Intranuclear cytoplasmic invaginations |i2.55| are common and suggest the diagnosis of BAC when numerous. Nucleoli, usually one or two, can vary from inconspicuous to prominent, depending on the cell type and degree of differentiation.

Abundant mucus in the background, when present, is a clue to the diagnosis. Psammoma bodies may be seen (|i2.18|, p 32).

A wide range of conditions, including pulmonary infarcts, bronchiectasis, asthma, viral pneumonia, and radiation or chemotherapy, among many others, can cause cellular atypia closely mimicking adenocarcinoma |i2.56|. In some cases, it may not be possible on cytologic grounds alone to differentiate benign reactive changes from adenocarcinoma, particularly BAC |i2.57|. BAC tends to shed more and better preserved cells; reactive conditions tend to shed sparse and degenerated cells. Cilia are an important benign feature. A discrete population of abnormal cells favors malignancy; a transition from reactive to atypical cells favors a benign diagnosis. Be particularly cautious in diagnosis of BAC in a patient with pneumonia, fever, or other condition known to be associated with reactive atypia in respiratory cells. With serial specimens, reactive atypia should diminish. The chest x-ray findings should be compatible with tumor to diagnose cancer.

The cytologic differential diagnosis of BAC vs ordinary bronchogenic carcinoma is largely presumptive: well-differentiated tumors, particularly papillary adenocarcinomas, often are presumed to be BAC. Squamous differentiation favors ordinary bronchogenic carcinoma. The differential diagnosis of BAC vs metastatic carcinoma can be impossible by cytology alone. Clinical correlation is required.

2.9.4 Large Cell Undifferentiated Carcinoma

Large cell undifferentiated carcinoma is easy to recognize as malignant but lacks light microscopic evidence of specific differentiation, although glandular, squamous, or neuroendocrine features are commonly demonstrable by using electron microscopy or immunocytochemistry.

The cells are relatively large and undifferentiated (ergo, the name). They can range from fairly uniform to bizarre. Single cells and syncytial-like aggregates with irregularly arranged, overlapped nuclei are present |i2.58|. By definition, neither glandular nor squamous features are seen.

The cytoplasm is abundant and varies from delicate (but not secretory) to dense (but not squamoid) to granular. The staining varies from basophilic to amphophilic to acidophilic. The cell borders can be well or poorly defined. Keratinization and mucin secretion are absent.

The nuclei are obviously malignant appearing. They are large and round to pleomorphic and have irregular to lobulated membranes. The chromatin can vary from fine to coarse and is irregularly distributed. Nucleoli can be prominent, multiple, and irregular. A diathesis usually is present in the background.

Germ cell tumors and the syndrome of undifferentiated carcinoma/poorly differentiated adenocarcinoma also should be considered in the differential diagnosis of large cell undifferentiated carcinoma, especially when the tumor occurs in a midline location in a young patient. Patients with germ cell tumors or the undifferentiated carcinoma/poorly differentiated adenocarcinoma syndrome may have elevated serum levels of β-human chorionic gonadotropin or α-fetoprotein. These diagnoses are important because patients may respond to appropriate therapy. Sarcoma, melanoma, and metastatic malignant neoplasms also can be considered in the differential diagnosis.

2.9.5 Giant Cell Carcinoma

If significant numbers of giant tumor cells are present, the tumor is designated giant cell carcinoma |i2.59|. This tumor is extremely aggressive. A spindle cell component also may be present (giant and spindle cell carcinoma). Giant cell change is common after radiation or chemotherapy. Exclude sarcoma.

2.9.6 Small Cell (Neuroendocrine) Carcinoma

Small cell carcinoma is one of the most aggressive of all cancers |i2.60|. It typically occurs in older patients who usually have a strong smoking history. Radiation and chemotherapy, rather than surgery, are the mainstays of therapy. Small cell carcinoma, also known as poorly differentiated neuroendocrine carci-

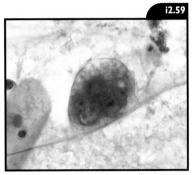

i2.59

Giant cell carcinoma

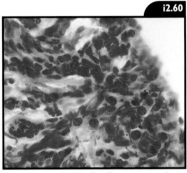

i2.60

Small cell carcinoma, tissue

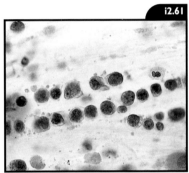

i2.61

Small cell carcinoma

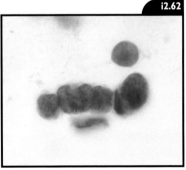

i2.62

Small cell carcinoma (oil)

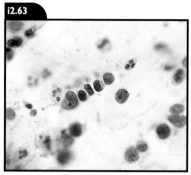

Small cell carcinoma—oat cell

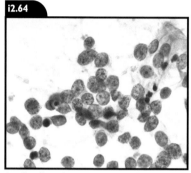

Small cell carcinoma—intermediate

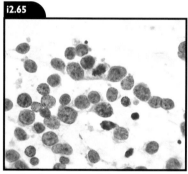

Small cell carcinoma—intermediate

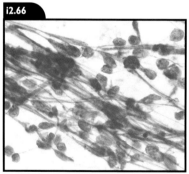

Small cell carcinoma—crush artifact

noma, is a specific category of tumor associated with Kulchitsky cell (neuroendocrine) differentiation. The tumor often produces polypeptide hormones and, hence, may be associated with various paraneoplastic syndromes.

General Features of Small Cell Carcinoma

The tumor cells are relatively small with high nuclear/cytoplasmic ratios. Although they can vary somewhat in size, marked pleomorphism is not a feature of pure small cell carcinoma. The cells tend to line up in strings or single files, particularly in sputum |**i2.61**|. Nuclear molding often is prominent |**i2.62**|. The chromatin is dark, and nucleoli are inconspicuous. In sputum, the tumor cells often are degenerated, and nuclear detail may be lacking, but in bronchial cytology, the cells are typically larger and better preserved. Sparse neurosecretory granules may be present in the cytoplasm, but their demonstration is not required to make the diagnosis. Because the cells are fragile, crush artifact (nuclear DNA streaming) is a characteristic feature, particularly in bronchial brush specimens.

Small cell carcinoma is divided, somewhat arbitrarily, into oat cell carcinoma, the classic type, and an intermediate type, which is probably the "real" small cell carcinoma (oat cells are due to degeneration). There are no significant biologic or therapeutic differences between these two cell types, and mixtures are common.

Small Cell Carcinoma, Oat Cell Type

Oat cell carcinoma is composed of lymphocyte-like tumor cells with high nuclear/cytoplasmic ratios |**i2.63**|. The cells range from one to two times the size of a lymphocyte. The nuclei vary from round to angular with irregular nuclear membranes; nuclear molding usually is prominent. The chromatin is intensely hyperchromatic to pyknotic ("ink dots"), especially in sputum. Nucleoli always are invisible or inconspicuous in classic oat cell carcinoma. The cytoplasm is scant and delicate, consisting of a thin basophilic wisp. A diathesis is characteristically present around the tumor cells. Crush artifact often is present, particularly in bronchial brush specimens.

Small Cell Carcinoma, Intermediate Type

The intermediate type of small cell carcinoma is composed of cells that are generally similar in appearance to those of oat cell carcinoma, except they are somewhat larger, ranging from about two to four times the size of a lymphocyte (up to twice the size of an oat cell) |**i2.64**|, |**i2.65**|. They also are more pleomorphic (including spindle and polygonal cells) with better preserved chromatin (similar to normal bronchial cells), more apparent (but not conspicuous) nucleoli, and more cytoplasm (but not abundant or dense). Crush artifact, a characteristic feature, is common, particularly in bronchial brush specimens |i2.66|.

Small Cell Carcinoma: Variants and Differential Diagnosis

Small cell carcinoma can have a large cell component (mixed small/large cell carcinoma) or show adenocarcinoma or squamous cell carcinoma (combined type). These variants are more common after therapy or in metastases. There is also a large cell neuroendocrine carcinoma.

Small cells with high nuclear/cytoplasmic ratios, prominent nuclear molding, inconspicuous nucleoli, and crush artifact characterize small cell carcinoma. If the tumor cells have abundant cytoplasm, prominent nucleoli, evidence of mucin or keratin production, or form glands, think of a diagnosis other than (pure) small cell carcinoma.

2.9.7 Adenosquamous Carcinoma

Cancer of the lung with well-defined adenocarcinomatous and well-defined squamous cell carcinomatous components, ie, adenosquamous carcinoma, has been considered relatively rare, particularly in histology. However, in cytology, tumors exhibiting at least a minor degree of dual differentiation are common. In fact, when studied carefully, mixed carcinomas are more common than pure forms of lung cancer.

A mixed adenosquamous carcinoma is a tumor that shows evidence of keratin and secretion, which are squamous and glandular features, respectively |i2.67|, |i2.68|. Squamous features include dense cytoplasm, distinct cell borders, rings, and pearls. Glandular features include nucleocytoplasmic polarity, acini, intracytoplasmic lumens, and mucin. Double carcinomas, with squamous cell carcinoma in one site and adenocarcinoma in another, could shed into sputum, creating the false impression of dual differentiation.

2.9.8 Carcinoid Tumors

Carcinoid tumors usually arise in a large bronchus, probably from Kulchitsky cells or their precursors. They are essentially identical to the similar neuroendocrine tumors occurring in the gastrointestinal tract, among other sites. Typical carcinoids, atypical carcinoids, and small cell carcinoma constitute a spectrum of related neuroendocrine tumors. Bronchial carcinoids rarely produce the carcinoid syndrome. Because the tumors usually are covered by intact bronchial mucosa, the tumor cells seldom exfoliate spontaneously into sputum, although diagnostic cells may be found in bronchial brush specimens (or FNA biopsy specimens).

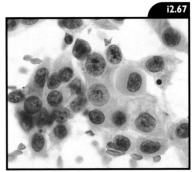
i2.67

Adenosquamous carcinoma

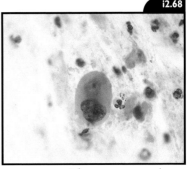
i2.68

Adenosquamous carcinoma

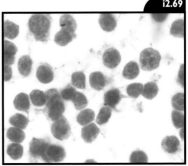
i2.69

Typical carcinoid

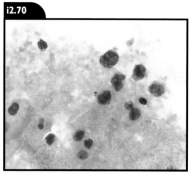

Non-Hodgkin lymphoma

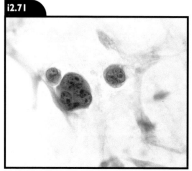

Hodgkin disease

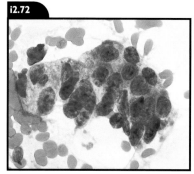

Metastatic colon carcinoma

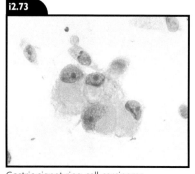

Gastric signet ring cell carcinoma

Typical carcinoids are characterized cytologically by cohesive, orderly, small sheets; clusters; rosettes; or chains of cells and single cells |i2.69|. They are small, round to oval, and monotonously uniform, resembling lymphocytes or plasma cells. The cytoplasm varies from scant to moderate in amount; it is delicate, basophilic, and poorly outlined. The nuclei are eccentrically located, round, and very uniform. The chromatin classically has a "salt and pepper" appearance, but the texture is variable. Nucleoli are usually small but may be conspicuous. There is no necrosis, and mitotic figures are rare. Occasionally, a few larger, atypical, or multinucleated cells are present ("endocrine atypia").

Spindle cell carcinoids usually occur in the lung periphery and are characterized by small spindle cells. Their nuclear and cytoplasmic features are otherwise similar to typical carcinoids.

Atypical carcinoids are intermediate in morphology and behavior between typical carcinoid and small cell carcinoma. Atypical carcinoids show more pleomorphism, hyperchromasia, mitoses, necrosis, and molding than typical carcinoids but less atypia, more cytoplasm, and more prominent nucleoli than small cell carcinoma. Atypical carcinoid tends to occur peripherally, while typical carcinoid and small cell carcinoma tend to arise centrally. In essence, the more the tumor resembles small cell carcinoma, the worse the prognosis.

2.9.9 Granular Cell Tumor

Granular cell tumors occur in the submucosa and usually do not spontaneously exfoliate cells, but they may be amenable to diagnosis by bronchial brushing (or FNA biopsy). The most characteristic feature is the abundant, coarsely granular cytoplasm. Ultrastructurally, the granules correspond to tertiary lysosomes. Nuclei usually are small and uniform but can be more variable.

2.9.10 Salivary Gland Analog Tumors

Adenoid-cystic carcinoma is a rare lung tumor that more commonly arises in the trachea than the bronchi. The tumor may be covered with tracheobronchial epithelium; therefore, the examination of sputum is usually negative, but the tumor may yield cells for diagnosis by bronchial brush or FNA biopsy.

The tumor is composed of small, bland, uniform, basaloid cells, most characteristically forming microcystic spaces containing hyaline basement membrane–like material that is metachromatic (magenta in Diff-Quik). The differential diagnosis includes well-differentiated adenocarcinoma, carcinoid, and small cell carcinoma.

Mucoepidermoid carcinoma shows clusters of malignant squamous cells and mucus-producing glandular cells; a third (intermediate or spindle) cell type may be seen in low- to intermediate-grade mucoepidermoid carcinoma. High-grade mucoepidermoid carcinomas are indistinguishable from ordinary mixed adenosquamous carcinoma.

2.9.11 Sarcomas and Rare Tumors

Any type of primary or metastatic sarcoma can occur in the lung; the basic cytomorphology can be spindle, round, or pleomorphic. Carcinosarcoma may shed sarcoma cells (eg, rhabdomyoblasts) plus carcinoma cells. Pulmonary blastoma is a biphasic malignant tumor of epithelium (adenocarcinoma) and mesenchyme (blastema cells). The malignant cells tend to be relatively small, and only the adenocarcinomatous component may be seen in some cases. Germ cell tumors also can occur.

2.9.12 Malignant Lymphoma

Primary malignant lymphoma of the lung is rare; large cell non-Hodgkin lymphoma is the most common primary type. Secondary involvement is more common. Cytologically, no true tissue aggregates are formed |i2.70|, and lymphoglandular bodies may be seen in the background. The cells show characteristic lymphoid cytology, particularly in Diff-Quik, and a limited range of maturation. Reed-Sternberg cells and variants in a benign, reactive background are characteristic of Hodgkin disease |i2.71|. Mycosis fungoides, leukemias, or myeloma also can be seen rarely.

2.9.13 Metastases

Metastatic adenocarcinoma is more common than primary adenocarcinoma of the lung. Virtually any malignant tumor can involve the lung, but the most common tumors are those of the gastrointestinal tract |i2.72|, |i2.73|, breast |i2.74|, and lymphoma/leukemia, among others |i2.75|, |i2.76|. Melanoma |i2.77| and sarcomas also frequently metastasize to the lung.

Metastatic carcinoma is more difficult to detect by exfoliative cytology than primary lung cancer because the cells may not exfoliate readily. Consider a metastasis when the cells do not resemble the usual forms of lung cancer. Compare the metastasis with the primary lesion, if possible. Metastatic tumor usually occurs in a clean background (ie, no tumor diathesis).

In some cases, it may be difficult to distinguish primary from metastatic lung cancer. The presence of multiple or bilateral nodules and a history of a morphologically compatible cancer strongly favor metastasis. Also consider that tumor cells deriving from primary lesions in the oral cavity or esophagus, not involving the lung, could be found in sputum. Tumors also can involve the lung by direct extension rather than metastasis.

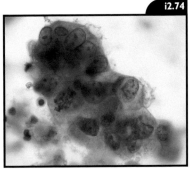

i2.74

Metastatic breast carcinoma

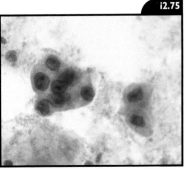

i2.75

Transitional cell carcinoma

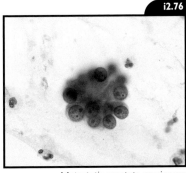

i2.76

Metastatic prostate carcinoma

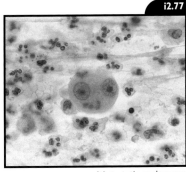

i2.77

Metastatic melanoma

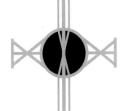

Cytology of body fluids encompasses effusion specimens from the pleural, abdominal, and pericardial spaces. The cytology of body cavity washings, which is morphologically quite similar to effusion cytology, is also considered. Synovial fluid cytology, also somewhat similar to effusion cytology, is discussed next. Finally, the cytology of nipple discharge is presented. The primary purpose of cytologic examination of these specimens is detection of malignancy, although it is also possible to diagnose a variety of benign diseases.

BODY CAVITY FLUIDS

Body cavities are lined by serous membranes: the pleura, pericardium, and peritoneum. These membranes are embryologically, microscopically, and immunologically identical. Each encloses a potential space normally containing only enough fluid to lubricate the membranes. Any excess amount of this fluid—an effusion—is always due to a pathologic process. An effusion can be a transudate, due to physicomechanical factors, such as congestive heart failure or cirrhosis, or an exudate, which implies damage to the serous membrane, due, for example, to inflammation or tumor. Malignant effusions are usually exudates.

3.1 Pleural Effusions

Pleural effusions can arise in the thorax (ie, a primary effusion, often due to pulmonary infection or infarction) or can be secondary to ascites. Right-sided pleural effusions resulting from abdominal disease commonly are due to cirrhosis, subdiaphragmatic or hepatic abscess, and Meigs syndrome (pleural effusion and ovarian fibroma). Pancreatitis is noteworthy for more often being associated with a left-sided pleural effusion. Among the most common sources of malignant pleural effusions are lung, breast, lymphoreticular system, and gastrointestinal (GI) tract cancers. Primary malignant tumors of the mesothelium, mesotheliomas, also can cause effusions. In many cases the primary site remains unknown.

3.2 Ascites

Ascites can result from a wide variety of disorders, ranging from cirrhosis to neoplasia. Malignant ascites commonly is associated with cancers of the ovary, breast, GI tract, or lymphoreticular system. In malignant ascites of unknown origin, consider the genital tract in women and the GI tract in men.

3.3 **Pericardial Effusions**

Many diseases, including infections and neoplasms, can cause pericardial effusions; most result in exudates. Infectious etiologies are more common in immunosuppressed patients. Malignant pericardial effusions often are due to carcinomas of the lung or breast, followed by lymphoma, sarcoma, and melanoma. Be cautious when evaluating pericardial effusions because they often contain extremely reactive mesothelial cells mimicking cancer.

3.4 **Special Types of Effusions**

3.4.1 Chylous Effusion

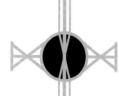

A chylous effusion is due to leakage or blockage of the thoracic duct (main lymph duct). It is classically milky white. True chylous effusions are rare, but causes include cancer (especially lymphoreticular malignancies), trauma, and tuberculosis.

Turbid effusions (due to tumor or WBCs) and pseudo-chylous effusions can be distinguished from true chylous effusions. The presence of neutral lipid distinguishes a true chylous effusion from its imitators.

3.4.2 Pseudochylous Effusions

Pseudochylous effusions classically have a metallic sheen, like gold paint, caused predominantly by cholesterol crystals. Although they are rare, pseudochylous effusions are associated with long-standing effusions, usually due to rheumatoid lung disease, tuberculosis, or myxedema. Cyst fluids also can have a pseudochylous appearance.

3.4.3 Bile-Stained Effusions

Bile-stained effusions are greenish. They are associated with cholecystitis, acute pancreatitis, and perforated viscus.

3.4.4 Bloody or Dark Brown ("Chocolate") Effusions

Bloody fluids can be due to such causes as a traumatic tap, bleeding, and malignancy. A traumatic tap tends to clear as the fluid is withdrawn. Benign and malignant effusions can be bloody; thus, the presence of blood is not diagnostic of malignancy. Conversely, many malignant effusions are not bloody. Rarely, melanin pigment produced by metastatic melanoma produces a dark brown effusion.

3.4.5 Air and Fluid

Air can be introduced into a body cavity through a penetrating wound (including surgery or even the paracentesis procedure itself) or bronchopulmonary fistula due to infection or tumor. Eosinophils are frequently present microscopically.

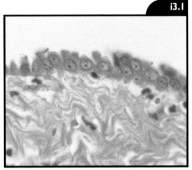

Serous membrane, tissue

3.4.6 Mucinous Effusions

Mucinous effusions ("jelly belly") can be due to pseudomyxoma peritonei caused by mucinous cysts of the ovary or appendix or colloid carcinomas (eg, stomach, breast, colon, or ovary). The cytology shows bland tumor cells, singly and in clusters, that may resemble reactive mesothelial cells or histiocytes.

3.4.7 Effusions of Unknown or Occult Etiology

When the cause of an effusion is unknown, suspect cirrhosis, carcinomatosis, or tuberculosis, among numerous other possibilities. In many cases, no cause can be found.

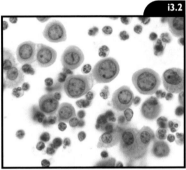

Reactive mesothelial cells

3.5 The Cells

3.5.1 Mesothelial Cells

Mesothelial cells are mesodermally derived epithelial cells. Normally, the mesothelium is a single layer of flat cells. However, when irritated, the mesothelium becomes hyperplastic, and the cells become plump and cuboidal with active nuclei |i3.1|. These reactive mesothelial cells can be confused with cancer. And therein lies the essence of the diagnostic dilemma in fluid cytology: distinguishing reactive mesothelial cells from cancer.

Mesothelial cells in fluid are predominantly single |i3.2| but also form small groups, including cell balls and papillae, that can mimic formations of tumor cells. Large groups of cells are suspicious for malignancy. Groups with lobulated, flower-like borders |i3.3|, |i3.4| favor mesothelial origin, while smooth, "community" borders favor carcinoma, although these outlines are not specific. A clear space, or "window" |i3.5|, between adjacent cells is characteristic of mesothelial cells but can sometimes be seen between malignant cells. Mesothelial cells frequently

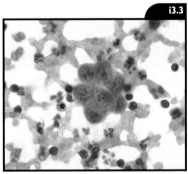

Reactive mesothelial cells

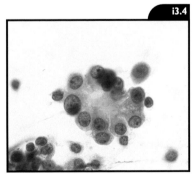

Reactive mesothelial cells

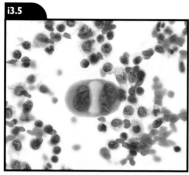

Mesothelial cells—"window"

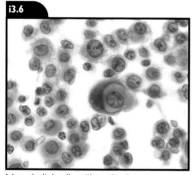

Mesothelial cells—"hugging"

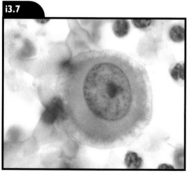

Mesothelial cells—"skirt" (oil)

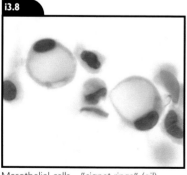

Mesothelial cells—"signet rings" (oil)

exhibit "molding," ie, adjacent cells compress one another. Orderly, mosaic-like sheets of cells, occasional cell-in-cell "bird's eyes," and "hugging" |i3.6| (in which two cytoplasmic "arms" reach out and embrace an adjacent cell) are also characteristic of mesothelial cells.

Mesothelial cells can range from small to large; occasionally, multinucleated giant cells are seen. Characteristically, the cytoplasm is dense in the center (endoplasm) and pale in the periphery (ectoplasm). The cell borders of mesothelial cells are not sharply demarcated but often appear to have a lacy "skirt" |i3.7|, due in part to surface microvilli. Occasionally, metachromatic red "whiskers," which are prominent microvilli, can be seen with the Diff-Quik stain. Mesothelial cells also can have blunt cytoplasmic processes, or blebs, that are degenerative in nature.

The cytoplasm is typically homogeneous and granular, with a ground-glass appearance. However, lipid, glycogen, and degenerative vacuoles are common nonspecific findings. Large degenerative vacuoles may cause a signet ring appearance |i3.8|, mimicking signet ring cell carcinoma (look for mucin).

The nuclei of mesothelial cells are usually single, but binucleation is common, and multinucleation also occurs. The nuclei are usually near the center of the cell but can be eccentric, especially if there is vacuolar cytoplasmic degeneration. The nuclei are usually round to oval, with well-defined, smooth nuclear membranes, fine chromatin, and inconspicuous nucleoli. However, reactive changes are common and may include nuclear enlargement and pleomorphism, slight nuclear membrane irregularity, chromatin clumping, and prominent nucleoli. Mitoses are not diagnostic of malignancy unless clearly abnormal.

Reactive mesothelial cells can mimic mesothelioma or metastatic carcinoma. Well-known causes of marked reactive changes include pulmonary embolism or infarct, active cirrhosis or hepatitis |i3.9|, uremia, pancreatitis, long-term dialysis, and radiation and chemotherapy |i3.10|. Although reactive atypia can be severe, it affects the cells more or less uniformly, resulting in the "sibling image" characteristic of benign cells. In contrast, a foreign population of cells usually indicates metastasis. Marked nuclear abnormalities (eg, pleomorphism, irregular membranes, chromatin clumping, multiple nucleoli or macronucleoli) suggest malignancy. Marked inflammation—common in benign effusions with reactive mesothelial cells—is unusual in malignant effusions. Be cautious when diagnosing malignancy in patients with conditions known to induce marked reactive changes. (See "Malignant Effusions," p 55.)

3.5.2 Histiocytes

Histiocytes usually are present in effusions |i3.11|. They can be particularly prominent in cancer, tuberculosis, and embolism.

Although it can sometimes be difficult to distinguish histiocytes from mesothelial cells, both cell types are benign.

Histiocytes are usually of moderate size but range from small to large; however, giant cell histiocytes are rare in effusions. Histiocytes occur singly or in loose sheets, without the molding, hugging, windows, or tight groups that are characteristic of mesothelial cells. The cytoplasm is usually delicately vacuolated or finely granular with indistinct cell borders. Phagocytosis (eg, RBCs, debris, hemosiderin, lipid, melanin) is a characteristic feature of histiocytes.

The nuclei are variably sized, round to oval or, classically, bean-shaped, and eccentrically located in the cytoplasm. Binucleation or multinucleation is common. The chromatin texture varies from fine to "salt and pepper" to coarse. In air-dried material, it has a characteristic "raked sand" appearance. Nucleoli are usually small and indistinct but can be prominent in reactive conditions. Mitotic figures can be seen.

3.5.3 Lymphocytes

Some lymphocytes usually are present in an effusion as a nonspecific finding. They can be numerous in a wide variety of conditions ranging from congestive heart failure and infections to carcinoma and malignant lymphoma.

3.5.4 Eosinophils

Eosinophilic effusions usually portend a good prognosis. Most are pleural and apparently result from allergic reactions to dust particles in the air, introduced by previous taps or pneumothorax. Other causes include pulmonary infarct, pneumonia, trauma, hydatid disease, Löffler syndrome, polyarteritis nodosa, dialysis, and asbestos; however, cancer (including Hodgkin disease) and tuberculosis are rare causes. In many cases, the cause is never identified. Eosinophils typically have bilobed nuclei, and, in contrast with neutrophils, the eosinophilic granules are large enough to be resolved individually with the light microscope |i3.12|. Charcot-Leyden crystals may be present.

3.5.5 Neutrophils

Neutrophilia is nonspecific and can have many causes, particularly infections. However, malignant effusions are seldom associated with acute inflammation.

3.5.6 Other Cells and Miscellaneous Findings

Lung, liver, skin, soft tissue, gut, etc, usually represent "pickups" from the needle. Rarely, they may indicate a fistula, which is more likely if inflammation, food, bacteria, etc, also are present.

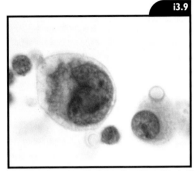
i3.9
Reactive mesothelial cells—hepatitis (oil)

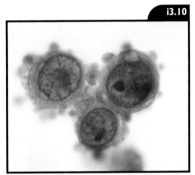
i3.10
Reactive mesothelial cells—chemotherapy

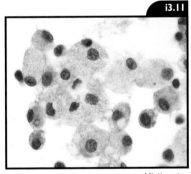
i3.11
Histiocytes

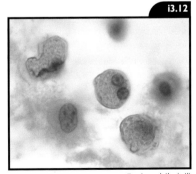
i3.12
Eosinophils (oil)

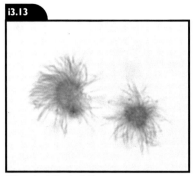

Ciliocytophthoria (oil)

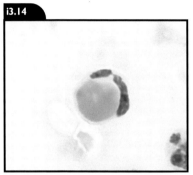

LE cell (oil)

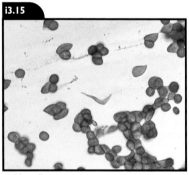

Sickle cell

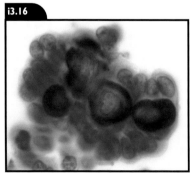

Psammoma bodies

Ciliocytophthoria is detached ciliated tufts of fallopian tube origin |**i3.13**|. This nonspecific finding is relatively common in peritoneal specimens from females. *Not a protozoan or parasite!*

Microorganisms of virtually every type have been described in effusions (see the Appendix).

Megakaryocytes are rarely observed in effusions but can be seen in any condition associated with extramedullary hematopoiesis, such as myeloid metaplasia, myeloproliferative disorder, anticoagulant therapy, and metastatic carcinoma. Megakaryocytes are large cells with single multilobated nuclei and granular, platelet-producing cytoplasm. Factor VIII expression is a potential aid in the differential diagnosis with carcinoma.

LE cells, although suggestive of systemic lupus erythematosus (ergo, LE cell), also can be seen in rheumatoid arthritis and drug reactions (eg, procainamide, hydralazine), as well as in multiple myeloma and Hodgkin disease. An LE cell is a neutrophil containing a hematoxylin body, which is a cytoplasmic inclusion of homogenized nuclear material |**i3.14**|. Look for them in an unexplained pleural effusion in a woman of childbearing age.

Sickle cells, sickle-shaped RBCs, can be seen in sickle cell anemia |**i3.15**|.

Curschmann spirals have been described in effusions, with and without obvious source of mucin (eg, adenocarcinoma).

Charcot-Leyden crystals are more likely to form with delayed processing and refrigeration of eosinophilic effusions.

Psammoma bodies are not diagnostic of malignancy. They are commonly found in benign conditions, eg, mesothelial hyperplasia and endosalpingiosis. Ovarian cancer is the most common malignancy with psammoma bodies in an effusion |**i3.16**|.

Collagen balls are cores of collagen usually covered with mesothelium. More common in peritoneal washes than in effusions, they can be seen in benign mesothelial proliferations and mesothelioma but are rare in adenocarcinoma |**i3.17**|.

3.6 Special Benign Effusions

3.6.1 Tuberculosis

A tuberculous effusion is typically turbid and yellow or may have a silky green, metallic sheen (pseudochylous effusion). Characteristically, lymphocytes are abundant (small T cells) and form groups, and mesothelial cells are conspicuously sparse or absent (due to fibrin trapping) |**i3.18**|. Histiocytes may be present, but giant cells, especially Langhans type, are rare. Flow cytometry may be helpful in the differential diagnosis with lymphoma (see p 60).

3.6.2 Rheumatoid Effusion

Rheumatoid effusions usually are associated with active arthritis. A pseudochylous appearance (metallic sheen) is classic. The cytologic picture reflects the histology of a rheumatoid granuloma, a diagnostic triad consisting of necrotic debris, epithelioid histiocytes, and multinucleated giant cells |i3.19|, |i3.20|. The epithelioid histiocytes are spindle or carrot-shaped cells that are frequently degenerated, with pyknotic nuclei and dense, blue to pink to orangeophilic cytoplasm, which can mimic keratinizing squamous cell carcinoma. Inflammation may be present, but mesothelial cells are sparse or absent. Rheumatoid granuloma is a rare condition in which bizarre cells can be present in a benign effusion; otherwise, bizarre-appearing cells usually indicate malignancy.

3.6.3 Endometriosis

Endometriosis can cause body cavity effusions with grossly bloody to chocolate brown fluid. The diagnostic microscopic triad is hemosiderin-laden macrophages, endometrial glands (small columnar cells similar in appearance to mesothelial cells), and endometrial stroma (similar in appearance to histiocytes or lymphocytes). Because the full triad may not be present, and because of the similarity of endometrial cells to mesothelial cells and histiocytes, endometriosis is difficult to specifically diagnose in a fluid; clinical history (and cell block) may help. Endometrial carcinoma can arise in endometriosis rarely.

3.7 Malignant Effusions

Malignancy is second only to congestive heart failure as a cause of effusions. Although most effusions in patients with cancer are malignant, oncology patients also can have benign effusions, eg, due to congestive heart failure or cirrhosis, as well as a reaction to radiation or chemotherapy. Virtually any malignancy can cause an effusion, but carcinomas of the lung, breast, ovary, and GI tract are common causes. Abdominal or pelvic malignancies usually cause ascites before causing a pleural effusion. Occasionally, a malignant effusion is the first sign of cancer (particularly lung and ovarian cancers, but rarely breast cancer because the primary tumor is usually clinically obvious).

A malignant effusion is usually a grave prognostic sign. However, certain subsets of patients, eg, women with peritoneal carcinomatosis, patients with lymphomas, and children with "small blue cell tumors," may respond to treatment.

Fluid cytodiagnosis can be very difficult, particularly when the cells are degenerated. A request to submit more mate-

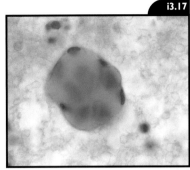

i3.17

Collagen ball

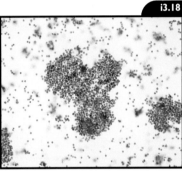

i3.18

Tuberculous effusion—lymphoid groups

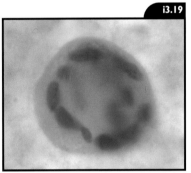

i3.19

Rheumatoid effusion

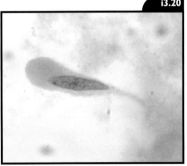

i3.20

Rheumatoid effusion

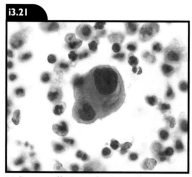

Malignant effusion—foreign cells

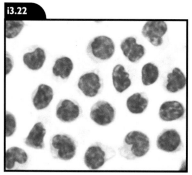

Lymphoma—single cells, small cleaved (oil)

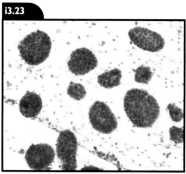

Adenocarcinoma—cell balls

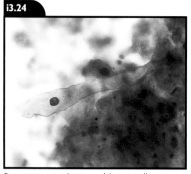

Squamous carcinoma—bizarre cell

rial, if the fluid reaccumulates, can be helpful. Benign atypia tends to resolve, in contrast with malignancy.

3.7.1 General Features of a Malignant Effusion

The key to diagnosis of a malignant effusion is the presence of a population of foreign cells |i3.21|. Foreign features include malignant atypia, particularly chromatin abnormalities, as well as mucin, melanin, or heavy keratinization. Mesothelioma may be an exception to this general diagnostic rule, because the cells are native rather than foreign and can be cytologically bland. Also, some other malignancies, such as metastatic breast cancer, can shed cytologically bland cells mimicking reactive mesothelial cells, making diagnosis difficult. Clinical history is the most important information to determine the primary site. For cases in which the primary site is unknown, consider ovary, lung, GI tract, and the lymphoreticular system.

3.7.2 Tumor Diagnosis

No single feature is diagnostic of malignancy.

Cell Groups

Tumors frequently exfoliate large groups, including cell balls, papillae, or glands. Benign mesothelial cells in effusions usually do not shed in large aggregates. Single tumor cells are typical of lymphoma (classic) |i3.22|, melanoma, sarcoma, and, occasionally, mesothelioma.

Group Contours

Clusters of adenocarcinoma typically have smooth outlines (community borders) |i3.23|, while mesothelial cell groups usually have knobby, flower-like outlines. Unfortunately, these contours are not specific.

Cell Shape

All cells tend to round up in fluid. Unusual or bizarre shapes are highly suggestive of malignancy |i3.24| (exclude rheumatoid effusion).

Cell Surface

Malignant cells usually have well-defined cell borders in contrast with mesothelial cells or, particularly, histiocytes. Cilia usually indicate benign cells; however, long microvilli mimicking cilia can be seen in mesothelial cells or certain malignancies, especially ovarian carcinoma, which very rarely has true cilia |i3.25|.

Cytoplasm

Secretory vacuoles (including intracytoplasmic lumens and signet ring cells |i3.26|) are virtually diagnostic of malignancy. Mucicarmine can be extremely useful in the diagnosis of adenocarcinoma. Degenerative vacuoles are a common, nonspecific finding. On the other hand, degenerative vacuoles are crystal clear because they contain only water and electrolytes. Other cytoplasmic products, including melanin, heavy keratin, and cross-striations, are also important diagnostically.

Nuclei

Malignant nuclei, of course, are the sine qua non of a diagnosis of malignancy |i3.27|. They are usually enlarged and pleomorphic, with high nuclear/cytoplasmic ratios. Irregular nuclear membranes; abnormal, coarse, irregular chromatin; and large or abnormally shaped nucleoli are important diagnostic clues. Hyperchromasia, however, may not be prominent because the cells can proliferate in body cavity fluids. Mitotic figures are not helpful in diagnosis unless they are clearly abnormal.

Background

Acute inflammation is unusual in cancer. Chronic inflammation or blood is common but nonspecific. Lipophages, which imply tissue destruction, are a warning to look for cancer.

3.7.3 Adenocarcinoma

Adenocarcinoma is, by far, the most common cause of a malignant effusion. Among the most useful features in diagnosis of adenocarcinoma are glandular acini, papillae, or cell balls; increased nuclear/cytoplasmic ratios; irregular nuclear membranes; abnormal chromatin; large or irregular nucleoli; and, particularly, secretory vacuoles with mucin. However, vacuolization, per se, is virtually meaningless.

General Patterns of Adenocarcinoma

Certain patterns of adenocarcinoma may suggest a site of origin. Cannonballs, which are very large balls of cells with smooth community borders, suggest breast cancer. Papillae, which are three-dimensional clusters longer in one direction than in the other two, suggest GI tract or ovarian cancer in ascitic fluids and lung |i3.28| or breast cancer in pleural fluids; also consider mesothelial hyperplasia and neoplasia. Signet ring cells suggest gastric or breast cancer. Intracytoplasmic lumens (targetoid secretory vacuoles) are characteristic of breast cancer, particularly lobular type. Extreme vacuolization is most characteristic of ovarian carcinoma but also can be seen in lung and pancreatic carcinomas, among others. A predominance of single tumor cells

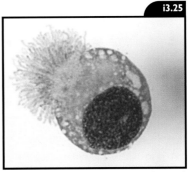
Ciliated ovarian carcinoma, rare (DQ, oil)

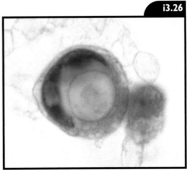
Signet ring cell carcinoma (oil)

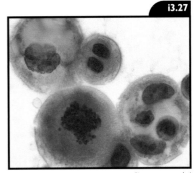
Malignant nuclei

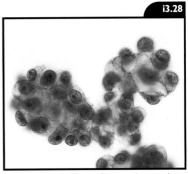
Papillary adenocarcinoma, lung

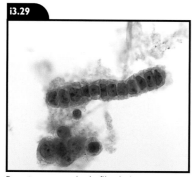

Breast cancer—single file chain

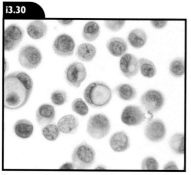

Breast cancer—intracytoplasmic lumens

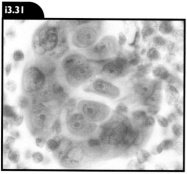

Non–small cell lung cancer

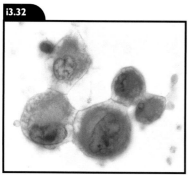

Renal cell cancer

suggests breast or gastric cancer (also lymphoma, sarcoma, melanoma). Single file chains of cells suggest breast |**i3.29**|, pancreas, or gastric carcinoma, as well as lung cancer (small cell) and mesothelioma. Bizarre or giant tumor cells are associated with carcinomas of the lung and pancreas but also can be seen in squamous cell carcinomas, sarcomas, and melanomas, among others. Rheumatoid effusion is a rare benign explanation for bizarre or giant cells in an effusion. Clear cells are associated with carcinomas of the kidney and ovary, as well as with germ cell tumors. Clear cells in fluids may have unexpectedly dense cytoplasm.

"Specific" Patterns of Adenocarcinoma

Breast Cancer: Breast cancer is the most common cause of malignant pleural effusions in women; most are ipsilateral to the primary tumor. The cells are usually fairly bland and uniform and may form aggregates or be predominantly single. Diagnostic clues are cannonballs, intracytoplasmic lumens |**i3.30**|, and single file chains of cells. Some cases are exceedingly difficult to diagnose because they closely mimic reactive mesothelial cells (mesothelial pattern). A positive mucicarmine stain implies cancer.

Lung Cancer: Lung cancer is one of the most common causes of malignant effusions. The common forms of lung cancer can be divided into small cell and non–small cell types. The non–small cell pattern typically shows large pleomorphic cells but can range from bland to bizarre. The cytoplasm is often vacuolated, sometimes markedly, but can be dense and squamoid or contain mucin (as a reflection of dual glandular and squamous differentiation) |**i3.31**|. See also "Small Cell Carcinoma," next page.

Renal Cancer: The tumor cells can exfoliate in papillary or acinar groups. The cytoplasm can be granular or clear (but is often dense in effusions) and is mucin-negative. Tumor cells with granular centers and clear periphery are particularly characteristic |**i3.32**|.

Gastric Cancer: Intestinal type sheds clusters of large, highly atypical cells; gastric type sheds single signet ring cells. Most gastric cancers are mucin-positive.

Colorectal Cancer: Colorectal carcinomas characteristically exfoliate papillary or acinar aggregates of tall columnar cells with nuclear palisading, highly irregular nuclear membranes, and apical cytoplasmic densities suggesting terminal bars |**i3.33**|. Signet ring cells also may be seen. Most cases are mucin-positive.

Pancreaticobiliary Cancer: Carcinomas of the pancreas and bile ducts are morphologically indistinguishable. The cells may be similar to those of non–small cell lung cancer, including cytoplasmic density, or ovarian cancer, with marked vacuolization. Single file chains of cells may be seen.

Ovarian Cancer: This is the most common cause of malignant ascites. There are three common types: mucinous (resembles endocervical cells or gastrointestinal malignancy), serous (resembles fallopian tube cells or reactive mesothelial cells/mesothelioma), and endometrioid (identical to endometrial carcinoma). However, ovarian carcinoma most often is characterized by markedly vacuolated tumor cells |i3.34|. The vacuoles are large and transparent. Psammoma bodies, if present, suggest an ovarian origin of a malignancy, but psammoma bodies are not necessarily associated with malignancy. The differential diagnosis includes non–small cell lung cancer, pancreatic carcinoma, and mesothelioma.

Pseudomyxoma Peritonei: The effusion fluid is characteristically composed of thick mucus (mucinous ascites, "jelly belly"). The mucinous tumor cells tend to be bland and present in a few cohesive sheets. Other cells (mesothelial cells, histiocytes, or leukocytes) are sparse or absent. The essence of the diagnosis is the presence of endocervical-like cells in mucous lakes.

Liver Cancer: Hepatocellular carcinoma is frequently associated with ascites because the tumor usually arises in the setting of cirrhosis. However, it is unusual to find tumor cells in the fluid. Tumor cells, if present, have malignant nuclear features, granular cytoplasm, and, possibly, evidence of bile production |i3.35|.

Thyroid Cancer: Papillae or microacinar complexes, intranuclear cytoplasmic invaginations, colloid and psammoma bodies may suggest thyroid cancer, but this is a rare cause of effusions, particularly as an unknown primary site.

Prostate Cancer: Prostate cancer is characterized by microacinar complexes and uniform tumor cells with prominent nucleoli.

3.7.4 Squamous Cell Carcinoma

Although squamous cell carcinoma is a common cancer, it rarely sheds diagnostic cells into an effusion. The tumor cells are characterized by thick dense cytoplasm with distinct cell borders. Clues to the diagnosis include cells with bizarre shapes (|i3.24|, p 56), rings of keratinization in the cytoplasm, and pearls |i3.36|. The differential diagnosis includes sarcomas and rheumatoid effusions. Also, benign squamous cells can be seen in a variety of conditions, including cysts, fistulas, and contamination.

3.7.5 Small Cell Carcinoma

Small cell carcinoma usually forms definite tissue aggregates with marked molding and, frequently, single file arrangements |i3.37|, |i3.38|. The cells range in size from lymphocytes to small mesothelial cells. Most cells are rounded or angular, but some may be elongated to spindle-shaped. The chromatin may appear somewhat coarse in effusion fluids. Similarly, although nucleoli are usually inconspicuous, they may be somewhat more prominent than usually expected. The differential diagnosis includes breast cancer (small cells, single file chains of cells; look

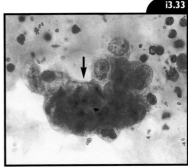

i3.33

Colon cancer—"terminal bar"

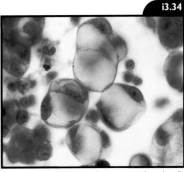

i3.34

Ovarian cancer—hypervacuolated cells

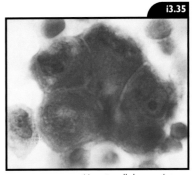

i3.35

Hepatocellular carcinoma

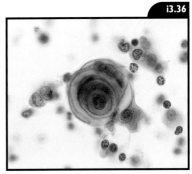

i3.36

Squamous cell carcinoma—pearl

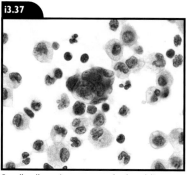

i3.37

Small cell carcinoma—marked molding

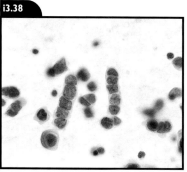

i3.38

Small cell carcinoma—single file chains

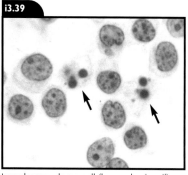

i3.39

Lymphoma—large cell (karyorrhexis, oil)

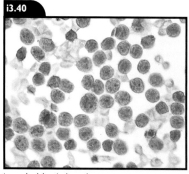

i3.40

Lymphoblastic lymphoma

for mucin secretion) and small blue cell tumors of childhood (small cell carcinoma is a tumor of older adult smokers).

3.7.6 Lymphoma/Leukemia

The most characteristic feature of lymphoreticular malignancies is that all the tumor cells are single; there are no true tissue aggregates. In general, the larger the cell type, the easier the diagnosis. Small cell and mixed lymphomas may be difficult to distinguish from reactive lymphocytosis. Anaplastic lymphoid cells may be difficult to recognize as lymphoid. In practice, it can be very difficult to diagnose lymphoma in an effusion fluid; flow cytometry can be very helpful.

The cells often have scant, delicate cytoplasm, with relatively high nuclear/cytoplasmic ratios, although in some large cell lymphomas, the cytoplasm can be more abundant. Nuclear abnormalities often are present, including prominent nucleoli and irregular nuclear membranes (eg, cleaves, nuclear knobs). Massive karyorrhexis ("mercury droplets") |i3.39| suggests lymphoma, especially high-grade, or previous therapy.

Small cleaved non–Hodgkin lymphoma is one of the most common lymphomas diagnosed in an effusion (|i3.22|, p 56). It may show significant size variation, including the presence of large cells. The nuclei of large cell lymphoma are larger than histiocyte nuclei and commonly have nuclear knobs. The amount of cytoplasm is variable. Lymphoblastic lymphoma |i3.40| is characterized by small to medium-sized cells with scant cytoplasm, fine chromatin, and inconspicuous nucleoli; nuclear membranes can be smooth or convoluted. Although it is rare to find diagnostic Reed-Sternberg cells in effusions due to Hodgkin disease, large Hodgkin cells may be seen |i3.41|. Unfortunately, they may be difficult to distinguish from large cells of non–Hodgkin lymphoma or metastatic carcinoma.

Air-dried, Diff-Quik–stained slides may be useful in classification. Cell blocks can be helpful for performing special stains. Immunocytochemistry and flow cytometry can be helpful in diagnosis and classification of these tumors. Most lymphomas in effusions are B-cell type. Marked chronic inflammation, eg, in tuberculosis, may be difficult to distinguish from malignant lymphoma. The presence of groups of lymphocytes trapped in fibrin exudate suggests an inflammatory condition (|i3.18|, p 55). A mixed pattern of chronic inflammatory cells, in which small lymphocytes predominate and plasma cells are present, also favors a reactive process. Eosinophils may be observed, rarely, in Hodgkin disease. Myeloma is characterized by mature or immature plasma cells, which may have cytoplasmic Russell or nuclear Dutcher bodies. Benign plasma cells may be numerous in a wide variety of diseases, ranging from congestive heart failure to cancer.

Leukemias are cytologically similar to lymphomas in fluid specimens, ie, they are composed of malignant hematopoietic cells in a dispersed, single cell pattern. Cytoplasmic features can be helpful in classification (best appreciated in Diff-Quik stain). For example, myelogenous leukemias may have cytoplasmic granules or Auer rods as evidence of granulocytic differentiation. The differential diagnosis of acute myelogenous leukemia includes large cell lymphoma, and the differential diagnosis of chronic myelogenous leukemia includes marked acute inflammation. Hairy cell leukemia is characterized by singly dispersed malignant cells with "hairy" cytoplasmic projections.

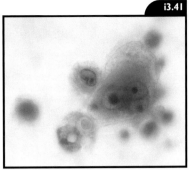

Hodgkin disease

3.7.7 Melanoma

The effusion fluid in metastatic melanoma may be dark brown or black. The cells are usually single and relatively large, with large, eccentrically located nuclei. Binucleation is common. The nuclei usually have very prominent nucleoli and frequently have intranuclear cytoplasmic invaginations. The presence of melanin pigment in malignant cells is diagnostic |i3.42|. Melanoma is notorious for its ability to mimic a wide variety of other neoplasms, as well as for late recurrences.

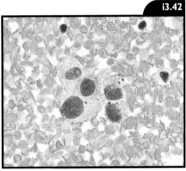

Melanoma—note pigment (DQ)

3.7.8 Carcinoid Tumors

The most characteristic pattern shows monotonously uniform, small, round tumor cells arranged in loose clusters or singly; short single file chains of cells with cellular molding may be seen. The nuclei are usually single and typically have a salt-and-pepper chromatin pattern; mitotic figures are rare. The cytoplasm is scant; neurosecretory granules may be demonstrated with special stains or immunocytochemistry. The differential diagnosis includes small cell carcinoma (a related neuroendocrine tumor) and small cell adenocarcinoma.

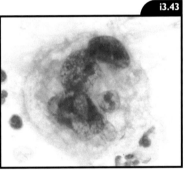

Pleomorphic sarcoma

3.7.9 Sarcomas and Rare Tumors

Effusions may develop in patients with sarcoma, but the primary tumor is usually well known clinically. The cells can vary from pleomorphic |i3.43| (eg, malignant fibrous histiocytoma) to relatively small and uniform (round cell sarcomas, eg, rhabdomyosarcoma) to spindle-shaped |i3.44| (spindle cell sarcoma, eg, leiomyosarcoma). The differential diagnosis includes mesothelioma, squamous cell carcinoma, and rheumatoid effusion. In fact, because there may be no obvious special differentiation and all cells tend to round up in fluids, the differential diagnosis may include practically any malignant tumor.

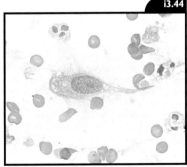

Spindle cell sarcoma

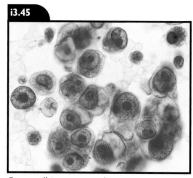

Germ cell tumor—seminoma

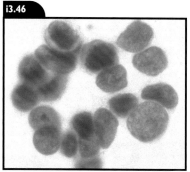

Neuroblastoma—rosette (oil)

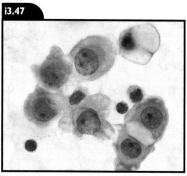

Mesothelioma

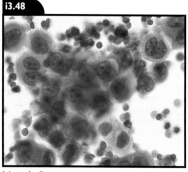

Mesothelioma

Germ cell tumors also can shed diagnostic cells into fluids |i3.45|. Consider a germ cell tumor when confronted with "big ugly tumor cells" in a young patient. The diagnosis is important because some patients will respond to therapy.

3.7.10 Malignant Effusions in Children

Pediatric effusions are usually benign. Among malignant effusions, most are small cell type, mostly lymphomas. The differential diagnosis of small blue cell tumors of childhood includes lymphoma/leukemia (exclusively single cells), Wilms tumor (small blastema cells, spindle cells), neuroblastoma |i3.46| (uniform small cells with molding, with or without rosettes, periodic acid–Schiff negative), Ewing sarcoma (uniform periodic acid– Schiff–positive cells), and embryonal rhabdomyosarcoma (pleomorphic small cells, plus elongated and strap-shaped cells; cross striations are rare but diagnostic). Distinguishing small cell malignancies from benign mononuclear inflammatory cells can sometimes be difficult.

3.8 Mesothelioma

Most mesotheliomas arise in the pleura but also can occur in the peritoneum, pericardium, or, rarely, the tunica vaginalis testis. The classic clinical history of pleural mesothelioma is one of asbestos exposure, persistent pleural effusions, chest pain, and evidence of pleural thickening. Most cases occur in men, usually between the ages of 50 and 70 years, but there is a wide age range. Mesothelioma characteristically grows by encasement (with superficial invasion of underlying viscera) but can form a dominant mass. Conversely, lung cancer usually forms a dominant mass but can grow by encasement ("pseudomesotheliomatous pattern"). Metastases occur with about the same frequency as non–small cell lung cancer, although brain metastases are rare in mesothelioma.

Fluid cytology is frequently the first diagnostic specimen. The fluid is characteristically highly viscous due to hyaluronic acid. The essence of the diagnosis of mesothelioma is that the malignant cells look like mesothelial cells (morphologic kinship) |i3.47|. There is no foreign population of tumor cells. Unfortunately, some mesotheliomas have subtle cytologic abnormalities, making them difficult to distinguish from benign or reactive mesothelial cells.

An important clue to the diagnosis of mesothelioma is the presence of "more and bigger cells in more and bigger clusters" |i3.48|. Single cells, however, are also usually present and may predominate in some cases |i3.49|.

Clusters of cells with irregular, knobby, flower-like outlines are characteristic of mesothelioma. The clusters tend to be larger and more complex than those in benign effusions. Cell clusters in adenocarcinoma usually have smooth community borders. Numerous cell-in-cell patterns and long chains of cells are common in mesothelioma compared with benign effusions.

The individual malignant mesothelial cells are usually larger and more variable than benign mesothelial cells. However, a relatively constant nuclear/cytoplasmic ratio is maintained, giving the overall impression of uniformity. Occasionally, giant tumor cells are seen, but frankly bizarre-appearing cells favor carcinoma.

Mesothelial cytoplasm is characteristically dense, particularly in the central perinuclear area (the endoplasm), but often fades to a delicate lacy appearance toward the edges (the ectoplasm). In contrast, adenocarcinoma usually has diffusely delicate, pale to foamy cytoplasm. Thin rings of keratinization may be observed in the mesothelial endoplasm. "Windows" |i3.50|, "skirts" |i3.51|, blebs, and cytoplasmic glycogen are more characteristic of mesothelioma than of adenocarcinoma.

Central or paracentral location of the nucleus in the cytoplasm favors mesothelial cell origin, while eccentric location is more characteristic of adenocarcinoma. The usual nuclear criteria of malignancy, ie, enlargement and pleomorphism with irregular membranes and abnormal chromatin, apply in diagnosis of mesothelioma, but these features may be subtle in some cases. Although prominent nucleoli can be seen in reactive mesothelial cells, macronucleoli are uncommon in benign effusions and may be the only malignant feature in some cases of mesothelioma. Mitotic figures are not helpful unless they are clearly abnormal.

Collagen balls |i3.52| may be seen with benign or malignant mesothelial proliferations but are rarely observed in adenocarcinoma. Psammoma bodies are more common in benign effusions and metastatic carcinoma. Lymphocytic infiltration may be extensive. Flocculent material, corresponding to hyaluronic acid, may be seen. "Asbestos bodies" are actually more commonly seen in lung cancer than in mesothelioma. The differential diagnosis of mesothelioma with papillary serous carcinoma of the ovary can be particularly difficult or impossible.

3.8.1 Special Studies

Adenocarcinomas of the lung typically produce epithelial mucin, stainable with mucicarmine. Mesotheliomas produce acid mucins, stainable with alcian blue and digested with hyaluronidase.

Mesothelioma is characterized ultrastructurally by long, slender, branching microvilli |i3.53|. Adenocarcinoma is characterized by short, stubby microvilli associated with rootlets and terminal webs, as well as true glands, often containing mucus.

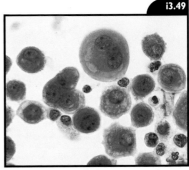
i3.49

Mesothelioma—note glycogen

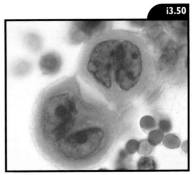
i3.50

Mesothelioma—"window" (oil)

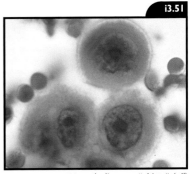
i3.51

Mesothelioma—"skirts" (oil)

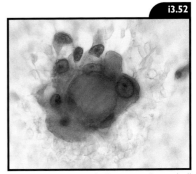
i3.52

Mesothelioma—collagen ball

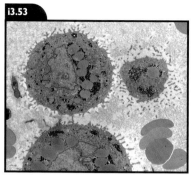
Mesothelioma—ultrastructure

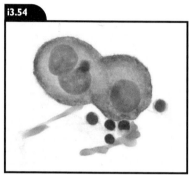
Mesothelioma—high molecular wt keratin

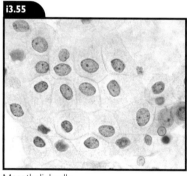
Mesothelial cells

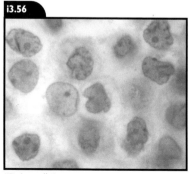
"Daisy cells"

Cytokeratins are found in mesothelioma and adenocarcinomas. However, high molecular weight keratins are more characteristic of mesothelioma |i3.54|. At least two epithelial markers should be negative before making a diagnosis of mesothelioma. Epithelial markers include CEA (in carcinomas of endodermal origin, eg, lung, GI tract), BerEp4, Leu M1, and B72.3 |t3.1|. Mesothelium-associated antibodies, eg, HBME1 and Calretinin, are now available but are not entirely specific for mesothelioma.

BODY CAVITY WASHINGS

Washings of body cavities consist of traumatically exfoliated sheets of mesothelial cells, WBCs, macrophages, blood, fibrin, and debris, often including glove powder. Other cells, eg, endometrial (including endometriosis) or fallopian tube (including endosalpingiosis) as well as psammoma bodies, may be seen in benign or malignant disease. Unsatisfactory specimens can result from inadequate cellularity or obscuring blood or debris.

3.9 **Mesothelial Cells**

Nonreactive mesothelial cells are polygonal cells with moderate amounts of delicate cytoplasm, yet they have prominent cell borders |i3.55|. They can form large orderly sheets, or mosaics, of cells reminiscent of the honeycomb arrangement characteristic of benign glandular cells. The nuclei are single, paracentrically located, and usually round to oval, with smooth to slightly irregular membranes, fine chromatin, and small nucleoli. The nuclei can vary slightly in size and shape. Occasionally, the cells have lobulated nuclear outlines, known as "daisy cells," which may be related to estrogen |i3.56|.

In response to a variety of conditions (eg, inflammation, trauma, radiation, or chemotherapy—as well as cirrhosis, uremia, and pancreatitis) the mesothelial cells may undergo reactive changes, identical to those previously described for reactive mesothelial cells in an effusion.

3.10 **Gynecologic Cytology in Peritoneal Washes**

There is a morphologic spectrum from reactive mesothelial cells to endosalpingiosis to "borderline" serous tumors to serous adenocarcinoma. The cells of any of these conditions can

t3.1 Characteristic Immunoreactions of Mesothelioma vs Adenocarcinoma*

	CEA	EMA	AE1	AE3	Other
Mesothelioma	−	+	+	+	−
Adenocarcinoma	+	+	+	−	+

* At least two epithelial markers should be negative in mesothelioma. Carcinoembryonic antigen (CEA) marks adenocarcinomas of endodermal origin (eg, lung, gastrointestinal tract). Epithelial membrane antigen (EMA) shows a "thick cell membrane" (mesothelioma) vs diffuse (adenocarcinoma) staining pattern. AE1, low molecular weight keratin, is expressed in both mesothelioma and adenocarcinoma. AE3, high molecular weight keratin, is characteristic of mesothelioma and unusual in adenocarcinoma. Other epithelial markers include BerEp4, Leu M1, B72.3.

appear quite similar to one another with only subtle differences. The differential diagnosis of reactive mesothelial cells with low-grade adenocarcinoma is based on finding orderly flat sheets of cells with smooth nuclear membranes and bland chromatin vs disorderly, three-dimensional clusters of cells with irregular nuclear membranes and abnormal chromatin. However, irregular nuclear membranes also can be seen in benign cells owing to osmotic or degenerative effects (ie, crenation) or daisy cells (described previously).

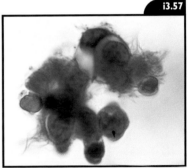
i3.57

Endosalpingiosis—cilia (oil)

3.10.1 Endosalpingiosis (Müllerian Glandular Inclusions)

Endosalpingiosis is ectopic benign epithelium, composed of cells morphologically identical to those lining the fallopian tube (the endosalpinx) |i3.57|. The cells form tightly cohesive aggregates and simple papillae of small cells, which may be associated psammoma bodies. Few or no single epithelial cells are present. Cilia are characteristic.

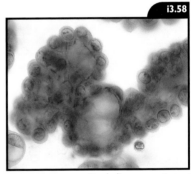
i3.58

Borderline serous tumor

3.10.2 Serous Cystadenoma and Cystadenofibroma

Papillary clusters of epithelial cells are similar to those described for endosalpingiosis. Psammoma bodies may be seen.

3.10.3 Borderline (Low Malignant Potential) Serous Ovarian Tumors

Ovarian serous tumors of low malignant potential, or so-called borderline tumors, are noninvasive histologically. Cytologically, these tumors are characterized by the presence of cohesive, often branching, papillary structures with smooth borders |i3.58|. Low-grade nuclear atypia, consisting of minor variation in size, irregular membranes, coarse chromatin, and occasional prominent nucleoli, and single cells may be seen, but mitoses are rare or absent. Psammoma bodies may be present. (Compare with serous carcinoma |i3.59|.)

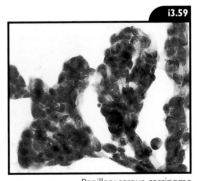
i3.59

Papillary serous carcinoma

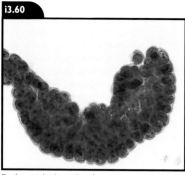

Endometriosis—glands

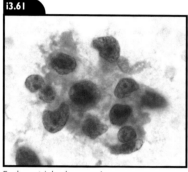

Endometrial adenocarcinoma

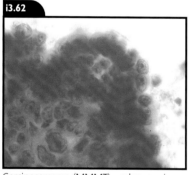

Carcinosarcoma (MMMT)—adenocarcinoma

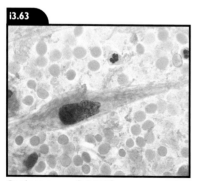

Carcinosarcoma (MMMT)—sarcoma

3.10.4 Ovarian Adenocarcinoma

Compared with borderline tumors, adenocarcinoma is characterized by a predominance of smaller, less cohesive clusters and papillae, with more irregular borders and an increase in single cells |i3.59|. The cells are larger and more atypical, and the cytoplasm is more abundant and usually vacuolated. Mitoses may be frequent. Psammoma bodies can be seen.

3.10.5 Endometriosis

Endometrial glandular |i3.60| and stromal cells and hemosiderin-laden macrophages characterize endometriosis. This triad is diagnostic, but it is unusual to find all three components in peritoneal washes.

3.10.6 Endometrial Adenocarcinoma

Papillary clusters or single atypical cells may be identified in patients with endometrial adenocarcinoma. High-grade cancers are obviously malignant |i3.61|. Low-grade tumor cells may resemble reactive mesothelial cells, forming loose, three-dimensional clusters of cells with delicate cytoplasm that is scant to abundant. The nuclei may have coarse chromatin and macronucleoli.

3.10.7 Malignant Mixed Mesodermal (Müllerian) Tumor

The majority of malignant mixed mesodermal (müllerian) tumors (MMMTs), also known as carcinosarcoma, show only adenocarcinomatous cells or adenocarcinoma |i3.62| plus sarcomatous |i3.63| cells. The minority show only sarcomatous cells.

SYNOVIAL FLUID

Synovial fluid is examined to facilitate diagnosis of inflammations, infections, crystals, and tumors.

3.11 The Cells

3.11.1 Synovial Cells

Synovial cells usually are present in synovial fluid but are sparse. They resemble reactive mesothelial cells with round to oval nuclei, fine chromatin, and moderate cytoplasm |i3.64|.

3.11.2 Inflammatory Cells

Inflammatory cells are normally scant. Increased numbers are seen in diverse conditions |**i3.65**|, |**i3.66**|, including arthritis, infection, trauma, and tumor. Numerous eosinophils, a rare finding, can be seen in parasitic infections, malignant effusions, after arthrography (in which air or contrast material was injected), or idiopathically.

3.11.3 Cartilage Cells (Chondrocytes)

Cartilage cells have a thick capsule-like structure surrounding granular or homogeneous cytoplasm |**i3.67**|. The nuclei are central, round, and often multiple. They have granular chromatin and prominent nucleoli. Chondrocytes are not normally present but can be seen following injury.

3.12 Diseases of Synovium and Joints

3.12.1 Rheumatoid Arthritis

Significant numbers of ragocytes or "RA cells" suggest a diagnosis of rheumatoid arthritis. Ragocytes are neutrophils with coarse cytoplasmic granulations; they are associated with rheumatoid arthritis but are not specific. In the background, marked chronic inflammation, cholesterol crystals, cellular debris, and protein precipitate are present, but synovial cells are sparse.

3.12.2 Degenerative Arthritis (Osteoarthritis)

The most characteristic feature of osteoarthritis is the presence of multinucleated cartilage cells, often in sheets or clusters, rather than singly. The background is particularly clean; few inflammatory cells and no ragocytes, crystals, or debris are present.

3.12.3 Systemic Lupus Erythematosus

The most characteristic feature of systemic lupus erythematosus is the presence of LE cells (see p 54), which are usually easy to find but are not completely specific.

3.12.4 Infectious Arthritis

Septic arthritis is characterized by abundant neutrophils. Organisms are frequently identifiable |**i3.65**|.

Tuberculous arthritis characteristically shows chronic inflammation, but acid-fast bacilli may be difficult to identify. The specimen can be cultured for definitive diagnosis.

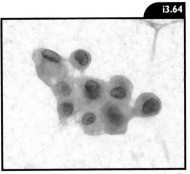

i3.64

Synovial cells

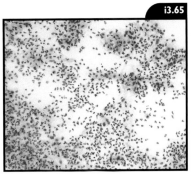

i3.65

Acute (septic) arthritis

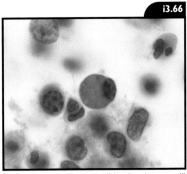

i3.66

Plasma cells, Russell bodies (Mott cell)

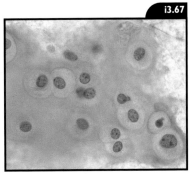

i3.67

Chondrocytes

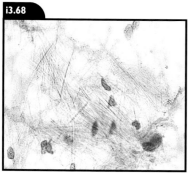

Gout

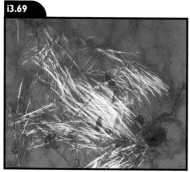

Gout with compensator

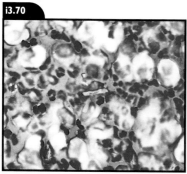

Pseudogout

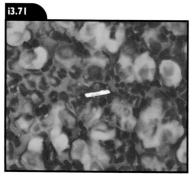

Pseudogout with compensator

Reiter syndrome is the triad of urethritis, arthritis, and conjunctivitis due to *Chlamydia* infection. Chronic inflammatory cells are present early; paradoxically, neutrophils appear later. Chlamydial cytoplasmic inclusions are found in synovial cells, best appreciated using Diff-Quik stain and a green filter. Prompt therapy with appropriate antibiotics prevents irreversible joint injury.

3.12.5 Traumatic Arthritis

Traumatic arthritis is a common cause of a hemorrhagic joint effusion. The findings are similar to septic arthritis, except that hemosiderin-laden macrophages and tissue fragments may be seen.

3.12.6 Villonodular Synovitis

Villonodular synovitis is inflammation, of unknown etiology, of the synovial membrane, usually involving the knee of young adult males. Multinucleated giant cells containing hemosiderin are characteristic but not specific.

3.12.7 Gout

Gout is an inherited disorder of purine metabolism characterized by hyperuricemia and deposition of urate crystals in and about the joints. Urate crystals are needle-shaped, with pointed ends, and about 5 to 10 µm long |i3.68|. By using compensated polarization, the crystals will show strong negative birefringence |i3.69|.

3.12.8 Pseudogout: Chondrocalcinosis

Pseudogout is an inherited disorder of pyrophosphate metabolism characterized by deposition of calcium pyrophosphate crystals in major joints. Calcium pyrophosphate crystals are rod-shaped or rhomboid crystals with square ends and about 5 µm long |i3.70|. By using compensated polarization, the crystals will show weak positive birefringence |i3.71|.

3.12.9 Tumoral Effusion

The most common types of tumors causing a synovial effusion are squamous cell carcinoma, adenocarcinoma, and lymphoma/leukemia. Lung is the most common source of metastatic carcinoma. Primary neoplasms, including osteosarcoma and giant cell tumor, also occur. Note that synovial sarcoma rarely arises in the joints. Diagnosis is usually easy, since the tumor cells are foreign to the joint space.

NIPPLE DISCHARGE

Discharges from the nipple can be normal or abnormal. Most abnormal nipple discharges are associated with benign conditions. Fibrocystic disease, physiologic disturbances, and papillomas are among the most common benign causes of abnormal breast discharges. Malignant nipple discharges are usually unilateral and bloody and occur in older patients. Note, however, that bloody nipple discharges can occur in benign conditions. Any patient with a suspicious breast mass or abnormal mammogram must be appropriately investigated regardless of the presence or absence of a nipple discharge.

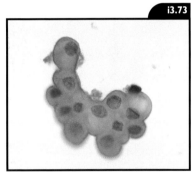

i3.72

Benign duct cells

3.13 The Cells

3.13.1 Duct Cells

Duct cells are normally small and occur singly or in small compact clusters |i3.72|. The nuclei have smooth nuclear membranes and are hyperchromatic with granular chromatin and inconspicuous nucleoli. The cytoplasm is scant and homogeneous. Good intercellular cohesion and uniformity of the cells are clues to a benign diagnosis.

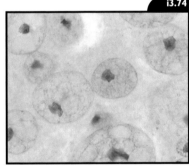

i3.73

Apocrine cells

3.13.2 Apocrine Metaplasia Cells

Apocrine cells have relatively abundant, finely granular cytoplasm that usually stains orange or occasionally blue with Papanicolaou stain |i3.73|. The nuclei are regular and hyperchromatic and may have prominent nucleoli.

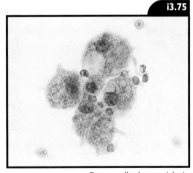

i3.74

Foam cells

3.13.3 Foam Cells

Foam cells are a common finding in nipple discharges. They are large, with abundant vacuolated cytoplasm due to lipid content |i3.74|. They usually appear singly but can form loose clusters. The nuclei are small and frequently degenerated. Foam cells can vary considerably in size and may exhibit binucleation or multinucleation. Hemosiderin indicates bleeding |i3.75|. The origin (duct vs histiocytes) is controversial.

i3.75

Foam cells, hemosiderin

3.13.4 Miscellaneous Cells

Squamous cells and anucleate squames from the nipple may be seen. Also, inflammatory cells, including neutrophils, lymphocytes, and histiocytes, as well as giant cells and necrotic cells, can occur in various diseases. Microcalcifications also can be seen.

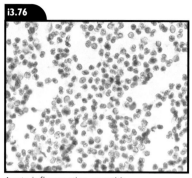

Acute inflammation, mastitis

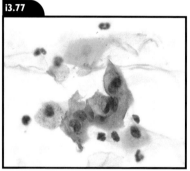

Lactating sinus granuloma

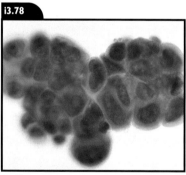

Papilloma

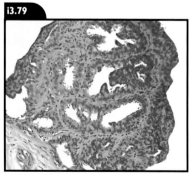

Intraductal papilloma, tissue

3.14 Abnormal Nipple Discharge

Most nipple discharge specimens have a variably stained proteinaceous background. In many cases, the smear is acellular. Foam cells or a few uniform duct cells are benign findings but do not exclude malignancy. Neutrophils correlate with clinical mastitis; RBCs correlate with discharges described clinically as bloody.

Ductal cells with atypia are suspicious for malignancy. Papillary aggregates, particularly if there is cytologic atypia, are also suspicious. These findings require further investigation.

3.14.1 Galactorrhea

Galactorrhea is abnormal milk secretion. The cytology shows foam cells in a lipoproteinaceous background. Blood usually is absent.

3.14.2 Duct Ectasia

Duct ectasia refers to duct obstruction and dilatation with accumulation of secretions. The discharge tends to be bilateral and to exit from multiple ducts. Multicolored sticky secretion is characteristic. The smear may be cellular with numerous foam cells, including large multinucleated forms, and small clusters of duct cells in a granular proteinaceous background.

3.14.3 Infection/Inflammation

A variety of infectious agents, ranging from virus to fungus to microfilaria, can be associated with an abnormal nipple discharge.

Bacterial infections are associated with acute inflammation. Bacteria may be identified |i3.76|.

Tuberculosis of the breast can mimic breast cancer clinically, including a breast mass and a bloody nipple discharge. The cytology may show epithelioid histiocytes, giant cells, foam cells, and necrotic material. Look for acid-fast bacilli and culture the secretion for definitive diagnosis.

Lactating sinus granuloma is associated with squames and foreign body giant cell reaction |i3.77|.

3.14.4 Intraductal Papilloma

A bloody discharge limited to a single duct is characteristic of an intraductal papilloma |i3.78|, |i3.79|. The cytology shows cohesive papillary clusters of ductal cells, which may show slight nuclear pleomorphism. In addition, foam cells and RBCs are frequently present. Apocrine cells suggest a benign diagnosis. Unfortunately, the differential diagnosis with papillary carcinoma |i3.80|, |i3.81| may be impossible in exfoliative cytology. Therefore, in practice, the presence of papillary clusters in a nipple discharge must be regarded as a suspicious finding.

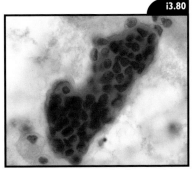

Papillary carcinoma

3.15 Breast Cancer

Carcinoma of the breast, whether in situ or invasive, can shed cells into the ductal system |i3.82|, |i3.83|. The cytology shows abnormal cells, singly or in crowded clusters. The cells typically have enlarged, pleomorphic, hyperchromatic nuclei, irregular nuclear membranes, coarse chromatin, and prominent nucleoli or macronucleoli. Papillary clusters or cell balls are abnormal and suggestive of malignancy. Loss of cohesion is also a feature suggestive of malignancy. The background can be clean, hemorrhagic, or necrotic (tumor diathesis). Benign foam cells may be present. A diagnosis of malignancy should be confirmed by biopsy (fine-needle aspiration or tissue) before undertaking definitive therapy.

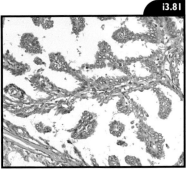

Papillary carcinoma, tissue

3.15.1 Paget Disease

Paget disease is involvement of the nipple ducts by an underlying breast cancer, which can be in situ or invasive. Paget disease presents as an eczematous, crusting, or ulcerating lesion of the nipple. There may be a nipple discharge, or the lesion can be directly sampled by scraping. The cytology shows Paget cells, which are large carcinoma cells with abnormal nuclei, prominent nucleoli, and abundant dense or vacuolated cytoplasm, that may contain mucin. A characteristic feature is the presence of cell-in-cell patterns. Melanoma is frequently mentioned in the differential diagnosis. However, melanoma of the nipple is exceedingly rare, and mucin positivity, if present, rules out this diagnosis.

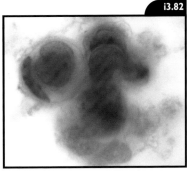

Breast carcinoma

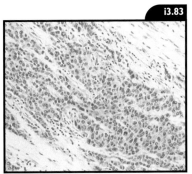

Breast carcinoma, tissue

CHAPTER FOUR

Gastrointestinal (GI) malignancies are common; only lung and breast cancers are more common noncutaneous malignancies. Except for oral and anal lesions, most GI cytology is obtained via an endoscope, by brushing (for lesions involving surfaces) or aspiration (for deep-lying lesions). Although most oral and anal cancers are squamous cell carcinomas that could be amenable to early detection via cytology, such specimens rarely are submitted to the laboratory. Unfortunately, endoscopy does not lend itself easily to mass screening. However, GI cytology is important in diagnosis of diseases in immunocompromised patients, including those with infections, lymphomas, and sarcomas. It also can be useful in surveillance of high-risk patients with ulcerative colitis or Barrett esophagus, looking for evidence of dysplasia. Histopathology and cytopathology are complementary diagnostic techniques. Advantages of cytology include the ability to sample wider areas, to select dyshesive neoplastic cells, to sample areas beyond a stricture, low cost, and rapid turnaround time.

ORAL CAVITY

Oral cancer occurs most commonly in older male patients. Risk factors include alcohol and tobacco abuse as well as a history of previous aerodigestive malignancy. Human papillomavirus may have a role in the development of some oral cancers. Any unhealing sore in the mouth is suspicious for malignancy. Leukoplakia ("white plaque") can be associated with malignancy, but the most common early sign of oral cancer is erythroplasia of Queyrat, which is a red, velvety lesion that represents an inflammatory reaction to the tumor. The vast majority of oral malignancies are squamous cell carcinomas, which can be detected via exfoliative cytology. However, a malignant diagnosis should be confirmed histologically before definitive therapy.

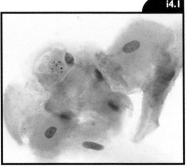

i4.1

Anucleate squames and superficial cells

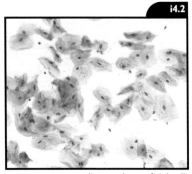

i4.2

Intermediate and superficial cells

4.1 **The Cells**

Anucleate squames and superficial squamous cells (identical to those in the Pap smear) predominate in cytologic samples from the lips, hard palate, gingiva, and dorsal tongue |**i4.1**|. Intermediate squamous cells predominate in samples from the remainder of the oral cavity, including the buccal mucosa |**i4.2**|. Barr bodies can be identified in 20% to 80% of squamous cells from normal females.

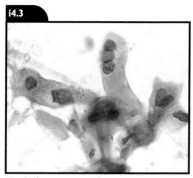

Atypical squamous cells

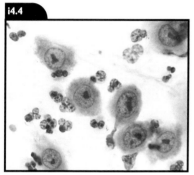

Pemphigus vulgaris

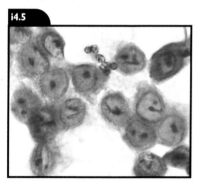

Pemphigus vulgaris

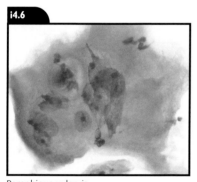

Pemphigus vulgaris

4.2 Benign Diseases

4.2.1 Hyperkeratosis, Parakeratosis, Atypical Parakeratosis

Chronic irritation of the squamous mucosa can cause abnormal keratinization (hyperkeratosis, parakeratosis, and atypical parakeratosis). Irritants include ill-fitting dentures, smoking, and poor dentition. Hyperkeratosis is characterized by the presence of anucleate squames, parakeratosis by miniature superficial cells, and atypical parakeratosis by pleomorphic parakeratotic cells.

4.2.2 Leukoplakia

Leukoplakia is a clinical term meaning "white plaque." It is usually caused by benign hyperkeratosis or parakeratosis but can be associated with dysplasia or cancer.

4.2.3 Inflammatory Atypia and Repair/Regeneration

Inflammation can cause reactive/reparative changes in the squamous cells, characterized by nuclear enlargement and multinucleation, increased nuclear/cytoplasmic ratios, and prominent chromocenters and nucleoli |i4.3|. The inflammatory component is variable. Occasionally, specific infectious agents, such as herpes or *Candida*, are identified. Saprophytic fungi, actinomyces, bacteria, and *Entamoeba gingivalis* can be seen without infection in patients with poor oral hygiene.

4.2.4 Pemphigus Vulgaris

Pemphigus vulgaris is an autoimmune disease of skin and mucous membranes; the mouth is frequently involved. The disease attacks intercellular junctions (desmosomes), causing a suprabasilar bleb or blister, with acantholysis and intercellular IgG deposition. The blisters break, resulting in painful ulcers. Tzanck (or acantholytic) cells are characteristic cytologic findings. These are atypical parabasal-sized cells, with cytologic features suggesting repair, but the cells are poorly cohesive |i4.4|. The cytoplasm is dense and may display characteristic perinuclear acidophilic staining |i4.5|. The nuclei are enlarged, with smooth but thick-appearing nuclear membranes. As in repair, the chromatin is pale and nucleoli are prominent (typically bar- or bullet-shaped). Normal mitotic figures can be seen. Occasionally, large or giant cells are present, particularly after therapy |i4.6|. There is a variable inflammatory infiltrate. The presence of cytologic atypia (eg, prominent nucleoli, mitotic figures) plus numerous single cells may suggest malignancy. Cytologic features such as the fine, pale chromatin favor a benign diagnosis.

4.2.5 Radiation

Radiation results in "macrocytes," ie, cytomegalic cells in which both the nucleus and the cytoplasm enlarge but the nuclear/cytoplasmic ratios remain relatively normal |i4.7|. Evidence of regeneration (eg, enlarged nuclei and cytoplasm, multinucleation, and prominent nucleoli) and degeneration (eg, nuclear pyknosis; karyorrhexis and karyolysis; cytoplasmic vacuolization and amphophilia) is also common. Similar changes (macrocytosis) can also be seen with chemotherapy or vitamin deficiency (folate, B$_{12}$).

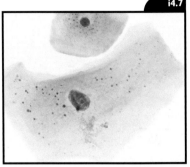

Radiation effect

4.3 **Malignant Diseases**

Oral cancer accounts for about 2% to 3% of noncutaneous cancers and 1% to 2% of cancer deaths. The vast majority are squamous cell carcinomas.

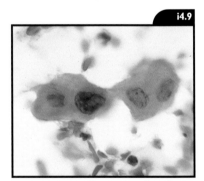

Squamous cell carcinoma

4.3.1 Squamous Cell Carcinoma

Most oral squamous cell carcinomas (SCCs) are well-differentiated and keratinizing tumors. In some cases, malignant cytologic features are subtle. Poorly differentiated SCCs also occur. The cells shed singly or in clusters. Keratinizing SCC is characterized by cellular pleomorphism (including snake-, tadpole-, and bizarre-shaped cells) and heavy cytoplasmic keratinization (thick, dense cytoplasm, often orangeophilic, with refractile rings) |i4.8|, |i4.9|, |i4.10|. Pearls are pathognomonic of keratinization. The nuclei are hyperchromatic and variable in size and shape. The chromatin is irregular and coarse to pyknotic. Nucleoli may be obscured by the dense chromatin. Anucleate "ghost" cells may be numerous. Nonkeratinizing SCC is characterized by more uniform cells, with less keratinization; pearls are absent by definition. The nuclei have more open chromatin and more prominent nucleoli than those of keratinizing SCC. Mitotic figures, rare in benign disease, may be seen. The background usually shows a tumor diathesis (ie, necrotic material, blood, and inflammation).

Squamous cell carcinoma

Squamous cell carcinoma, tissue

4.3.2 Other Tumors

A wide variety of other benign and malignant tumors can occur in the mouth. They can arise from lymphoid tissue (eg, tonsils), minor salivary glands, or soft tissue. Melanoma can also occur in the oral cavity.

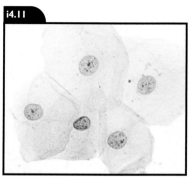

Squamous cells

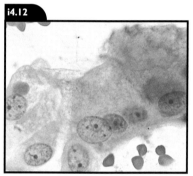

Glandular cells

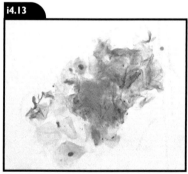

Hyperkeratosis

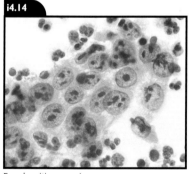

Esophagitis—repair

ESOPHAGUS

The esophagus has a rich vascular and lymphatic supply, and, unlike most of the rest of the GI tract, there is no serosal lining to act as a barrier to the spread of inflammation, infection, or cancer. Therefore, lesions of the esophagus can readily disseminate to surrounding vital structures.

4.4 The Cells

4.4.1 Squamous Cells

Most of the esophagus is lined by a nonkeratinized, stratified, squamous epithelium. Cytologically, most of the exfoliated cells are intermediate cells with a few superficial cells |i4.11|. Parabasal cells can be seen in inflammation, ulcer, or excessively vigorous abrasion.

4.4.2 Glandular Cells

Although the esophagus does have submucosal glands, the cells are usually inaccessible to exfoliative cytology. However, gastric-type glandular cells often are obtained near the gastroesophageal junction |i4.12|. Otherwise, glandular cells in an esophageal specimen may indicate Barrett esophagus. Respiratory cells (including ciliated cells and alveolar macrophages or even tumor cells) also can be seen as swallowed or "pickup" contaminants.

4.5 Benign Diseases

4.5.1 Leukoplakia

Leukoplakia is a nonspecific clinical term for a white plaque. Causes include hyperkeratosis |i4.13|, parakeratosis, atypical parakeratosis, condyloma, dysplasia, and cancer. The cytology varies accordingly.

4.5.2 Esophagitis and Ulcers

Esophagitis, with or without ulceration, can be due to a wide variety of causes, including irritants (eg, alcohol, smoking, lye, hot drinks), reflux, hiatal hernia, Crohn disease, radiation/chemotherapy, infectious agents (eg, fungus, virus), or other sorts of injury (eg, trauma, uremia). Esophagitis is also a common early manifestation of AIDS. The differential diagnosis includes malignant ulceration.

Reactive/reparative cells, with enlarged, reactive nuclei, vesicular chromatin, prominent nucleoli, and increased nuclear/ cytoplasmic ratios are typical of esophagitis or esophageal ulceration |i4.14|. Nuclear and cytoplasmic degenerative changes, including karyorrhexis, karyopyknosis, and cytoplasmic vacuolization, may be seen. Inflammation, including neutrophils, is present in the background of the smear. Eosinophils have been associated with reflux esophagitis |i4.15|. Reactive mesenchymal cells may be obtained from the base of an ulcer |i4.16|. Hyperkeratosis may occur in chronic esophagitis. Eventually, the squamous epithelium may be replaced by gastric or intestinal-type glandular epithelium (ie, Barrett esophagus).

"Atypical" (reactive) cells in a "dirty" (inflammatory) background may suggest malignancy. Factors favoring a benign process include cellular cohesion, orderly cellular arrangements, maintained nuclear/cytoplasmic ratios, fine chromatin, and smooth nuclear membranes.

4.5.3 Barrett Esophagus

Barrett esophagus is defined as columnar epithelium lining the lower esophagus. It is thought to be a protective metaplastic reaction of the esophageal mucosa to gastric reflux. Heredity, smoking, and alcohol abuse also may be predisposing factors. The disease occurs predominantly in white males. Adenocarcinoma (Dawson syndrome) develops in about 10%.

In essence, the cytologic diagnosis of Barrett esophagus consists of identifying glandular cells in an esophageal specimen |i4.17|. Gastric, intestinal, or goblet cells may be seen. Benign glandular cells exfoliate in large, cohesive, honeycombed sheets. Villous arrangements are characteristic of intestinal-type epithelium. The nuclei are usually bland and uniform. The background may be clean or inflammatory. Reactive/reparative changes, including nuclear enlargement and pleomorphism, prominent nucleoli, and mitotic figures, as well as degenerative changes, may occur |i4.18| (see p 80).

4.5.4 Radiation and Chemotherapy

Radiation or chemotherapy commonly causes clinical esophagitis with dysphagia and substernal burning. The morphologic changes can mimic cancer. The clinical history is important in diagnosis.

The cytology of radiation change is similar to that described in the Pap smear, exemplified by macrocytes, with nuclear and cytoplasmic enlargement and maintained nuclear/ cytoplasmic ratios. Hypochromatic or hyperchromatic degenerated nuclei with "thickened" or wrinkled membranes can be

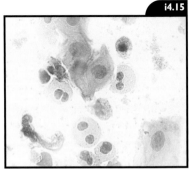
i4.15

Reflux esophagitis—eosinophils

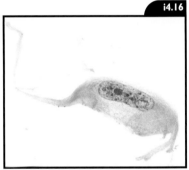
i4.16

Reactive mesenchymal cell

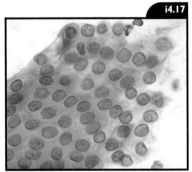
i4.17

Barrett esophagus

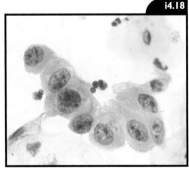
i4.18

Barrett esophagus

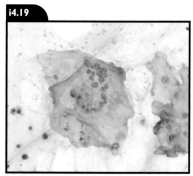

Radiation effect

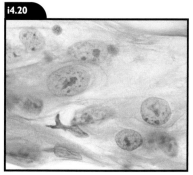

Chemotherapy effect

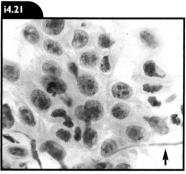

Candidiasis

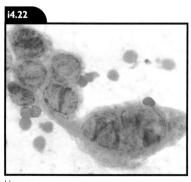

Herpes

seen. Multinucleation also occurs |i4.19|. Nucleoli are usually inconspicuous. The cytoplasm may be vacuolated and stains polychromatically (pink and blue). Multinucleated giant cell histiocytes may be seen. Chemotherapy can cause similar changes, but nuclear hyperchromasia, prominent nucleoli, and high nuclear/cytoplasmic ratios are more common than in radiation effect |i4.20|.

4.5.5 Infections

Bacterial Esophagitis

Bacterial esophagitis, though uncommon, may occur in immunocompromised patients or as a secondary infection, eg, of herpetic ulcers. Bacteria, inflammation, debris, and possibly reparative cells are seen cytologically.

Candida

Esophageal candidiasis in immunocompromised patients is the most common cause of infectious esophagitis. Esophageal candidiasis may be an early sign of AIDS and is used as a diagnostic criterion for that disease. *Candida* infection also is associated with antibiotic therapy or esophageal abnormality (eg, achalasia, stricture, neoplasm). It is typically associated with a pseudomembrane covering the mucosal surface.

Cytologically, invasive infection is characterized by the presence of significant numbers of *Candida* organisms (budding yeasts, pseudohyphae) accompanied by necrotic debris, inflammatory cells (mostly neutrophils), reactive/reparative cells |i4.21|, and anucleate squames. Special stains, eg, Gomori methenamine silver, may help identify the organisms.

Herpes

Factors predisposing to herpetic esophagitis include immunocompromised state, cancer, chemotherapy, achalasia, and trauma (including intubation).

Herpes simplex and varicella-zoster viral changes are morphologically indistinguishable. The cytology shows the usual cellular features, including multinucleation, molding, and margination (the three Ms) with ground-glass chromatin and, sometimes, acidophilic intranuclear inclusions |i4.22|. Ulceration may produce reactive and reparative epithelial atypia with an inflammatory or necrotic background mimicking malignancy. Bacterial or fungal superinfection may occur.

Other Infections

Cytomegalovirus infection usually occurs in immunocompromised patients. The diagnostic cells (big cells with a large intranuclear inclusion surrounded by a halo and satellite nuclear and cytoplasmic inclusions) may be sparse.

Human papillomavirus (HPV) is the primary cause of squamous papillomas and flat condylomas of the esophagus. Koilocytes are pathognomonic of HPV infection (see Chapter 1).

4.6 Malignant Diseases

Squamous cell carcinoma is the most common malignant tumor of the esophagus; adenocarcinoma is second but increasing in frequency, and other tumors (eg, melanoma, soft tissue tumors, and metastases) are rare. Plummer-Vinson syndrome (sideropenic dysphagia); alcohol abuse; smoking; diet (excess nitrites or deficiencies of vitamins or trace metals); esophagitis, including Barrett esophagus; or previous head and neck malignancies are predisposing factors. HPV is probably not significantly associated with esophageal carcinoma in the United States. Most patients have dysphagia, but unfortunately, by the time dysphagia develops, the cancer is often far advanced.

4.6.1 Squamous Cell Carcinoma

Esophageal SCC occurs most commonly in black men, usually older than 50 years of age, predominantly in the midesophagus. Because the tumors are frequently detected late, the prognosis is grim. Esophageal balloon cytologic screening of high-risk populations could help decrease the mortality.

SCC of the esophagus ranges from well-differentiated to poorly differentiated. The tumor can be keratinizing or nonkeratinizing.

Keratinizing SCC is characterized by marked cellular pleomorphism (including spindle, caudate, and bizarre cells) and marked keratinization |i4.23|, |i4.24|. The nuclei are pleomorphic and densely hyperchromatic. Nuclear/cytoplasmic ratios are low in some cells, high in others. The tumor shows definite evidence of keratinization, eg, cytoplasmic orangeophilia, refractile keratin rings, and intercellular bridges. Pearls are pathognomonic of keratinization.

Nonkeratinizing SCC sheds more uniform cells than keratinizing SCC, approximating the size of parabasal cells |i4.25|, |i4.26|. The cells have enlarged, moderately hyperchromatic nuclei with irregular nuclear membranes and high nuclear/cytoplasmic ratios. Nuclear chromatin is more open and nucleoli are more prominent than in keratinizing SCC. The cytoplasm is dense and often stains cyanophilic to basophilic. An occasional orange, dyskeratotic cell (ie, single cell keratinization) may be seen, but

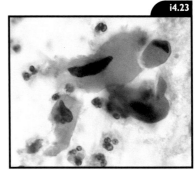
i4.23
Keratinizing SCC

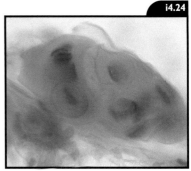
i4.24
Keratinizing SCC

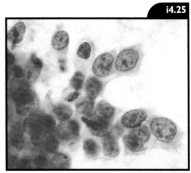
i4.25
Nonkeratinizing SCC

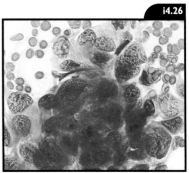
i4.26
Nonkeratinizing SCC

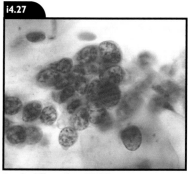

Poorly differentiated SCC

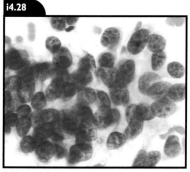

Adenocarcinoma

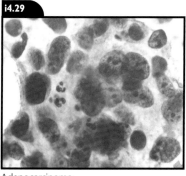

Adenocarcinoma

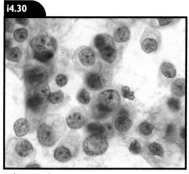

Adenocarcinoma

pearls are not present. A tumor diathesis (cytoplasmic debris, inflammation, and necrosis) is typically found in the background.

When very poorly differentiated, the malignant squamous cells have a basaloid appearance with small hyperchromatic nuclei and scant cytoplasm |i4.27|, which may be difficult to distinguish from small cell (neuroendocrine) carcinoma or poorly differentiated adenocarcinoma. Spindle squamous cell carcinoma also can arise in the esophagus.

Degenerative vacuolization of the cytoplasm can mimic secretory vacuoles of adenocarcinoma. Benign reactive and reparative atypia, as well as radiation or chemotherapy effects, can mimic SCC. Disorderly cellular arrangements, numerous single atypical cells, irregular nuclei, coarse chromatin, and high nuclear/cytoplasmic ratios are among the most reliable diagnostic features of cancer.

4.6.2 Adenocarcinoma

Adenocarcinoma occurs most commonly in the distal esophagus, is usually associated with Barrett esophagus, and, therefore, occurs predominantly in white males, particularly those who smoke cigarettes or abuse alcohol.

Esophageal adenocarcinoma is usually a relatively well-differentiated cancer, similar to adenocarcinoma of the stomach (although signet ring morphology is rare) |i4.28|, |i4.29|, |i4.30|. Cell balls, microacini, or papillae are characteristic cytologic findings; such cell groups that are disorderly and poorly cohesive suggest malignancy. The individual cells are characterized by nucleocytoplasmic polarity and high nuclear/cytoplasmic ratios. Nuclear atypia ranges from subtle "thickening" and irregularity of the membrane with fine chromatin in well-differentiated tumors to large irregular nuclei with coarse, dark, irregular chromatin, prominent nucleoli, and obvious malignant features in poorly differentiated carcinomas.

The cytoplasm is granular or vacuolar, mucin content is decreased, and cell borders are indistinct. Cellular molding may occur. An occasional larger, or even giant, tumor cell may be present. A tumor diathesis may be seen in the background.

Benign reactive/reparative atypia can be quite marked, with large nuclei and macronucleoli, and difficult to distinguish from adenocarcinoma. Orderly groups, cohesion, smooth nuclear membranes, and fine chromatin favor a benign reactive process.

Glandular Dysplasia in Barrett Esophagus

Glandular dysplasia usually is characterized by crowded, enlarged, elongated, hyperchromatic nuclei, increased nuclear/cytoplasmic ratios, and loss of nuclear polarity, reminiscent of endocervical dysplasia and adenocarcinoma in situ |i4.31|. A less common pattern is reminiscent of atypical repair/regeneration and is characterized by less crowded, frankly malignant appearing nuclei with marginated chromatin, prominent nucleoli, and increased nuclear/cytoplasmic ratios. Both patterns show loss of cytoplasmic mucin. In contrast with frankly invasive cancer, single atypical cells tend to be sparse in dysplasia.

4.6.3 Small Cell (Neuroendocrine) Carcinoma

Primary small cell (neuroendocrine) carcinoma of the esophagus is rare |i4.32|. Most cases of small cell carcinoma actually arise in the lung and spread to the esophagus. The cytology is similar to that of pulmonary small cell carcinoma. The differential diagnosis also includes poorly differentiated squamous carcinoma or adenocarcinoma, carcinoid, and lymphoma.

4.6.4 Rare Tumors

A variety of other tumors, eg, granular cell tumors |i4.33|, benign and malignant smooth muscle tumors, lymphoma, and melanoma, occur rarely in the esophagus. Salivary gland–type adenocarcinomas, such as adenoid cystic and mucoepidermoid carcinomas, are other rare tumors. Except for melanoma, most of these tumors arise in the submucosa and are unlikely to be diagnosed by exfoliative cytologic methods, unless they are ulcerated.

STOMACH

For descriptive purposes, the stomach is divided into the cardia (immediately adjacent to the esophagus), fundus (above the gastroesophageal junction), body (largest portion), and pyloric area (which joins the duodenum at the pyloric sphincter). Cells from the oral cavity or respiratory tract, as well as food particles, may be seen as contaminants.

4.7 The Cells

The entire surface of the stomach is lined by mucous cells |i4.34|. Although the fundus and body also contain chief and parietal cells, these deep lying cells are seldom sampled by exfoliative cytology. Kulchitsky (neuroendocrine) cells also are present but cannot be specifically recognized without special stains.

4.7.1 Mucous Cells

Mucous cells, usually the predominant cell type in gastric specimens, are tall columnar cells, with uniform basal nuclei, fine

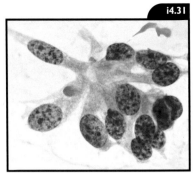
Barrett dysplasia

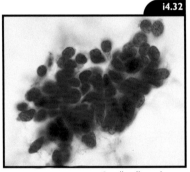
Small cell carcinoma

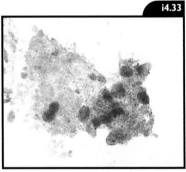
Granular cell tumor

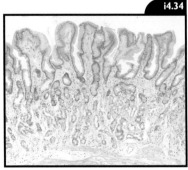
Stomach, tissue

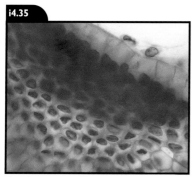

Gastric mucous cells

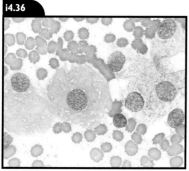

Chief cells (blue); parietal cells (pink)

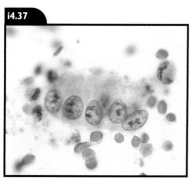

Reactive gastric cells

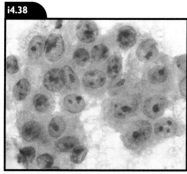

Repair

chromatin, and small nucleoli |**i4.35**|. The cytoplasm is finely granular or multivacuolated with apical membrane densities (microvilli). The cells form orderly honeycombs, palisades, or rosettes. Single cells and naked nuclei may be present. Goblet cells with large, single, mucin vacuoles indicate intestinal metaplasia.

4.7.2 Chief Cells

Chief cells contain relatively coarse, basophilic zymogen granules and are similar in appearance to acinar cells of the pancreas or salivary gland |**i4.36**|. The cytoplasm also can be vacuolated due to leaching of the zymogen granules. The nuclei are round and smooth with fine chromatin.

4.7.3 Parietal Cells

Parietal cells secrete intrinsic factor (to absorb vitamin B_{12}) and hydrochloric acid. They are typically pyramidal or flask-shaped and are larger than chief cells |**i4.36**|. The cytoplasm is finely granular and characteristically stains intensely eosinophilic but may be vacuolated and pale. The nuclei can have moderately coarse chromatin and prominent nucleoli.

4.7.4 Reactive/Reparative Cells and Degeneration

Reactive/reparative and degenerative changes are commonly observed in gastric specimens, particularly in chronic gastritis or gastric ulcers, and can mimic malignancy |**i4.37**|, |**i4.38**|. Chemotherapy can induce particularly marked reactive changes. Nuclear enlargement and pleomorphism, with coarse, dark chromatin and prominent or irregular nucleoli, can be seen in benign reactive/degenerative conditions. Although benign cells can be somewhat crowded, they usually lack significant nuclear molding, piling up, or loss of polarity. Other features favoring a benign process include good intercellular cohesion, orderly cellular arrangements, flat sheets of cells with little crowding, few single cells, maintained nuclear/cytoplasmic ratios, smooth nuclear membranes, and fine chromatin. Inflammation usually is present. Degeneration often causes nuclear pyknosis or karyorrhexis and cytoplasmic vacuolization. Naked nuclei are common.

4.8 Benign Diseases

4.8.1 Intestinal Metaplasia

Intestinal metaplasia—intestinalization—is a diagnostic feature of chronic atrophic gastritis or gastric atrophy, as may be seen in, eg, pernicious anemia (B_{12} deficiency), folate deficiency, and radiation. Although intestinal metaplasia is benign, it is the milieu in which most gastric cancers arise.

Intestinal metaplasia is characterized cytologically by cohesive orderly sheets of absorptive or mucous cells and scattered goblet cells (with large secretory vacuoles) |i4.39|, |i4.40|. The pale goblet cells contrast with the darker staining surrounding cells, producing a Swiss cheese appearance. The nuclei are usually bland and uniform, although mild reactive changes may be seen. Absorptive cells are tall columnar with finely granular cytoplasm and may have a striated border (due to microvilli).

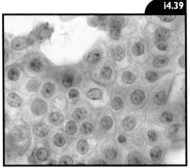
Intestinal metaplasia

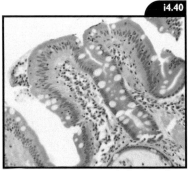
Intestinalization, tissue

4.8.2 Chronic Gastric Ulcer

Gastric cytology often is used to differentiate benign from malignant ulcers. Benign ulcers may show cells deriving from repair/regeneration, with reactive nuclear atypia, mitoses, and necrosis. *Helicobacter pylori* may be identified (see "Organisms," below). Benign and malignant ulcers can be associated with inflammation, degeneration, siderophages, and debris and occur in intestinal metaplasia. Malignant ulcers show typical malignant cytologic features.

4.8.3 Granulomatous Gastritis

Granulomas (loose aggregates of epithelioid histiocytes with or without giant cell histiocytes) may indicate any of a wide variety of diseases, including Crohn disease, tuberculosis, sarcoid, fungal infections, or a response to peptic ulceration or cancer.

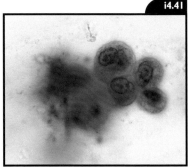
Gastric polyp—reactive type cells

4.8.4 Gastric Polyps

There are two basic kinds of gastric polyps: hyperplastic polyps characterized cytologically by reactive gastric cells |i4.41| and adenomas characterized cytologically by dysplastic gastric cells.

4.8.5 Organisms

Candida and *Actinomyces* are usually contaminants, but can grow on ulcers.

Helicobacter (Campylobacter) pylori is associated with chronic gastritis, gastric or duodenal ulcers, and gastric cancer, and, unusually, is found on normal mucosa. The organisms are tiny curved or spiral-shaped bacteria, about 1 to 3 μm long, found in the mucus surrounding glandular cells |i4.42|.

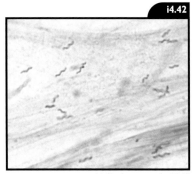
Helicobacter pylori (oil)

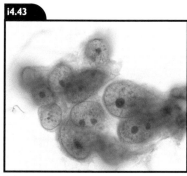

Adenocarcinoma

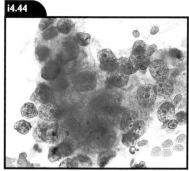

Adenocarcinoma

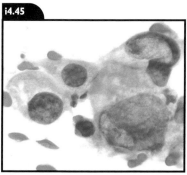

Adenocarcinoma

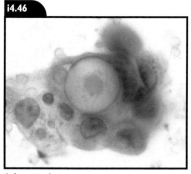

Adenocarcinoma

4.9 Malignant Diseases

For unknown reasons, the incidence of gastric cancer has been decreasing in the United States. Environmental and dietary factors are suspected in the etiology (eg, high salt, nitrites). There may well be a causative association with *H pylori* infection. Gastric cancer is more common among blacks than whites and people with blood group A.

Gastric cancers often are ulcerated but also may be flat or polypoid. The great majority of gastric cancers are adenocarcinomas. The prognosis is poor unless disease is detected early. Other malignancies, such as leiomyosarcoma and malignant lymphoma, also occur in the stomach.

4.9.1 Adenocarcinoma

Adenocarcinoma occurs in two basic cytologic patterns: intestinal and gastric types; a mixture can also be seen. Fungating growth is more common with the intestinal type; infiltrating linitis plastica is more common with the gastric type; either can be excavating. Malignant ulcers tend to occur on the greater curvature of the stomach in older patients with hypochlorhydria. The ulcer is often relatively large and has heaped-up margins.

Intestinal-Type Adenocarcinoma

The intestinal type of gastric cancer is associated with intestinal metaplasia and dysplasia of the gastric epithelium. The malignant cells resemble colonic carcinoma; they are usually abundant and can range from well-differentiated to poorly differentiated. The cells form loosely cohesive, disorderly sheets, papillae, or acini, with many single cells.

The malignant nuclei tend to have either fine pale chromatin and prominent single nucleoli |i4.43| or coarse hyperchromatic chromatin with multiple smaller nucleoli |i4.44|. The nuclei have irregular nuclear membranes. The cytoplasm is granular or vacuolated |i4.45|. A characteristic "terminal bar–like" edge, corresponding to the striated microvillous border, is characteristic of the intestinal-type cancer |i4.46|. A tumor diathesis with necrotic debris and acute inflammatory exudate is common but nondiagnostic. A colloid variant shows malignant cells floating in pools of mucus.

Gastric-Type Adenocarcinoma

The gastric type of stomach cancer is, in essence, a signet ring cell adenocarcinoma but also may show a mixture of poorly differentiated, pleomorphic cells with scant to abundant cytoplasm. This type of cancer is not significantly associated with intestinal metaplasia or glandular dysplasia. Since the overlying mucosa may not be ulcerated, false-negative diagnoses may occur in exfoliative cytology.

The cells are found predominantly singly or in small, loose clusters. Glandular groupings or papillae are absent or rare. The cells tend to be rounded rather than columnar and relatively small and uniform. The nuclei have fine chromatin and prominent nucleoli and are round or, most characteristically, indented by mucin vacuoles, resulting in classic signet ring cells |i4.47|. The background is usually relatively clean or mucoid.

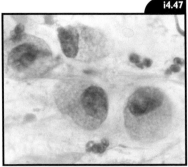
Signet ring cell carcinoma

Gastric Dysplasia

Adenocarcinoma of the stomach, particularly the intestinal type, is thought to be preceded by dysplasia/carcinoma in situ. The morphology is similar to dysplasia involving Barrett esophagus (|i4.31|, p 81), intestinal adenomas, and inflammatory bowel disease, as well as endocervical adenocarcinoma in situ.

Early Gastric Cancer

Early gastric cancer, or superficial cancer, is restricted to the mucosa or submucosa without penetration of the muscularis propria, although regional lymph node metastases may be present. These cancers can be minute (less than 5 mm). The cytology reflects the intestinal or gastric type of adenocarcinoma. When detected early, cure is possible.

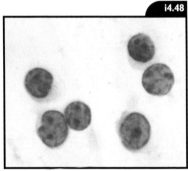
Large cell gastric lymphoma (oil)

4.9.2 Malignant Lymphoma

The GI tract, particularly the stomach, is the most common extranodal site of origin of malignant lymphoma, which is the second most common gastric malignancy (albeit a distant second to adenocarcinoma). The prognosis is considerably better than for adenocarcinoma.

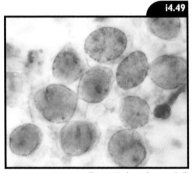
Large cell gastric lymphoma (oil)

Gastrointestinal lymphomas usually occur in middle-aged to elderly patients. Predisposing factors include celiac disease, chronic inflammatory bowel disease, immunocompromised state (eg, AIDS), and other conditions, including chronic gastritis associated with *H pylori*. The signs and symptoms of gastrointestinal lymphomas are usually indistinguishable from carcinomas occurring at the same site. Ulcerated lesions, in particular, can mimic adenocarcinoma clinically.

Nearly all gastrointestinal lymphomas are non-Hodgkin type, and most are of B-cell origin. Aggressive diffuse large B-cell lymphomas, including immunoblastic lymphoma, are most common |i4.48|, |i4.49|, |i4.50|. Low-grade lymphomas developing in mucosa-associated lymphoid tissue ("MALTomas") are characterized by indolent growth, a tendency to remain localized for long periods, and then dissemination to regional lymph nodes and other mucosal (MALT) sites. MALTomas may be related to *H pylori* infection (T-cell–driven B-cell proliferation with clonal expansion) and, remarkably, possibly may be reversed with antibi-

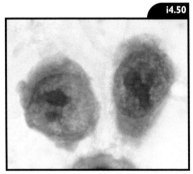
Immunoblastic lymphoma (oil)

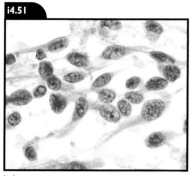

Leiomyosarcoma

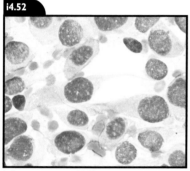

Leiomyosarcoma (DQ)

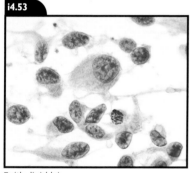

Epithelioid leiomyosarcoma

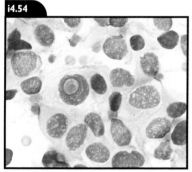

Epithelioid leiomyosarcoma—nuclear pseudoinclusions (DQ)

otic therapy. Small, noncleaved (Burkitt, non-Burkitt types) non-Hodgkin lymphomas are more common in the iliocecal area.

Tumors causing ulceration are more amenable to diagnosis by exfoliative cytology. The most characteristic cytologic feature of malignant lymphoma is lack of cellular cohesion: no true tissue aggregates are formed. The cells, even from large cell lymphomas, can be unexpectedly small owing to degeneration. The nuclei may be hyperchromatic, nuclear membrane irregularities are common, and nucleoli may be prominent. Cytoplasm is scant. Inflammation and debris can mask the single tumor cells. Plasmacytoid differentiation is common in gastrointestinal lymphomas and should not be diagnosed as plasmacytoma or myeloma unless the entire lesion is composed of neoplastic plasma cells.

The differential diagnosis includes benign lymphoid cells of chronic inflammation or pseudolymphoma. Pseudolymphoma, like follicular cervicitis seen in the Pap smear, is characterized by a "range of maturation" of the lymphoid cells, with a predominance of small "mature" lymphocytes; mature plasma cells; and tingible body macrophages. The cytologic diagnosis of low-grade MALTomas is difficult, and many cases of "pseudolymphoma" are actually MALTomas. Careful marker studies (usually of tissue) may be required for final diagnosis.

4.9.3 Gastrointestinal Stromal Tumors

Gastrointestinal stromal tumors can show smooth muscle or neural differentiation (or both, or neither) with spindle or epithelioid cells. Many show smooth muscle differentiation. They do not exfoliate unless ulcerated. Smooth muscle tumors are classically spindle cell neoplasms |i4.51|, |i4.52|; malignant tumors usually have large, hyperchromatic nuclei and mitoses. Contractile filaments may be seen in some cells. Differential diagnostic problems include separating benign from malignant tumors: markedly atypical cells can occur in benign bizarre leiomyomas; leiomyosarcomas can be cytologically bland. Benign reactive myofibroblasts from chronic ulcers can be cytologically atypical.

Leiomyoblastoma is thought to be an epithelioid smooth muscle |i4.53|, |i4.54| or possibly neural tumor. It occurs predominantly in the stomach. The cells are round and found in loose groups and singly. The nuclei are centrally located and round; the cytoplasm is vacuolated. The cells also may have a signet ring appearance. Nuclear pseudoinclusions may be seen.

4.9.4 Miscellaneous Tumors

Squamous cell carcinoma, adenosquamous carcinoma, large cell undifferentiated carcinoma, and small cell (neuroendocrine) carcinoma all can arise in the stomach but are rare. Carcinoid is the second most common epithelial tumor of the stomach. Gastric carcinoids are often multiple. Small cell carcinoma occurs rarely, but metastasis from the lung must be excluded. Sarcomas, germ cell tumors (eg, choriocarcinoma), and other tumors can arise rarely in the stomach. Melanoma and carcinomas of the breast and lung are the most common malignancies to metastasize to the stomach.

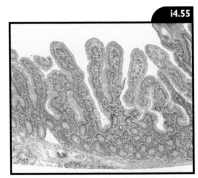

Small intestine, tissue

Small Intestine

Most pathologic conditions of the small intestine diagnosed cytologically involve the duodenum, particularly the descending portion, which contains the ampulla of Vater with the common bile duct |i4.55|. (See also "Extrahepatic Biliary Tract," p 92.) Neoplasms of the small intestine are unusual, but malignant tumors are somewhat more common than benign ones.

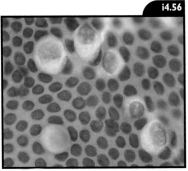

Normal intestinal cells

4.10 The Cells

4.10.1 Normal

The small intestinal mucosal lining is composed principally of absorptive and goblet cells. The mucosa of the small intestine is characterized cytologically by honeycombed sheets of absorptive cells with pale goblet cells interspersed (Swiss cheese appearance) |i4.56|. The cells are tall columnar and usually well preserved in brush specimens. The nuclei are basal and round to oval and have smooth membranes, fine chromatin, and small nucleoli. The cytoplasm of absorptive cells is finely granular or vacuolar and has a striated, microvillous, apical border |i4.57|. Goblet cells contain large mucin vacuoles. A few inflammatory cells may be present in the background.

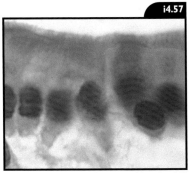

Absorptive cells, striated border (oil)

4.10.2 Reactive and Degenerative Changes

Due to ulceration or inflammation, the small intestinal cells may undergo reactive/reparative or degenerative changes |i4.58|. These cells often are poorly preserved; naked nuclei, nuclear pyknosis, and karyorrhexis are common. The cytoplasm may take on a squamoid appearance, and sometimes intercellular bridges are seen. Also, highly reactive spindle myofibroblasts may be obtained from the base of an ulcer, which must be differentiated from spindle cell tumors, eg, leiomyosarcoma. Evidence of inflammation or necrosis may be seen in the background.

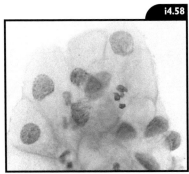

Reactive glandular cells

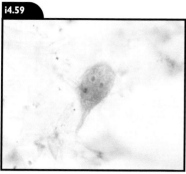

Giardia lamblia (oil)

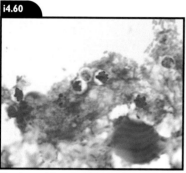

Cryptosporidium (acid-fast, oil)

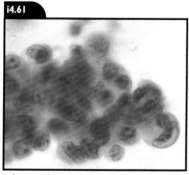

Adenocarcinoma

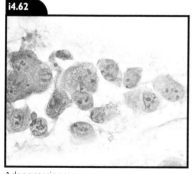

Adenocarcinoma

4.11 Infections

4.11.1 *Giardia lamblia*

Giardia lamblia is a pear-shaped organism, possessing a terminal flagellum, that resembles *Trichomonas* |i4.59|. The organism has two nuclei, each containing a prominent chromocenter (looks like a "smiley face"). *Giardia* can be particularly well-demonstrated ("pretty") in cytologic specimens.

4.11.2 Cryptosporidiosis

Cryptosporidiosis usually occurs in immunocompromised patients, particularly those with AIDS. It causes a profuse watery diarrhea. *Cryptosporidium* is a round, nonbudding, acid-fast protozoal organism, about 2 to 4 μm in diameter, that may resemble platelets (which tend to clump) or yeasts (which may bud) |i4.60|.

4.12 Malignant Diseases

4.12.1 Adenocarcinoma

Adenocarcinomas arising in the small intestine are similar to those of the colon. Adenocarcinomas of the ampulla of Vater are morphologically identical to those of the bile ducts and pancreas.

Adenocarcinomas of the ampulla of Vater or duodenum are usually well-differentiated. The cells are relatively large and are present singly, in loose sheets, or in small crowded clusters |i4.61|, |i4.62|. The nuclei are usually enlarged, pleomorphic, and hyperchromatic with irregular nuclear membranes and prominent nucleoli. The cytoplasm is relatively abundant with well-defined, irregular cell borders, particularly in well-differentiated tumors, and may show squamoid features, particularly in less-differentiated tumors. Anaplastic giant or spindle cells may be seen in some cases.

Distinguishing these often very well-differentiated tumors from reactive atypia in benign cells can be difficult. For a firm diagnosis of malignancy, numerous cells should be present, including single cells, with features described above. An important diagnostic feature, even in well-differentiated carcinomas, is the presence of irregular nuclear membranes. Also, abnormalities of the arrangement of the cells (eg, too crowded or too loose, loss of polarity) are associated with malignancy.

4.12.2 Malignant Lymphoma

Malignant lymphomas of the small bowel are similar to those of the stomach, except that a significant number (about one third) are T-cell type, often high-grade, which is rare elsewhere in the GI tract. The differential diagnosis includes metastatic carcinoma, eg, of the breast.

4.12.3 Carcinoid Tumors

Carcinoids are potentially malignant neuroendocrine tumors. Carcinoids are usually single but can be multiple, particularly when part of multiple endocrine neoplasia syndromes. Carcinoids often are associated with hormone production, frequently more than one, and may produce recognizable clinical syndromes due to hormone secretion, eg, Zollinger-Ellison (ulcerogenic) syndrome due to gastrin. However, the typical carcinoid syndrome, associated with serotonin production, is rare. More commonly than hormonal syndromes, local disease causes obstruction with jaundice, pancreatitis, and hemorrhage. Most small bowel carcinoids occur in the ileum; the duodenum is the next most common site.

Carcinoids characteristically display monomorphic plasmacytoid cells, present singly and in loose aggregates. Small spindle cells also may be seen. There are few mitotic figures and no necrosis. The nuclei are usually round and monomorphic with typical salt-and-pepper chromatin and inconspicuous nucleoli. Naked nuclei are common and may resemble lymphocytes. The cytoplasm is pale and granular and moderate in amount. Neurosecretory granules can be demonstrated with special stains or specifically identified via immunocytochemistry.

COLON AND RECTUM

Colorectal carcinoma is the second leading cause of cancer death in America (after lung cancer). Unfortunately, colonic cytology does not easily lend itself to mass screening.

4.13 The Cells

Histologically, the colorectal mucosa forms straight, nonbranching, test tube–like glands |**i4.63**|, |**i4.64**|. The epithelium is composed of absorptive cells and is rich in goblet cells. Occasional lymph follicles with germinal centers may be seen.

Cytologically, in brush specimens, the cells are exfoliated in relatively large, cohesive, orderly, honeycombed sheets with distinct edges. Glandular lumens of the colonic crypts may be seen |**i4.65**|. The cells are tall columnar with basal nuclei and apical cytoplasm |**i4.66**|. The nuclei are round and uniform and

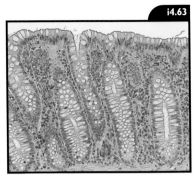
i4.63

Colon, tissue

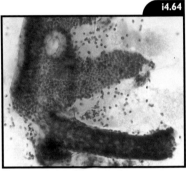
i4.64

Normal colonic epithelium

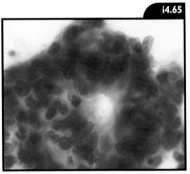
i4.65

Normal colon cells

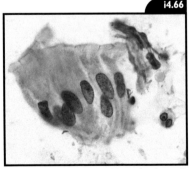
i4.66

Normal colon cells

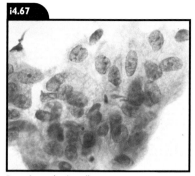

Reactive colonic cells

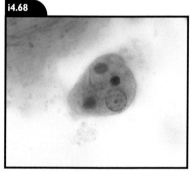

Entamoeba histolytica

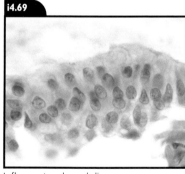

Inflammatory bowel disease

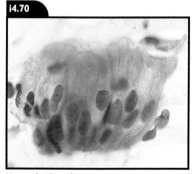

Hyperplastic polyp

have smooth membranes, fine even chromatin, and inconspicuous nucleoli. Absorptive cells have granular cytoplasm and a prominent striated, terminal bar–like apical border—a characteristic feature that is maintained in well-differentiated malignancy. Goblet cells, with large, pale, mucin vacuoles, are interspersed among the absorptive cells. The background may contain a few neutrophils, chronic inflammatory cells, macrophages, anal squamous cells, mucus, and possibly undigested food and debris.

In response to inflammation or ulceration, the cells may undergo reactive changes |i4.67| accompanied by a dirty inflammatory background, which may mimic malignancy. Squamous metaplasia, with marked reactive atypia, also can occur, eg, in diverticulitis, which could be mistaken for squamous cell carcinoma.

4.14 Benign Diseases

4.14.1 Infectious Colitis

Infectious colitis is characterized by the presence of acute or chronic inflammation and reactive or degenerated epithelial cells. A specific infectious agent (eg, ova, parasites) sometimes can be identified.

Bacillary dysentery is characterized by pus, blood, and many bacteria.

Ameba (Entamoeba histolytica) is characterized by ingested RBCs |i4.68|.

Cytomegalovirus infection is associated with immunosuppression. Diagnostic cells (enlarged cells—cytomegaly—with large nuclear inclusion and satellite nuclear and cytoplasmic inclusions) are few and single.

4.14.2 Chronic Idiopathic Inflammatory Bowel Disease

Chronic idiopathic inflammatory bowel disease, ie, Crohn disease and ulcerative colitis, are characterized cytologically by reactive/reparative epithelial cells |i4.69| and an increased number of neutrophils. Although granulomas are typically associated with Crohn disease, they are not specific and can be seen in diseases such as ulcerative colitis and tuberculosis. Specific forms of colitis, such as amebic colitis, must be excluded before accepting a diagnosis of chronic idiopathic inflammatory bowel disease. Patients are at increased risk of developing colorectal adenocarcinomas. Dysplasia is a precancerous change that identifies patients at highest risk for developing cancer. Malignant lymphomas, mostly extraintestinal, also occur in these patients.

4.14.3 Adenoma

Adenomas include adenomatous polyps and villous adenomas but not hyperplastic polyps |i4.70|, |i4.71|, |i4.72|. Patients with adenomas are at increased risk of developing adenocarcinoma. The risk increases with the size and type of adenoma; villous adenomas are higher risk than adenomatous polyps. Any degree of neoplastic change, from low-grade dysplasia to invasive carcinoma, can occur in these polyps.

The cells exfoliate in crowded sheets. Goblet cells and mucin are typically decreased. The nuclei are enlarged, oval to elongated, slightly irregular, hyperchromatic, and crowded with increased nuclear/cytoplasmic ratios. Nucleoli vary from inconspicuous to prominent. Mitotic figures can be seen, but none are abnormal in benign adenomas. No diathesis is present.

4.15 Malignant Diseases

4.15.1 Adenocarcinoma

The smears are cellular, with numerous single, atypical cells. Groups are small, crowded, and disorderly and may form microacinar glandular arrangements |i4.73|. The cells vary from tall columnar with elongated, cigar-shaped nuclei (when well-differentiated) to rounded cells with irregular nuclei (when poorly differentiated). The nuclei are enlarged and pleomorphic, with irregular nuclear membranes; abnormal, coarse, dark chromatin; and prominent nucleoli. The cytoplasm is granular, with variable degrees of mucin vacuolization. Better differentiated tumor cells may have a terminal bar–like edge on the apical border, corresponding ultrastructurally to microvilli with long rootlets |i4.74|. A diathesis is present in the background. Some cases show tumor cells floating in abundant mucus ("colloid or mucinous carcinoma"). Signet ring cell carcinoma is rare but occurs more commonly in younger patients.

Dysplasia and Carcinoma In Situ

Dysplasia is characterized by abnormalities of the nucleus with enlargement, irregularity, loss of polarity, and prominent nucleoli. However, cohesiveness and uniformity of the cells are relatively maintained. Adenocarcinoma is characterized by more single cells, more cytologic atypia, more disorderly cellular arrangements, and a diathesis. Low-grade dysplasia may be difficult to distinguish from reactive changes; high-grade dysplasia may be difficult to distinguish from invasive carcinoma.

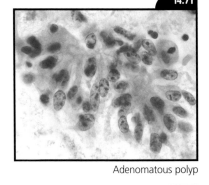
i4.71
Adenomatous polyp

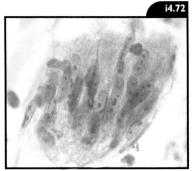
i4.72
Villous adenoma

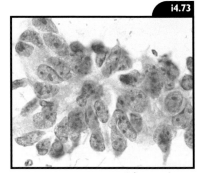
i4.73
Adenocarcinoma

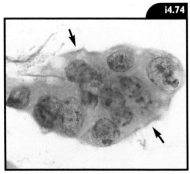
i4.74
Adenocarcinoma—"terminal bars"

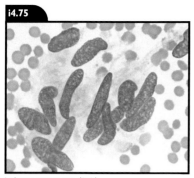

Leiomyosarcoma (DQ)

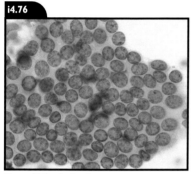

Normal bile duct cells

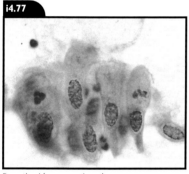

Reactive/degenerative changes

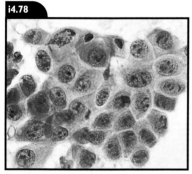

Reactive/reparative changes

4.15.2 Miscellaneous Tumors

The large intestine may be involved by carcinoids, malignant lymphoma, and soft tissue tumors such as leiomyosarcoma |i4.75|. They are usually more amenable to diagnosis by endoscopic fine-needle aspiration biopsy than surface exfoliative cytology.

EXTRAHEPATIC BILIARY TRACT

Cells from the biliary tract can be obtained by endoscopic retrograde cholangiopancreatography, percutaneous transhepatic cholangiography, or intraoperatively. Cytologic examination of material obtained from T tubes or drains is not recommended because the cells are usually markedly degenerated.

4.16 The Cells

4.16.1 Normal

The cells deriving from the pancreatic ducts and biliary tract are cytologically similar. The specimens are often of low cellularity. Regular honeycomb arrangements |i4.76| and orderly palisades of medium-sized columnar cells are characteristic. Single cells tend to round up. The nuclei are round to oval and basally located. The nuclei have smooth membranes and fine, evenly distributed chromatin and may have small nucleoli. The cytoplasm is pale, delicate, and scant to moderate in amount. Goblet cells also can be seen. Greenish brown, granular bile pigment is commonly present in the background.

4.16.2 Reactive and Degenerative Changes

In response to inflammation, gallstones, manipulation, instrumentation, or catheters, the biliary tract epithelium may undergo significant reactive or degenerative changes |i4.77| that can be suggestive of malignancy |i4.78|. Benign, reactive/reparative cells can show marked variation in nuclear size and enlargement up to four or five times normal. Nucleoli can become prominent and may be single or multiple. Normal mitotic figures can be seen. Squamous metaplasia may occur.

In contrast with cancer, reactive cells occur in well-ordered cohesive clusters or sheets, with minimal nuclear crowding or overlap, and have smooth nuclear membranes, less abnormal chromatin, and adequate cytoplasm (thus, normal nuclear/cytoplasmic ratios).

4.17 Benign Tumors

Several benign or low-grade malignant tumors can occur in and around the biliary tract, including islet cell tumors, carcinoids, paragangliomas, and Brunner gland neoplasms. These typically grow in a submucosal location, making diagnosis by exfoliative cytology difficult.

Granular cell tumor is more common in blacks, young adults, and, particularly, females. It is characterized by large single cells with coarsely granular cytoplasm (due to lysosomes) (see |i4.33|). The tumor may be associated with marked hyperplasia and atypia of the overlying mucosa (pseudoepitheliomatous hyperplasia), which could result in an erroneous diagnosis of malignancy.

4.18 Malignant Tumors

Carcinomas arising anywhere in the pancreaticobiliary ductal-type epithelium, including the gallbladder, are morphologically similar |i4.79|. Most of these cancers show glandular differentiation, but in addition, squamoid features are also common |i4.80|, particularly in tumors that are other than very well-differentiated. In fact, combined adenosquamous differentiation is a characteristic feature of neoplasms arising in this type of epithelium. Pure squamous cell carcinoma, however, is rare.

The cytology shows the usual features of adenocarcinoma, including single cells, nuclear enlargement and irregularity, abnormal chromatin, and prominent nucleoli. Abnormal mitotic figures may be seen. The cytoplasm varies from delicate and vacuolated to dense and squamoid. Signet ring cells or malignant giant and spindle cells may be present. Blood, bile, inflammation, and necrosis may be seen in the background. However, a similar background also can be found in benign disease, eg, cholelithiasis (gallstones).

Pancreaticobiliary carcinomas sometimes can be extremely well-differentiated |i4.81|. The cells may appear deceptively bland and uniform. There are three important clues to a malignant process: abnormalities of cellular arrangement (cells too crowded or too loose), irregular nuclear membranes, and increased mitotic activity |i4.82|. In practice, biliary cancer is possible to diagnose but impossible to exclude by exfoliative cytology.

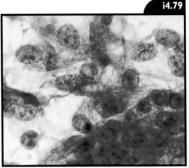

i4.79

Bile duct carcinoma

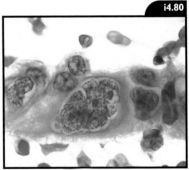

i4.80

Carcinoma with squamoid cytoplasm

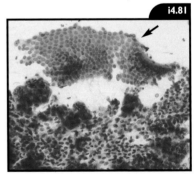

i4.81

Well-differentiated AdCA—benign cells

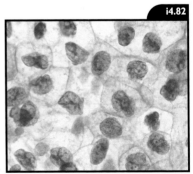

i4.82

Well-differentiated carcinoma

Urine

n ⋈

Urothelium, or transitional epithelium, lines most of the collecting and storage system of the urinary tract, including the renal pelvis, ureter, bladder, and part of the urethra (particularly in males) |i5.1|. Transitional epithelium maintains a barrier between the urine (which is toxic) and the blood, and it is able to stretch, especially in the bladder, to accommodate urine. To perform these two functions, transitional cells have asymmetric cell membranes (the outer lamina is thicker and denser than the inner), and there are intracytoplasmic fusiform vesicles, continuous with the surface, that provide membrane as the cell stretches. The cells are welded together by numerous tight junctions, making the epithelium watertight.

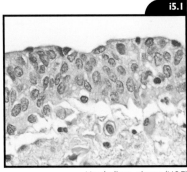
i5.1

Urothelium, tissue (H&E)

5.1 Urinary Tract Cytology

Tumors of the urinary tract are relatively inaccessible to direct biopsy and are often multifocal. Since urine is easily obtained and washes over the entire mucosal surface, urine cytology is, in theory, the perfect specimen to examine to detect a tumor. Unfortunately, interpretation of urine cytology is difficult, and both false-negative and false-positive results are very well known. Moreover, lesions cannot be localized by urine cytology alone.

Diagnostic accuracy increases with the grade of the tumor. Urinary cytology usually can detect carcinoma in situ (CIS) and high-grade neoplasms. Low-grade noninvasive papillary tumors are the sources of most false negatives. Reactive and degenerative changes due to conditions such as inflammation, stones, prostatic hyperplasia, and therapy are responsible for most false-positives. However, lesions may be detected by cytology long before they can be seen cystoscopically, resulting in apparent false-positives (false false-positives).

Clinical history is, as always, important in proper evaluation of the specimen and should include previous diagnoses, therapy, or surgery; recent instrumentation (including catheterization); history of stones; method of specimen collection; cystoscopic findings; and any other pertinent clinical data. The most common symptoms of patients with bladder cancer are hematuria (gross or microscopic) or cystitis-like symptoms (frequency, urgency, pain), but these symptoms are nonspecific.

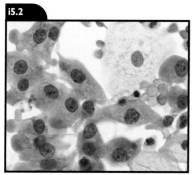

Transitional cells (compare squamous cell)

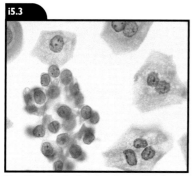

Transitional cells (basal and superficial)

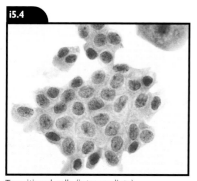

Transitional cells (intermediate)

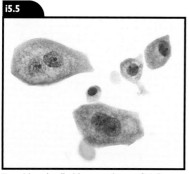

Transitional cells (deep and superficial)

5.2 The Cells

5.2.1 Transitional Cells

Transitional cells are among the most pleomorphic benign epithelial cells in the body, ranging from basal cells, somewhat larger than a lymphocyte (~ 10 μm), to giant multinucleated superficial (umbrella) cells (≥ 100 μm), perhaps the largest benign epithelial cells in humans |i5.2|, |i5.3|, |i5.4|, |i5.5|. Due to expansion and contraction, the cells vary from triangular to polyhedral to rounded, or caudate to columnar. Single, mononuclear, parabasal-sized cells usually predominate in voided specimens. Multinucleated umbrella cells, groups of cells, and pseudopapillary aggregates are observed more commonly in catheterized samples, including washes and brushes, owing to mechanical avulsion. All transitional cells may contain glycogen, and superficial cells also may contain mucin. Glycogen may be washed out during processing, resulting in a clear appearance of the cytoplasm.

5.2.2 Deep Transitional Cells (Basal and Intermediate)

Basal and intermediate transitional cells are cytologically similar and considered together as deep transitional cells. The cytoplasm is moderately dense, with well-defined, often scalloped, cell borders. Diffuse fine vacuolization is characteristic; coarse degenerative vacuoles are also common. Transitional cells take the Papanicolaou stain variably, usually staining blue to gray but occasionally red to orange.

The nuclei are usually centrally located. They are larger than those of intermediate squamous cells. The nuclear shape varies from oval to slightly triangular or polyhedral. Binucleation is common. The chromatin is evenly distributed and ranges from finely granular to "salt-and-pepper" coarseness; it usually appears bland in well-preserved cells. However, polyploidy and hyperchromasia are common and result in "big dark" nuclei that do not necessarily indicate dysplasia or neoplasia. One or two conspicuous nucleoli are characteristic, especially in washes.

5.2.3 Superficial Transitional Cells (Umbrella Cells)

Superficial transitional cells, or umbrella cells, resemble other transitional cells, but are larger, usually about the size of a mature squamous cell. They have a rounded (convex) luminal surface and a scalloped (concave) border, where they cover the underlying cells like an umbrella. The cytoplasm is abundant, and there are frequently two to three or more nuclei that can vary moderately in size. In addition, giant forms, with up to dozens of nuclei, are sometimes seen |i5.6|. Giant umbrella cells are more common in specimens from the ureter or renal pelvis but also can occur in the bladder. They frequently are associated with instrumentation and are benign.

5.2.4 Columnar Cells

Although rare in voided urine, columnar-shaped transitional cells are a normal and relatively common finding in specimens obtained by bladder wash |i5.7|. Columnar transitional cells also can derive from the urethra, particularly in males, as well as from cystitis cystica. Columnar transitional cells often have a thin cytoplasmic tail. They can be single or form small groups. Columnar transitional cells also can be seen in well-differentiated papillary neoplasms. Other possible sources of columnar-shaped cells include genital tract contamination, renal tubular cells, and cystitis glandularis.

5.2.5 Reactive and Degenerative Transitional Cells

Reactive and degenerative changes are common in transitional cells and can be due to a wide variety of conditions, including inflammation and infection |i5.8|, stones, prostatic hyperplasia, radiation and chemotherapy, drugs, catheterization, or instrumentation. Umbrella cells, in particular, may become frankly bizarre appearing. The nuclei increase in size and number and become more pleomorphic, and the nuclear/cytoplasmic ratios may be slightly increased. Normal mitotic figures can be seen. Coarse dark chromatin and prominent nucleoli can mimic high-grade transitional cell carcinoma (TCC). Margination of the chromatin, karyolysis, and karyorrhexis are common degenerative changes. However, in benign changes, the nuclear membranes remain relatively smooth, the chromatin often has a smudgy quality, and the nuclear/cytoplasmic ratios are relatively maintained. Prominent nucleoli and cytoplasmic vacuolization are common in reactive transitional cells and high-grade TCC but are usually not seen in low-grade TCC.

5.2.6 Significance of Papillary Clusters

Transitional epithelium exfoliates easily; thus, the slightest trauma to the mucosa, including catheterization, bladder washing, and stones, as well as prostatic hyperplasia, can result in detachment of "papillary" tissue fragments (pseudopapillae). Reactive and degenerative changes also can occur in the cells. These findings can mimic papillary TCC. Therefore, "papillary clusters" should be interpreted cautiously in such cases, unless there is clear-cut evidence of malignancy. However, when papillary clusters are present in a spontaneously voided urine specimen |i5.9|, without a history of recent instrumentation, stones, etc, further

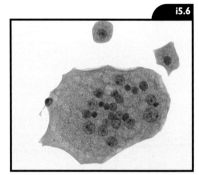
Giant umbrella cell

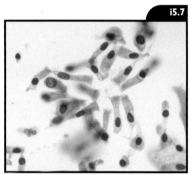
Columnar transitional cells

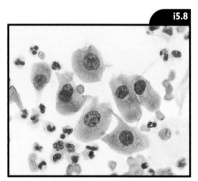
Reactive transitional cells—cystitis

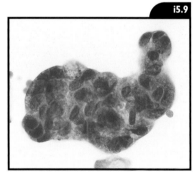
Papillary cluster, voided urine (exclude TCC)

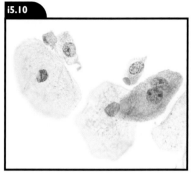

Squamous metaplasia (cf transitional cells)

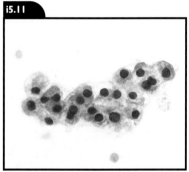

Renal tubular cells

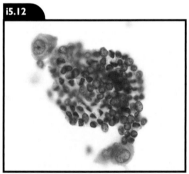

Prostatic cells (cf transitional cells)

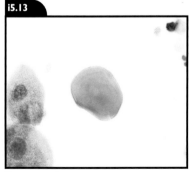

Corpus amylaceum

investigation is warranted to rule out papillary TCC, even when the cells appear normal.

5.2.7 Squamous Cells and Squamous Metaplasia

Voided urine, particularly from females, often contains squamous cells from the genital tract as contaminants. However, squamous epithelium is normally present in the urethra of men (distal) and women (almost entire). Moreover, squamous metaplasia (fully mature, nonkeratinized squamous epithelium) of the trigone is essentially normal in women. It also occurs in newborn boys and some healthy men, as well as in men treated with estrogen. In addition to hormones, chronic inflammation or irritation (eg, stones, schistosomiasis, indwelling catheters) can cause squamous metaplasia.

In urine cytology, squamous metaplastic cells are usually mature intermediate or superficial squamous cells identical to those seen in the Pap smear |i5.10|. Squamous cells are larger than deep transitional cells and have smaller nuclei with lower nuclear/cytoplasmic ratios. The cytoplasm of squamous cells is thin and usually stains pink or blue compared with the denser, gray-blue vacuolated cytoplasm typical of transitional cells.

5.2.8 Miscellaneous Findings

Inflammatory and Blood Cells

The urine is normally free of inflammatory cells and RBCs; their presence may indicate urinary tract disease, including inflammation, malignancy, or trauma.

Renal Tubular Cells

Renal tubular cells can be seen in renal disease ranging from nephritis to transplant rejection to renal cell carcinoma. Benign tubular cells are small columnar cells, usually recognized in small sheets or casts |i5.11|. Reactive and degenerative changes are common.

Prostatic and Seminal Vesicle Cells

Prostatic cells form small sheets or clusters of cuboidal cells with uniform small round nuclei but somewhat hyperchromatic chromatin |i5.12|. Small nucleoli may be seen in prostatitis, but macronucleoli suggest prostatic adenocarcinoma.

Seminal vesicle cells, although rarely found in urine, can be strikingly atypical in appearance, particularly in older men. Diagnostic clues are golden brown cytoplasmic pigment, dense smudgy chromatin, and presence of sperm or corpora amylacea.

Corpora Amylacea and Psammoma Bodies

      Corpora amylacea are concentrically laminated |i5.13| (usually noncalcified) bodies from the prostate. The differential diagnosis is psammoma bodies, which, unlike corpora amylacea, are always calcified and often surrounded by epithelial cells.

Globular or Hyaline Inclusion Bodies

      Little red or blue droplets are commonly seen in the cytoplasm of cells in the urine |i5.14|. These inclusion bodies are a nonspecific finding associated with degeneration that may represent giant lysosomes but are specifically not viral in origin. They are more common in voided than catheterized specimens and are abundant in ileal conduit urine. Similar inclusions also can be seen occasionally in nonurine specimens (eg, sputum, breast cysts).

Other Findings

      Sperm, crystals |i5.15|, casts |i5.16|, and various organisms, as well as extraneous material such as glove powder and lubricant (amorphous purplish glop), all can be seen from time to time in urine cytology.

5.3 Basic Specimens

      "Clean catch" voided urine is recommended for screening purposes. Three specimens are recommended for optimum sensitivity. First morning voided urine, although theoretically more cellular, is not a good specimen owing to degenerative changes. Similarly, urine from a collection bag should not be submitted for cytologic examination. Simple catheterization increases the cellularity over voided urine specimens, and the specimen may be somewhat better preserved. However, it makes the diagnosis of low-grade lesions more difficult because of diagnostic problems related to pseudopapillary clusters and may miss lesions in the urethra. Bladder washes are used when there is a high clinical suspicion of malignancy. Fresh specimens are preferred, and the Papanicolaou stain usually is used.

5.4 Benign Diseases of the Urinary Tract

5.4.1 Stones (Urinary Tract Lithiasis)

      Urinary tract lithiasis (stones) can cause marked cytologic atypia |i5.17| and high cellularity, mimicking TCC. Mechanical avulsion of pseudopapillary groups of transitional epithelium can

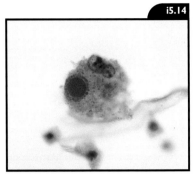
Nonspecific inclusion bodies

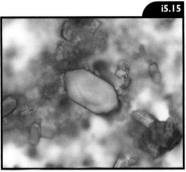
Crystals—triple phosphate

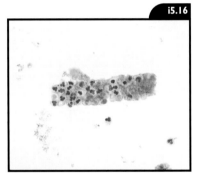
Cast—WBC cast

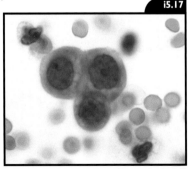
Stone atypia (oil)

99

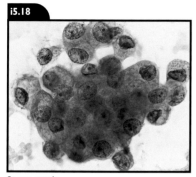

Stone atypia

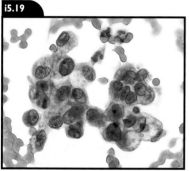

Indwelling catheter atypia

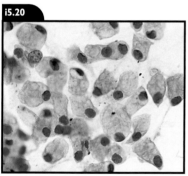

Cystitis glandularis

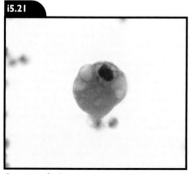

Cytomegalovirus

mimic neoplastic papillae. Cytologically, nuclear enlargement and pleomorphism, with increased nuclear/cytoplasmic ratios, coarse dark chromatin, prominent nucleoli, mitotic figures, inflammation, blood, and necrosis all can be seen in lithiasis |i5.18|. Be cautious diagnosing cancer in the presence of stones. Indwelling catheters can also cause similar changes |i5.19|.

5.4.2 Cystitis

Cystitis usually is caused by fecal flora, particularly *Escherichia coli.* The diagnostic features are neutrophils, histiocytes, RBCs, and necrotic debris. There may be an increased number of transitional cells with reactive and degenerative changes that can mimic cancer. Thus, caution is warranted in diagnosis. On the other hand, the presence of inflammation by no means excludes cancer. With prolonged chronic inflammation, a progression from Brunn nests (solid buds of transitional cells) to cystitis cystica (small cysts lined with transitional cells) to cystitis glandularis |i5.20| (cysts lined with metaplastic glandular cells) may occur.

5.4.3 Tuberculosis

Tuberculosis of the urinary tract is usually secondary to tuberculosis of the kidney. Clusters of epithelioid histiocytes, which may have spindle or carrot shapes, are diagnostic of a granuloma. The nuclei are round to oval with fine chromatin, and the cytoplasm is finely vacuolated to fibrillar with indistinct borders. Multinucleated giant cell histiocytes also may be identified. Acid-fast bacilli or positive urine cultures confirm the diagnosis. Mild to marked reactive epithelial atypia also may be seen, which could suggest malignancy. Similar findings can occur in patients treated with bacillus Calmette-Guérin (BCG) for TCC (see p 104) or following bladder surgery.

5.4.4 Fungus

Fungal infections of the urinary tract usually occur in immunosuppressed or diabetic patients but also can occur in some patients taking broad-spectrum antibiotics. Most of the common types of fungi can cause infection, including *Blastomyces, Crypto-coccus, Aspergillus,* or *Candida* (more commonly a contaminant from the female genital tract). A neutrophilic inflammatory response may be seen. Culture the specimen for definitive diagnosis.

5.4.5 Schistosomiasis

Schistosomiasis is rare in the United States but more common in Egypt or among immigrants. Schistosomal ova, usually *Schisto-*

soma hematobium, can sometimes be found in the urine. Chronic infection may result in squamous cell carcinoma of the bladder. The ova resemble large uric acid ("lemon drop") crystals and are identified by their characteristic lateral or terminal spine.

5.4.6 Cytomegalovirus

In the past, urine was more commonly examined for detection of cytomegalovirus. Because infected cells derive mostly from the renal tubules, diagnostic cells in urine are sparse. Cytomegalovirus is potentially fatal in infants or immunosuppressed patients; however, otherwise healthy adults may simply be carriers.

The classic diagnostic features are large single cells, large basophilic nuclear inclusion with halo, and thick-appearing nuclear membrane, with or without small round intracytoplasmic or intranuclear satellite inclusions |i5.21|.

5.4.7 Human Polyoma Virus

Human polyoma virus, also known as BK virus, is a member of the Papovavirus family. These are DNA viruses also related to progressive multifocal leukoencephalopathy, JC, and human papilloma viruses. Some infected patients are immuno-compromised, but others are otherwise apparently healthy. The infection can be asymptomatic or associated with hematuria, and spontaneously resolves, without sequelae, within a few months.

The number of diagnostic cells varies from sparse to abundant. Infected cells have enlarged dark nuclei and scant cytoplasm, mimicking cancer, particularly CIS (known as "decoy cells") |i5.22| and sometimes have short, cytoplasmic tails ("comet cells") |i5.23|. The most characteristic feature is the presence of a large, round, homogeneous, opaque blue-black inclusion in the nucleus. There may be a very thin halo between the inclusion and a "thickened" nuclear membrane. The viral inclusion can leach out, leaving a coarse chromatin network or a bland, washed-out appearance ("viral look") |i5.24|. In contrast with cancer |i5.25|, the infected nuclei appear smudgy, and the cells are usually sparse and singly dispersed, rarely forming clusters. The differential diagnosis also includes cytomegalovirus infection.

5.4.8 Other Viruses

Human papilloma virus causes condylomas, which can occur in the bladder, but more commonly represent genital tract contamination (see "Condyloma," p 110).

Herpes can infect transitional cells and is diagnosed by the usual criteria (the 3 Ms: multinucleation, molding, margination, with ground-glass chromatin and sometimes intranuclear inclusions).

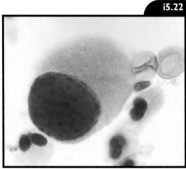
i5.22
Decoy cell (oil)

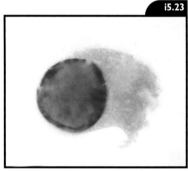
i5.23
Comet cell (oil)

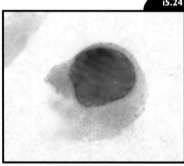
i5.24
Decoy cell—"viral look" (oil)

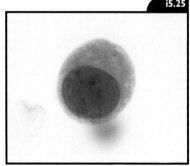
i5.25
High-grade TCC (oil)

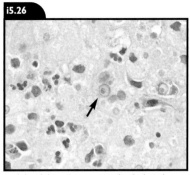

Malakoplakia, tissue—MG body (H&E)

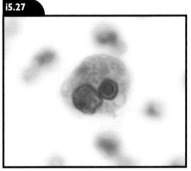

Malakoplakia—MG body (oil)

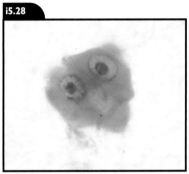

Lead poisoning—nuclear inclusions

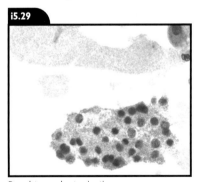

Renal transplant rejection

5.4.9 Malakoplakia

Malakoplakia is a rare, chronic granulomatous disease |i5.26| that typically occurs in middle-aged women but can affect any age and either sex. Immunodeficiency, due to defective phagocytosis or phagolysosomes, results in incomplete digestion of bacteria, which become mineralized, and leads to formation of characteristic Michaelis-Gutmann (MG) bodies |i5.27| in the histiocytes (of von Hansemann). These cytoplasmic inclusion bodies are about 5 to 10 μm in diameter, round, laminated, and usually basophilic. They are periodic acid–Schiff positive and contain iron and calcium. They are rare in voided urine but may be seen after biopsy or in bladder washes. The typical "bull's eye" appearance is best appreciated in larger inclusions. Granulomas composed of epithelioid histiocytes, lymphocytes, plasma cells, and, occasionally, multinucleated giant cells are seen.

5.4.10 Intravenous and Retrograde Pyelogram Effect

Within a few days after exposure to certain radiologic contrast materials ("dyes"), the transitional cells may be altered. Pseudopapillae may be shed. Reactive changes and degenerative changes mimicking malignancy may be seen; however, the nuclear/cytoplasmic ratio remains within normal limits. Colorless to pale yellow free dye occasionally can be seen as spheroid globules or rectangular plates.

5.4.11 Heavy Metal Poisoning (Bismuth, Lead)

In heavy metal poisoning, eg, lead poisoning in children, the renal tubular cells may contain red intranuclear inclusions that resemble viral inclusions or macronucleoli |i5.28|. These nuclear inclusions are homogeneous but irregular in outline, have a well-defined halo, and stain acid-fast positive.

5.5 Renal Transplant

One of the most important features for diagnosis of renal allograft rejection is an increased exfoliation of renal tubular cells. They occur singly or in small clusters, tubules, or sheets of cells that may be attached to a cast |i5.29|. Mitotic figures may be seen. Lymphocyturia, particularly reactive plasmacytoid lymphocytes with enlarged nuclei and prominent nucleoli, is an early and important sign of rejection. Hematuria, macrophages, casts, amorphous debris, and oxalate crystals are other features. Cytologic changes due to radiation or chemotherapy may be superimposed. Suspect rejection if the urine becomes cellular compared with the patient's own baseline. The differential diagnosis includes an inflammatory process in the urinary tract.

5.6 Cellular Reaction to Therapeutic Agents

5.6.1 Chemotherapy

Some chemotherapeutic agents (eg, cyclophosphamide, busulfan) can cause significant cytologic atypia that can mimic malignancy; other drugs (eg, thiotepa) cause less atypia, more reminiscent of reactive changes. Some drugs are administered intravesically and act locally (eg, mitomycin, thiotepa). Others may be given systemically and concentrate in the urine (eg, cyclophosphamide, busulfan).

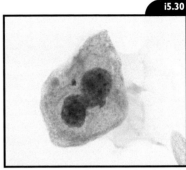
Chemotherapy effect (cyclophosphamide)

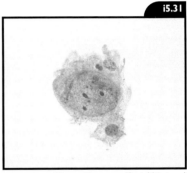
Chemotherapy effect (thiotepa)

Cyclophosphamide

Cyclophosphamide (Cytoxan) is concentrated in the urine, where it can cause severe hemorrhagic cystitis. Epithelial necrosis is followed by atypical repair and regeneration. Markedly atypical cells with increased nuclear/cytoplasmic ratios and bizarre shapes may be seen |i5.30|. The nuclei may be enlarged and hyperchromatic with granular to smudgy chromatin and irregular macronucleoli, mimicking high-grade TCC. Cytoplasmic vacuoles may contain debris or WBCs. There is a dirty inflammatory background.

Busulfan

Busulfan (Myleran) causes changes that are similar to those caused by cyclophosphamide and can mimic high-grade TCC.

Thiotepa, Mitomycin, and Others

Thiotepa and mitomycin cause increased cellular exfoliation, which usually diminishes after several weeks. Persistence of increased cellularity suggests persistent tumor.

Thiotepa and mitomycin cause reactive changes |i5.31| affecting mostly superficial umbrella cells. The nuclei are enlarged and round to oval; they have smooth nuclear membranes and multiple small nucleoli and usually are not hyperchromatic (unless degenerated). The cytoplasm is vacuolated and frayed, but the nuclear/cytoplasmic ratios are within normal limits.

Bizarre cells, as seen with cyclophosphamide therapy, are absent or rare. Significant cytologic atypia or frankly malignant-appearing cells should be carefully investigated.

Cyclosporine

Cyclosporine, used as an immunosuppressant, can cause nephrotoxic adverse effects, resulting in increased exfoliation of

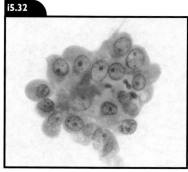

Radiation cystitis

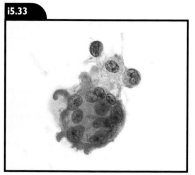

BCG therapy

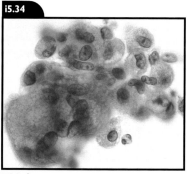

BCG therapy

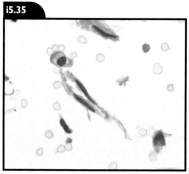

Thermal artifact

renal tubular cells, including papillary tissue fragments. The tubular cells can show cytoplasmic "inclusions" (giant mitochondria) and vacuolization. Microcalcifications also can occur.

5.6.2 Radiation

Radiation effects are generally similar to those described in the Pap smear. Reactive and degenerative changes are common and could be mistaken for malignancy |i5.32|. The most reliable criterion of radiation effect is marked enlargement of the cell, or cytomegaly, ie, macrocytes. The nuclei and cytoplasm enlarge in concert, so that the nuclear/cytoplasmic ratio is maintained. Multinucleation and macronucleoli may be seen. The chromatin is usually fine and even, although hyperchromasia, pyknosis, or karyorrhexis can occur. Cytoplasmic vacuolization and polychromasia or eosinophilia are also characteristic. The background of the smear contains debris, inflammatory cells, and proteinaceous material.

5.6.3 Bacillus Calmette-Guérin

BCG is used to treat bladder cancer, particularly CIS. BCG (an attenuated tubercle *Mycobacterium*) causes the epithelium to denude and granulomas to form in the stroma |i5.33|, |i5.34|. Neutrophils predominate early; later, lymphocytes, histiocytes, and giant cells appear. BCG also can cause mild epithelial atypia, but there is no significant nuclear pleomorphism, prominent nucleoli, or cytomegaly.

5.6.4 Laser Therapy/Cauterization

In response to laser therapy or cauterization, the transitional cells may show striking spindle artifact, probably a result of heat |i5.35|.

5.7 Urinary Tract Cancer

Bladder cancer is more common in men than women, in whites than blacks, and is rare before 40 years of age. The most common presenting symptom is painless hematuria. Nonspecific cystitis-like symptoms (eg, frequency, urgency, dysuria) occur late and may indicate invasive disease. Urothelial cancer is often multifocal, representing a field defect rather than a clonal proliferation. Risk factors include environmental and industrial carcinogens (eg, aniline dyes), cigarette smoking, certain drugs (eg, chemotherapeutic agents, phenacetin, opium), chronic irritation (eg, stones,

t5.1 Approximate Diagnostic Equivalents

Traditional	Revised*
Papilloma	Benign papilloma
TCC I	Benign papilloma
TCC II	TCC, low-grade
TCC III	TCC, high-grade

TCC, transitional cell carcinoma.
*Used in this discussion.

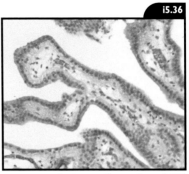

Benign papilloma, tissue (H&E)

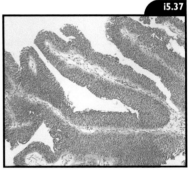

Low-grade TCC, tissue (H&E)

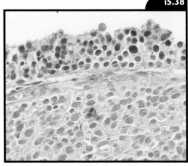

High-grade TCC, tissue

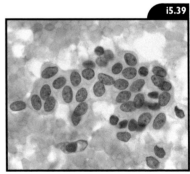

Benign papilloma, cytology

indwelling catheters, schistosomiasis), and previous history of bladder tumor.

Cytology can detect most high-grade TCCs, including CIS, but commonly fails to detect well-differentiated papillary transitional cell neoplasms. However, diagnostic accuracy improves if papillary lesions lined with nearly normal appearing cells are considered benign papillomas, and all transitional cell tumors composed of malignant-appearing cells, whether papillary or not, are considered TCCs |t5.1|.

Low-grade transitional cell neoplasms frequently recur but rarely develop into aggressive cancer. However, these patients are at higher risk of developing aggressive cancer and should be closely followed up. In contrast, high-grade carcinomas are aggressive, whether papillary or not. Patients who die of TCC usually present initially with high-grade lesions.

In summary, although low-grade transitional cell neoplasms are difficult or impossible to diagnose cytologically, these lesions are seldom fatal. CIS and high-grade invasive cancer are the dangerous lesions, and they can usually be readily detected cytologically |i5.36|, |i5.37|, |i5.38|.

5.7.1 General Principles of Cytologic Diagnosis

The higher the grade and the more extensive the tumor, the greater the ability to make a cytologic diagnosis. Important cytologic features of malignancy include crowded disorganized tissue fragments, enlarged nuclei, increased nuclear/cytoplasmic ratios, coarse chromatin, and macronucleoli. Spindle cells may be a clue to the diagnosis of low-grade neoplasms. Hyperchromasia, per se, and nuclear size alone are not good diagnostic criteria; degenerated or polyploid nuclei can stain dark, and it is the nuclear/cytoplasmic ratio rather than absolute nuclear size that is more important in diagnosis. Mitotic figures and necrosis are factors that correlate with poor prognosis. The differential diagnosis includes atypia due to trauma (including stones, catheterization), inflammation, and radiation or chemotherapy.

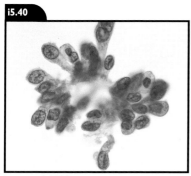

Low-grade TCC

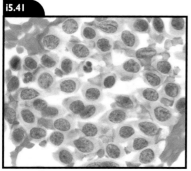

Low-grade TCC

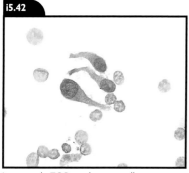

Low-grade TCC—columnar cells

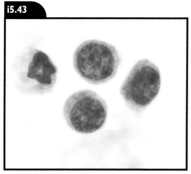

Low-grade TCC (oil)

5.7.2 Papilloma (Well-Differentiated Papillary Transitional Cell Neoplasm)

Well-differentiated papillary transitional cell neoplasms, or papillomas (amalgamating traditional benign papillomas and grade I papillary TCC), are composed of normal or nearly normal appearing cells, making cytologic diagnosis difficult or impossible |i5.39|.

Loose clusters and papillary-like aggregates commonly occur in these papillomas but must be differentiated from instrumentation and stone artifact. True papillary fronds (with fibrovascular cores) are diagnostic of papillary neoplasia but are rarely observed and are not essential for diagnosis.

Columnar, elongated, or spindle cells may be seen. The cells and their nuclei are larger than normal deep (not superficial) transitional cells. The cell borders are often indistinct. The cytoplasm is dense and homogeneous rather than vacuolated. The nuclei are eccentric and may have irregular membranes, such as notches or creases. The chromatin is fine and evenly distributed. Nucleoli, if present, are small. RBCs commonly are observed in the background.

Reactive transitional cells often have prominent nucleoli and vacuolated cytoplasm—features usually not associated with low-grade transitional cell neoplasms but seen in high-grade TCC (which has classic malignant features).

5.7.3 Transitional Cell Carcinoma, Low-Grade

Increased cellularity is a common, and suspicious, finding for low-grade TCC in voided urine specimens, which are usually sparsely cellular. The malignant cells often form loose or abnormally crowded cellular clusters or papillae |i5.40|. Although the cells may be smaller than those of papillomas, they have higher nuclear/cytoplasmic ratios. The nuclei are eccentrically located. Nuclear membrane irregularities usually are present and diagnostically important. The chromatin is more granular than normal but remains evenly distributed. Nucleoli are usually invisible or small, although some nuclei may have prominent nucleoli. The cytoplasm typically appears dense and homogeneous rather than vacuolated |i5.41|.

Although the cells appear more atypical than those of papilloma, significant pleomorphism, irregular chromatin distribution, and numerous large nucleoli are not seen. Mitotic figures may be observed. Focal evidence of glandular or squamous metaplasia as well as columnar, elongated, or spindle cells |i5.42| can occur. Small, pyknotic cells warn that TCC may be present.

High nuclear/cytoplasmic ratios, irregular nuclear membranes, and dense homogeneous cytoplasm are three key features in the diagnosis of low-grade TCC. In papillary aggregates, benign cells can be *more* pleomorphic than those of low-grade TCC; therefore, look carefully at the single cells in the background to help diagnose low-grade TCC |i5.43|.

5.7.4 Transitional Cell Carcinoma, High-Grade

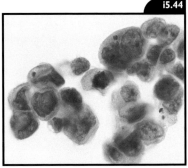

High-grade TCC

The cells of high-grade TCC are obviously malignant appearing, including pleomorphic and bizarre cells, with high nuclear/cytoplasmic ratios |i5.44|, |i5.45|, |i5.46|, |i5.47|. The nuclei display classic malignant features, including irregular nuclear membranes; abnormal coarse, dark, irregular chromatin; and prominent nucleoli. Mitotic figures are frequent and may be atypical. In contrast with well-differentiated neoplasms, the cytoplasm is frequently vacuolated. Glandular |i5.48| or squamous |i5.49| differentiation is more common in high-grade carcinomas. Spindle |i5.50| and giant |i5.51| cells also can be seen.

Reactive transitional cells also can have large nucleoli and cytoplasmic vacuolization, like high-grade TCC, but the reactive cells lack malignant features. Compared with low-grade TCC, high-grade TCC has more obvious malignant features. The best diagnostic criteria for high-grade TCC are enlarged nuclei with increased nuclear/cytoplasmic ratios; irregular nuclear membranes; coarse, dark chromatin; and macronucleoli.

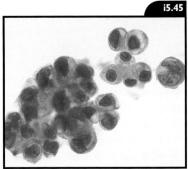

High-grade TCC

Pitfalls in diagnosis of transitional cell neoplasia include reactive umbrella cells, pseudopapillary fragments, stone atypia, ureteral or pelvic cells, ileal conduit cells, radiation or chemotherapy effect, viral changes (especially polyomavirus), hyperplasia or papilloma, and drugs.

5.7.5 Carcinoma In Situ of the Transitional Epithelium

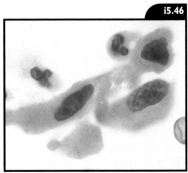

High-grade TCC (oil)

CIS is, by definition, a nonpapillary or flat lesion composed of high-grade tumor cells closely resembling those seen in invasive TCC. CIS is the usual source of deeply invasive cancers that can be lethal. In sharp contrast with CIS of the uterine cervix, CIS of the urothelium does not require a full thickness of anaplastic cells but rather is diagnosed by the "worst" cells present.

Cystoscopically, the CIS lesion may not be visible or only appears red, like cystitis. Urine cytology has an important role in diagnosis of this disease: CIS usually can be readily detected by cytology, although cytology cannot reliably determine whether the disease is in situ or invasive, nor can it localize lesions. Also, a positive cytologic diagnosis may precede by months or even years a positive histologic diagnosis, resulting in an apparent false-positive cytologic diagnosis ("false false-positive").

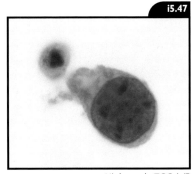

High-grade TCC (oil)

In essence, the diagnosis consists of finding many cells with marked atypia (similar to those of high-grade TCC) |i5.52|. The cells exfoliate readily and appear singly or in small clusters.

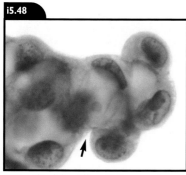

TCC—glandular differentiation, mucin

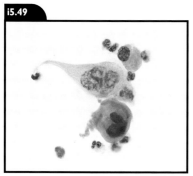

TCC—squamous differentiation

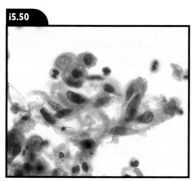

TCC—spindle cells

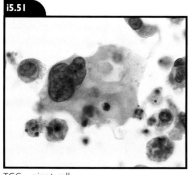

TCC—giant cell

t5.2 Cytologic and Cystoscopic Diagnosis

Cytology	Cystoscopy	Likely Diagnosis
–	–	No tumor
–	+	Low-grade papillary neoplasm
+	–	Carcinoma in situ or upper tract tumor
+	+	High-grade invasive cancer

Note: If cytology is positive but cystoscopy is negative, close follow-up is indicated.

The nuclei are hyperchromatic with coarse chromatin, and there is a moderate amount of delicate cytoplasm. The background is clean. Larger, more pleomorphic cells, more prominent nucleoli, and a diathesis favor invasive cancer; smaller, more uniform cells, with fewer nucleoli, and a clean background favor in situ carcinoma. Invasion can be suspected, but not excluded, by cytology.

5.7.6 Cystoscopy

Cystoscopy and cytology are complementary procedures. The low-grade papillary lesions that may be difficult to diagnose cytologically are usually easy to detect by cystoscopy; the papillae are literally waving at the observer through the cystoscope. In contrast, the high-grade flat CISs, which are much more ominous, are usually easy to detect cytologically but may be missed cystoscopically, because they are mistaken for hyperemia, cystitis, or even normal mucosa |t5.2|.

5.7.7 Ileal Conduit Urine

Ileal conduit urine is monitored to detect recurrence of tumor in the ureter or renal pelvis after cystectomy. Ileal conduit urine is usually highly cellular. The cells are characteristically markedly degenerated and resemble macrophages. Degenerated nuclei may appear hyperchromatic due to karyorrhexis and pyknosis. Many of the cells contain red or blue cytoplasmic inclusions. Debris, cytoplasmic fragments, granular deposits, bacteria, and crystals are found in the background. A few RBCs and WBCs are expected, but if increased, they may indicate infection. Cancer cells have the same morphology as in other urine specimens, but they may be difficult to find.

5.7.8 Carcinoma of the Upper Urinary Tract (Renal Pelvis and Ureter)

About 5% to 10% of urothelial tumors occur in the upper urinary tract (renal pelvis and ureter). Most of the tumors are papillary transitional cell neoplasms. Unfortunately, ureteral or renal pelvis specimens are among the most difficult types of urinary tract specimens to interpret.

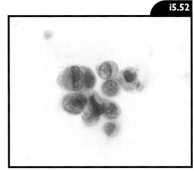
Carcinoma in situ

Voided Urine

High-grade cancer usually can be diagnosed, but low-grade tumors of the upper urinary tract are difficult to detect; neither can be localized by urine cytology alone. The tumors may shed diagnostic cells intermittently, and the cells may be markedly degenerated. Otherwise, the cytologic criteria for diagnosis of tumors of the upper urinary tract in voided urine are similar to those for bladder tumors.

Retrograde Catheterization With Brush or Lavage

By using retrograde catheterization, with brushing or lavage, cytologic specimens can be directly obtained. Many tumors, particularly when high-grade, can be accurately diagnosed, but low-grade tumors of the upper urinary tract are diagnostically difficult.

Transitional cells from the upper urinary tract are typically larger and more variable than those from the bladder. They can be polyploid and may have "atypical" nuclei (multiple, enlarged, hyperchromatic, sometimes with prominent nucleoli). The cells often appear in tight "papillary" clusters due to instrumentation. Lithiasis also can be associated with papillary clusters made up of atypical cells. These features easily could be mistaken for malignancy; therefore, diagnostic conservatism is warranted. Look for clear-cut malignant changes (eg, high nuclear/cytoplasmic ratios, nuclear hyperchromasia with coarse chromatin, nuclear membrane irregularities, macronucleoli, and diathesis) to diagnose malignancy. The higher the grade of the tumor, the more cells, the more atypia, and the more single cells. On the other hand, if *only* small, bland, uniform cells are present, without umbrella cells, a low-grade transitional cell neoplasm is suggested. The differential diagnosis, as usual, includes stone, inflammatory, reactive, and degenerative atypia, as well as therapeutic effects.

5.7.9 Squamous Lesions of the Urinary Tract

Leukoplakia

Leukoplakia, a clinical term meaning "white plaque," usually corresponds to squamous metaplasia and hyperkeratosis and is associated with chronic irritation (eg, stones, schistosomiasis, bladder obstruction).

The diagnostic cells of hyperkeratosis are anucleate squames. Leukoplakia must be differentiated from contaminating squames and from keratinizing squamous cell carcinoma of the bladder, which can be extremely well-differentiated.

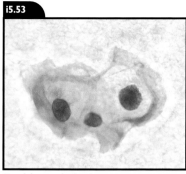

Condyloma—koilocytes

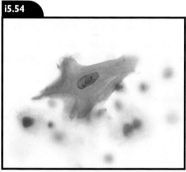

SCC—well-differentiated

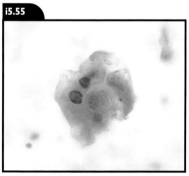

SCC—keratinizing

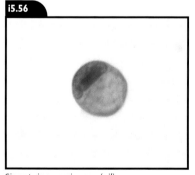

Signet ring carcinoma (oil)

Condyloma

Condylomas of the bladder often are associated with genital condylomas, and genital contamination of the specimen must be excluded before accepting this diagnosis. Koilocytes are diagnostic (see p 12) but may be poorly preserved in urine specimens |i5.53|.

Squamous Cell Carcinoma

Squamous cell carcinoma (SCC) is rare (≤ 5%) in the United States but is more common than TCC in Egypt, where SCC is associated with schistosomiasis (usually *S hematobium*). In contrast with TCC, women are affected as commonly as men. SCC has a poor prognosis even when well-differentiated, which it often is, particularly when associated with schistosomiasis. Very well-differentiated tumors may be difficult to diagnose |i5.54|.

Anucleate squames, or ghosts, may be the only cytologic findings in the urine. Nucleated cells have abnormal, hyperchromatic, coarse to pyknotic chromatin that is often degenerated. Single cells are common. Marked nuclear pleomorphism, membrane irregularities, and chromatin clumping and clearing are common. Macronucleoli may be seen in well-preserved nuclei. The cytoplasm is relatively abundant and dense and stains cyanophilic to red-orange |i5.55|. Intercellular bridges, pearls, spindle cells, or keratohyaline granules may be seen. A dirty background (diathesis) is common and is a poor prognostic sign.

The differential diagnosis includes leukoplakia, secondary SCC (especially from the cervix), and TCC with squamous differentiation. Nonkeratinizing SCC is cytologically similar to high-grade TCC.

5.7.10 Primary Adenocarcinoma

Adenocarcinoma accounts for less than 2% of primary urinary tract cancers. There are two basic morphologies: colonic type, which is more common, and signet ring cell type, which is rare.

The cytology shows clusters of tumor cells characterized by nuclear crowding and pleomorphism. Abnormal chromatin and prominent nucleoli may be seen. The cytoplasm is vacuolated, and mucin may be demonstrated by special stains. Signet ring adenocarcinoma is characterized by the presence of malignant signet ring cells in pools of mucus |i5.56|. The differential diagnosis includes TCC with glandular differentiation, renal cell carcinoma, and metastatic adenocarcinoma.

5.7.11 Small Cell (Neuroendocrine) Carcinoma

Small cell (neuroendocrine) carcinoma of the urinary tract is a rare primary tumor that is essentially similar to the much more common small cell carcinoma of the lung. The cells are present singly or in clusters; clusters exhibit nuclear molding. The cells are small with high nuclear/cytoplasmic ratios, hyperchromatic nuclei, and coarse chromatin |i5.57|. Neuroendocrine differentiation may be demonstrable by special studies, eg, immunocytochemistry. The differential diagnosis includes high-grade TCC composed of small cells and metastatic small cell carcinoma. Wilms tumor also may shed "small blue cells" into the urine but is usually a tumor of childhood.

5.7.12 Lymphoreticular Malignancies

Primary lymphoma of the urinary tract is rare; secondary involvement is more common. Cells derived from leukemia or plasmacytoma also can be found occasionally in the urine.

The cells of lymphoma/leukemia are usually smaller than those of epithelial malignancies. The most characteristic feature is the absence of true tissue aggregates. The morphology depends on the type of tumor, but the cells have high nuclear/cytoplasmic ratios and coarse to vesicular chromatin and may have prominent nucleoli |i5.58|. Plasmacytoma/myeloma shows mature or immature plasma cells. Hodgkin disease can be diagnosed by the presence of Reed-Sternberg cells. The differential diagnosis includes severe chronic inflammation and follicular cystitis.

5.7.13 Secondary Tumors of the Urinary Tract

Renal Cell Carcinoma

Renal cell carcinoma (RCC) is rarely first diagnosed in urine specimens, and, unfortunately, by the time diagnostic cells appear in the urine, the disease is usually far advanced. The diagnostic cells may be very degenerated, usually appear singly, and vary from sparse to abundant. The cells typically have large, eccentric, round to oval, hyperchromatic nuclei with prominent nucleoli |i5.59|. Clear (ie, finely vacuolated), granular, or spindle-shaped cells may be observed, but even clear cells appear more dense and granular than expected owing to degeneration. The malignant cells may be lipid positive (eg, oil red O), but lipid is not specific for renal cancer or even malignancy. Markedly reactive cells from renal infarct can mimic RCC |i5.60|.

Prostatic Adenocarcinoma

The most characteristic cytologic feature of prostatic carcinoma is the presence of prominent nucleoli in relatively uniform malignant glandular cells |i5.61|. When these cells are found in urine, the disease is usually advanced. Poorly differenti-

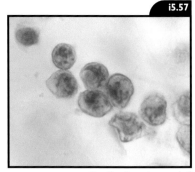
i5.57

Small cell carcinoma (oil)

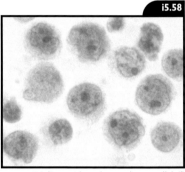
i5.58

Malignant lymphoma, large cell (oil)

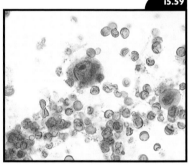
i5.59

RCC

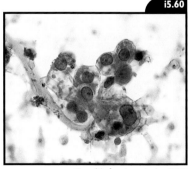
i5.60

Renal infarct—mimics RCC

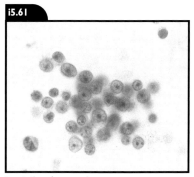

Prostatic adenocarcinoma

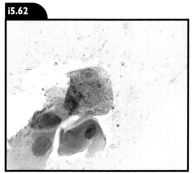

Malignant melanoma

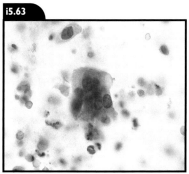

Colorectal carcinoma

ated prostate cancers may be difficult to distinguish from poorly differentiated TCC.

Melanoma

Primary melanoma of the urinary tract is rare; secondary involvement is more common. Melanoma cells tend to be found singly and typically have eccentric, large, vesicular nuclei with macronucleoli and, occasionally, intranuclear cytoplasmic invaginations |i5.62|. Melanin pigment may be observed, which must be distinguished from hemosiderin or lipofuscin.

Other Metastases

Tumors of the female genital tract, colon and rectum |i5.63|, and prostate may involve the bladder by direct extension. Testicular tumors also have been diagnosed in the urine. The tumors are usually high-grade and may be difficult to distinguish from TCC. Distant metastases, especially from lung and breast cancer, occasionally can be diagnosed in urine specimens.

Cerebrospinal Fluid

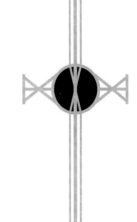

Cerebrospinal fluid (CSF) examination is part of a complete neurologic evaluation. CSF usually is obtained by lumbar puncture but also can be obtained from the lateral ventricles of the brain or the cisterna magna. CSF cytology is primarily useful in diagnosing tumors and infections, but CSF also can be sent for cell counts, chemical analysis, and culture. Clinical history, including the clinical diagnosis, signs, symptoms, and pertinent laboratory and radiologic findings, must be provided for accurate diagnosis.

Cytologic diagnosis of CSF may be difficult because only a small volume of fluid is submitted, the fluid is often sparsely cellular, and the cells tend to degenerate rapidly. Therefore, CSF specimens should be processed as soon as possible. The specimen must be concentrated, eg, by cytocentrifugation. Evaluation with both Diff-Quik and Papanicolaou stains is recommended.

6.1 CSF Physiology

CSF is formed in the cerebral ventricles and circulates over the surface of the brain and spinal cord in the subarachnoid space. CSF is continually produced by the choroid plexus of the ventricles and absorbed by arachnoid granulations of the meninges into the venous system, with complete turnover every 5 to 7 hours. The choroid plexus and vascular endothelium are the anatomic basis for the blood-brain barrier.

The normal CSF pressure is 100 to 200 mm H_2O in the lateral recumbent position, but CSF pressure varies with venous pressure and posture. CSF pressure is elevated in infections, hemorrhage, and tumors. Low pressure may be caused by hypotension or shock.

CSF is normally clear and colorless (like water) and sparsely cellular, containing only a few lymphocytes and monocytes. The protein concentration is normally very low. A high protein level is associated with infections or tumors and is usually proportional to the WBC count. The CSF glucose level is normally about two thirds that of the serum, ie, about 50 to 80 mg/dL (2.8-4.4 mmol/L). The combination of increased protein and decreased glucose suggests tumor or mycobacterial or fungal infection.

6.2 CSF Cytology

CSF cytologic findings are often nonspecific or normal, even in the face of serious central nervous system (CNS) disease.

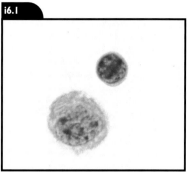

Lymphocyte, monocyte (P, oil)

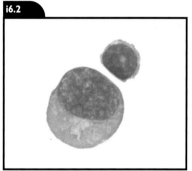

Normal and reactive lymphocytes (DQ, oil)

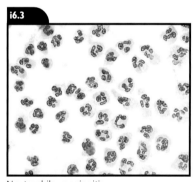

Neutrophils, meningitis

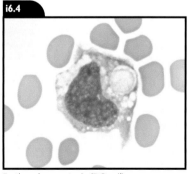

Erythrophagocytosis (DQ, oil)

However, CSF cytology can be useful in the diagnosis of meningitis, secondary malignancies, including carcinomas and lymphomas/leukemias, and some primary tumors. To be detected, a lesion must communicate with the CSF and exfoliate diagnostic cells. Thus, lesions deep in the brain or benign lesions, such as meningiomas, are unlikely to shed diagnostic cells into the CSF. However, even a single abnormal or alien cell can be a significant finding in CSF cytology.

6.2.1 Normal Cytology of CSF

Blood Cells

CSF normally contains few cells; those that are normally present are almost exclusively mononuclear WBCs (ie, lymphocytes and monocytes). In adults, the normal cell count is 0 to 5/µL (higher in children, up to ~ 30/µL in neonates). Thus, 1 mL of normal CSF from an adult could contain up to 5000 WBCs. However, in practice, total cell counts in the range of 20 to 70 are common, and many specimens are essentially acellular.

Lymphocytes normally outnumber monocytes by at least 2 to 1 |i6.1|. Lymphocytosis is seen in viral meningitis, tuberculosis, and fungal infections, as well as in carcinomatous or granulomatous meningitis.

Monocytes are bone marrow–derived and identical in appearance to those in the peripheral blood |i6.1|. Monocytosis is associated with the same conditions as lymphocytosis.

A mixed population of mononuclear cells suggests a benign, reactive, inflammatory infiltrate. Reactive or atypical lymphocytes |i6.2| can be seen in infections (particularly viral), multiple sclerosis, radiation, and chemotherapy. The differential diagnosis is lymphoma/leukemia.

Neutrophils, in small numbers, can be seen in CSF from patients without evidence of meningeal disease, although even a rare neutrophil may be abnormal, particularly in adults. However, when neutrophils are numerous, an acute process, particularly bacterial meningitis, should be suspected |i6.3|.

RBCs are not normally present in CSF, but a few are commonly observed due to microtrauma while obtaining the specimen. When numerous, the differential diagnosis is pathologic bleeding vs traumatic tap; also, a neoplasm must be excluded. Blood from a traumatic tap tends to clear in succeeding tubes. With bleeding, histiocytes appear, and erythrophagocytosis |i6.4| and hemosiderin deposition occur. RBCs from a traumatic tap also will be accompanied by WBCs. As a rule of thumb, there is normally about 1 WBC per 700 RBCs from the peripheral blood.

Macrophages, or histiocytes, are derived from transformed monocytes and are associated with destructive processes involving the CNS, including trauma, infarction, infections, foreign bodies (eg, shunts, reservoirs), invasive procedures, and surgery. Macrophages also are associated with benign cysts, histiocytoses, storage diseases, and neoplasms. Cytoplasmic inclusions may aid in the differential diagnosis. For example, lipid (eg, deriving from myelin) may be seen in the macrophage cytoplasm (lipophage) after various kinds of parenchymal destruction, including trauma and infarcts, as well as in abnormalities of myelin metabolism (eg, Tay-Sachs disease). Blood or blood pigment, such as hemosiderin, may be seen in histiocytes after cerebral hemorrhage (siderophages) |i6.5|. Siderophages can persist for months. Atypical histiocytes may be seen in Langerhans histiocytosis (formerly, histiocytosis X) and malignant histiocytosis (see p 126).

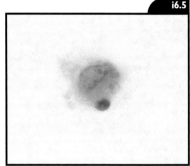
Siderophage (oil)

Plasma cells are not normally present in CSF. Although they could be seen in any chronic inflammatory process, they are particularly characteristic of multiple sclerosis and neurosyphilis. Immature or mature forms occur in plasma cell neoplasms.

Eosinophils are not normally found in the CSF |i6.6|. They are associated with foreign material (eg, shunts, intrathecal therapy, or contrast media), hypersensitivity and allergy, infections (particularly parasitic), leukemias, lymphomas (particularly Hodgkin disease), and, occasionally, primary or metastatic tumors. Sometimes they are idiopathic.

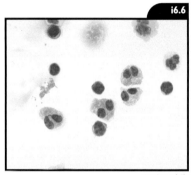
Eosinophils

6.2.2 CNS Cells

Neurons or neuroglia (astrocytes and oligodendrocytes) may be found after a procedure that penetrates the brain substance (eg, ventricular tap) or in some diseases. Normal cells of the CNS usually are found singly; clusters of cells in CSF are suspicious for malignancy. All cells in fluids have a tendency to round up. Degenerative vacuolization is also common, which may result in a signet ring appearance. Mitotic figures are most commonly associated with reactive processes, particularly in macrophages or monocytes and, therefore, are not diagnostic of malignancy, unless they are clearly abnormal.

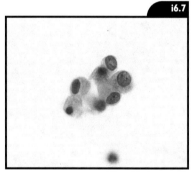
Choroid plexus cells

Ependymal and choroid plexus cells |i6.7|, |i6.8| line the cerebral ventricles and, therefore, are much more commonly observed in ventricular or cisternal fluids than in lumbar punctures. They are more commonly seen in patients with hydrocephalus and after trauma, instrumentation, surgery, or infarction. Choroid plexus cells are morphologically similar to ependymal cells, although cilia, if present, indicate an ependymal origin. Both cell types are uniform, small cuboidal to columnar cells that may resemble histiocytes and often form loose clusters or microacini. The cytoplasm is transparent, moderately abundant, and basophilic, with indistinct cell borders. They may become pleomorphic due to chronic

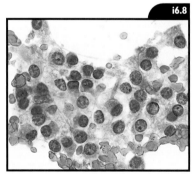
Choroid/ependymal cells

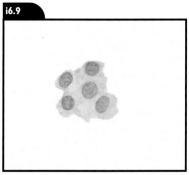

Leptomeningeal cells

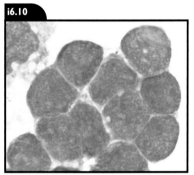

Undifferentiated leptomeningeal cells (DQ, oil)

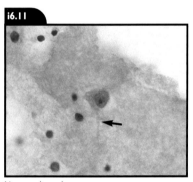

Neuron (axon)

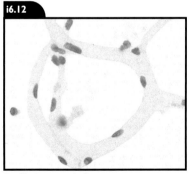

Capillaries, ventricular trap

irritation, mimicking tumor cells. Apart from their potential to be mistaken for tumor, choroid/ependymal cells have little diagnostic significance.

Pia-arachnoid, or leptomeningeal, cells |**i6.9**| are the counterpart of mesothelial cells in other body cavities. They are practically indistinguishable from monocytes, except that they may form sheets. They are rarely seen, but meningeal irritation causes increased exfoliation. When irritated, the reactive cells resemble macrophages and may have cytoplasmic pigment granules.

Undifferentiated leptomeningeal cells |**i6.10**| may be seen in neonates with hydrocephalus, often related to intraventricular brain hemorrhage associated with prematurity. They form clusters of immature blast-like cells, with round to oval, occasionally indented nuclei containing fine even chromatin and single small nucleoli. These primitive cells could easily be mistaken for those of "small blue cell" tumors, such as lymphoblasts or medulloblasts. Lymphoblasts are not cohesive; medulloblasts are usually larger but otherwise quite similar. Hemosiderin-laden macrophages, associated with hemorrhage, provide a benign diagnostic clue.

Neurons are triangular cells with prominent nucleoli and axons |**i6.11**|. *Astrocytes* are spindle cells with multiple branches. These cells are seen more commonly in ventricular or cisternal fluids than in lumbar punctures.

6.2.3 Miscellaneous Elements in CSF

Nonneoplastic cellular elements, such as skin and its appendages, capillaries |**i6.12**|, skeletal muscle, adipose tissue, fibrous tissue, and cartilage |**i6.13**|, can be found in CSF specimens as "pickup" contaminants. If bone marrow is inadvertently sampled, hematopoietic cells and megakaryocytic giant cells may be seen. Giant cells and epithelioid histiocytes also may be seen in granulomas (including foreign body reactions |**i6.14**|, sarcoid |**i6.15**|), as well as in malignancy. Squamous cells are usually contaminants but can arise from squamous cell carcinoma, craniopharyngioma (usually accompanied by marked chronic inflammation), or epidermal inclusion cysts.

Noncellular elements, including corpora amylacea, which concentrate around the ventricles and pial surfaces of the elderly, and psammoma bodies or calcospherites, which are normally found in the choroid plexus, also can be seen occasionally in CSF. Starch granules are common contaminants of cytologic specimens, usually deriving from glove powder. Macrophages ingesting these particles may resemble the cells of signet ring carcinoma. Protein appears as amorphous gray to blue to eosinophilic precipitate that may be somewhat fibrillar.

6.3 Reactive Conditions: Hemorrhage, Inflammation, Infection

A wide variety of conditions, such as trauma (including CNS instrumentation or surgery), neoplasms, and infections, can result in reactive changes in the CSF. Reactive changes usually result in increased numbers of normal cell types, such as leptomeningeal cells and monocytes.

6.3.1 Hemorrhage

Hemorrhage is characterized by fresh and old blood, erythrophagocytosis, and siderophages (see p 116).

6.3.2 Meningitis

The classic signs and symptoms of meningitis are fever, headache, and stiff neck. The disease can range from relatively mild and self-limiting (particularly viral meningitis) to life-threatening (particularly bacterial meningitis).

Bacterial Meningitis

Bacterial meningitis is characterized by cell counts of 30,000 to 50,000/µL or greater, with more than 90% neutrophils. In essence, the cytology shows frank pus, ie, neutrophils, fibrin, macrophages, degenerating cells, and cell debris, and sometimes bacteria |i6.16| (including *Neisseria meningitidis*, the "meningococcus," *Haemophilus influenzae*, and *Streptococcus pneumoniae*, the "pneumococcus"). There is a rapid decrease in the total cell count with therapy.

In patients with a brain abscess, the CSF is usually clear and colorless, the total cell count is usually less than 1000/µL, and the cytology is similar to that of chronic meningitis. When there is a brain mass and CSF cytology shows inflammation, debris, and fibrin, a neoplasm must be excluded. The primary cytologic differential diagnosis is with tuberculous meningitis.

Tuberculous Meningitis

The CSF cytology in tuberculous meningitis is similar to that of viral meningitis.

Viral Meningitis

In viral meningitis, the total cell count is generally less than 1000/µL, with a mixed picture composed predominantly of small mature lymphocytes, but also including reactive or atypical lymphocytes, monocytes, and plasma cells. The atypical lymphocytes are predominantly T cells, in contrast with lymphomas,

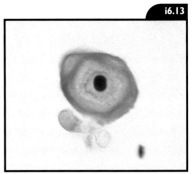
i6.13
Cartilage, mature chondrocyte

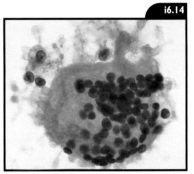
i6.14
Foreign body giant cell (shunt)

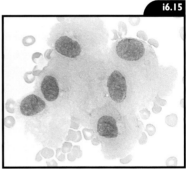
i6.15
Epithelioid histiocytes (sarcoid)

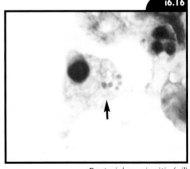
i6.16
Bacterial meningitis (oil)

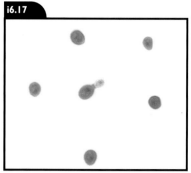

Cryptococcus

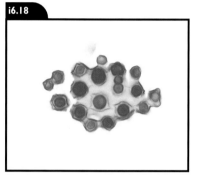

Cryptococcus (mucicarmine stain)

which are more commonly of B-cell origin. Characteristic viral inclusions are rarely observed in CSF specimens.

Fungal Infections

Cryptococcus is the most common fungal organism seen in CSF. It usually is found in immunosuppressed patients, such as transplant recipients and patients with lymphoma/leukemia or AIDS, but occasionally is seen in otherwise apparently healthy patients. The yeasts range from 5 to 15 μm in diameter, have a refractile center and mucoid capsule, and are characterized by teardrop-shaped budding |i6.17|. Mucicarmine stain highlights the mucoid capsule |i6.18|; Gomori methenamine silver stains the organism itself. The inflammatory reaction varies from none (in which case the poorly stained organisms may be overlooked or mistaken for starch granules) to marked reactive lymphocytosis (mimicking lymphoma/leukemia).

Toxoplasma

Mononuclear pleocytosis with increased CSF protein, in the absence of bacteria or fungus, strongly suggests toxoplasmosis. Trophozoites and cysts can be identified rarely with Romanovsky (eg, Diff-Quik) stains.

Lyme Disease

Clinical manifestations of Lyme disease are variable but may include skin rash, neurologic symptoms (meningitis, polyneuropathy), and arthritis. Lyme disease is due to the deer tick (*Ixodes dammini*)–borne spirochete (*Borrelia burgdorferi*). The CSF cytology ranges from normal to marked lymphocytic pleocytosis with immunoblasts and plasma cells associated with foamy macrophages. Markedly atypical plasmacytoid mononuclear cells together with mitotic figures may suggest non-Hodgkin lymphoma.

Other Infections

Blastomyces and *Histoplasma* are relatively common infectious agents. Others include *Coccidioides, Actinomyces, Aspergillus,* Phycomycetes (*Mucor*), and *Penicillium.* Spores, rather than hyphae, usually are seen. Cysticercus (larvae of the tapeworm, *Taenia solium*), *Angiostrongylus,* and other roundworms, as well as ameba such as *Naegleria fowleri,* cause nonspecific pleocytosis, in which eosinophils may be prominent.

CSF Manifestations of AIDS

CSF findings in AIDS are usually nonspecific, eg, mild pleocytosis. However, CSF examination can be helpful in diagnosing CNS infections, such as cryptococcosis, as well as malignant lymphomas (usually large B-cell type, including immunoblastic lymphoma, or Burkitt/non-Burkitt types). Note that the CSF of patients with AIDS is potentially infectious.

Mollaret Meningitis

Mollaret meningitis is a disease characterized by recurrent self-limited episodes of aseptic meningitis that may be associated with a virus, such as herpes. CSF shows marked pleocytosis, including lymphocytes and neutrophils, and large "Mollaret cells," which are probably nothing more than reactive monocytes.

6.4 Central Nervous System Tumors

Most CNS tumors diagnosed by CSF cytology are secondary lesions. CNS (or "brain") tumors, whether benign or malignant, often elicit characteristic reactive changes, including increased protein, decreased glucose, and increased cellularity, although tumor cells are not necessarily identified. Lymphoma/leukemia, carcinomas, and melanomas are the most likely metastatic lesions to shed diagnostic cells. Cells of nonlymphoid malignancies are usually relatively large; thus, large cells are suspicious for malignancy. They usually have hyperchromatic nuclei (Papanicolaou stain) and dark blue cytoplasm (Diff-Quik). Mitotic figures occasionally may be observed. The differential diagnosis includes monocytes and benign reactive lymphocytes, as well as blasts arriving from the peripheral blood in patients with leukemia (traumatic tap). Phagocytosis is evidence against a malignant diagnosis.

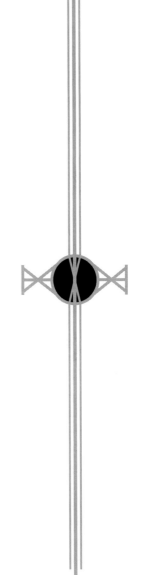

6.5 Primary Tumors of the Central Nervous System

Other than medulloblastoma, it is unlikely for primary brain tumors to shed diagnostic cells into the CSF.

6.5.1 Gliomas

Gliomas are, by far, the most common primary CNS tumors in children and adults and include astrocytomas (and glioblastoma multiforme), ependymoma, choroid plexus papilloma, and oligodendroglioma. In children, the majority of gliomas occur in the brain stem (posterior fossa). In adults, most gliomas arise supratentorially. Only a minority of gliomas (usually high-grade advanced tumors) shed diagnostic cells, even when they are in contact with CSF. Still, astrocytoma is the most common primary

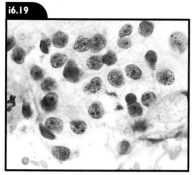

Astrocytoma

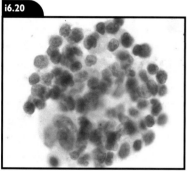

Astrocytoma

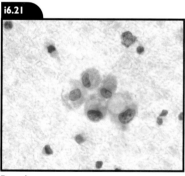

Ependymoma

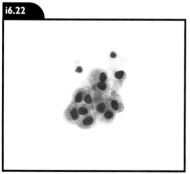

Choroid plexus papilloma

CNS neoplasm detected in the CSF of adults. The main differential diagnosis is with metastatic epithelial malignancy. Dyshesive cells with scant wispy cytoplasm characterize gliomas, while carcinoma tends to shed larger cells in more cohesive groups with more abundant and denser cytoplasm.

Astrocytoma

The cells of astrocytoma tend to form loose clusters. Tumor cell exfoliation, pleomorphism, nuclear atypia, and cytoplasmic density increase with the grade of the tumor |i6.19|, |i6.20|. Anaplastic small and giant tumor cells may be seen in high-grade tumors and glioblastoma multiforme. Spindle cells with fibrillar cytoplasm are typical of astrocytomas. Gemistocytic astrocytomas have dense, granular, eosinophilic cytoplasm and eccentric nuclei. Cell debris, blood, inflammatory cells, and protein precipitate may be seen in the background. Necrosis is associated with glioblastoma multiforme. The differential diagnosis includes reactive/degenerative astrocytes for low-grade tumors and metastatic carcinoma for high-grade lesions. Wispy cytoplasm vs cytoplasmic specialization (mucin, keratin, melanin) is helpful in differential diagnosis.

Oligodendroglioma

Oligodendroglioma, though rare, is the most common primary brain tumor of middle age and usually occurs in the white matter of cerebral hemispheres. There is often central cystic necrosis, and calcification occurs in most cases. Psammoma bodies also may be seen. The cells are usually round and uniform and form clusters and, rarely, rosettes. The nuclei are round and eccentrically located and have a "salt-and-pepper" chromatin pattern and small nucleoli. The cytoplasm is delicate. The classic "fried-egg" appearance of tissue is not seen in cytology.

Ependymoma

Ependymoma is the most common primary spinal cord tumor, but it also occurs in the fourth ventricle, predominantly in children and adolescents. The cells resemble normal ependymal cells; if they are numerous in the absence of hydrocephalus, suspect tumor |i6.21|.

6.5.2 Choroid Plexus Tumors

Choroid plexus papillomas and carcinomas are rare. They occur in the ventricular cavities and readily exfoliate cells into the CSF, even when benign. The diagnosis of choroid plexus papilloma is based on finding papillae and rosettes composed of choroid/ependymal type cells |I6.22|. Choroid plexus carcinoma occurs in young children and resembles metastatic papillary carcinoma, an unlikely diagnosis in children.

6.5.3 Neural Crest Tumors

Neural crest tumors include medulloblastoma |i6.23|, |i6.24|, retinoblastoma |i6.25|, pineoblastoma, neuroblastoma, and primitive neuroectodermal tumor. The cytology of these tumors is characterized by cohesive small blue cells with high nuclear/cytoplasmic ratios, nuclear molding, hyperchromasia, and inconspicuous nucleoli. Rosettes are also characteristic but rarely seen in CSF. The specific type of neural crest tumor cannot be determined by CSF examination alone. However, the clinical history, particularly the site of the tumor, may allow the specific diagnosis to be made. For example, medulloblastoma is the most common primary CNS tumor in children and usually arises in the cerebellum.

6.5.4 Midline Tumors

Most primary midline brain tumors occur in boys, with the exception of pituitary adenomas, which usually occur in adults. These tumors are seldom diagnosable by exfoliative CSF cytology, except after surgery, but may be encountered in fine needle aspiration biopsies.

Pituitary Adenoma

Pituitary adenomas may be associated with a variety of endocrine abnormalities. The cells are present singly, in papillary clusters, or in small honeycomb sheets. The cytoplasm is variable in amount and staining reaction, depending on the specific type of adenoma. The nuclei are usually round to oval, with salt-and-pepper chromatin and small nucleoli. Rarely, psammoma bodies may be seen.

Craniopharyngioma

Craniopharyngioma, although rare, is one of the most common suprasellar tumors in children. Craniopharyngioma is a cystic neoplasm that derives from the embryonic craniopharyngeal canal (Rathke pouch). The cytology is characterized by abundant squamous material, including anucleate squames, typical or atypical |i6.26| squamous cells, and pearls, accompanied by an intense inflammatory reaction to the keratin, including foreign body giant cells, calcification, and cholesterol crystals.

Pineal Gland Tumors

Tumors of the pineal gland may obstruct the cerebral aqueduct, producing hydrocephalus, which compresses the midbrain and results in aberrant eye movements. These clinical findings are relatively specific for a tumor in the pineal area. Germ cell tumors are the most common tumors to arise in the pineal gland. Pineal gliomas are similar to other gliomas. Primary tumors

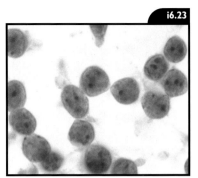
Medulloblastoma (oil)

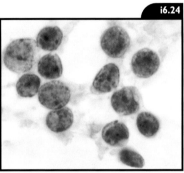
Medulloblastoma (oil)

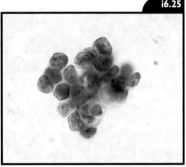
Retinoblastoma

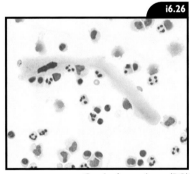
Craniopharyngioma (DQ)

of the pineal gland, ie, pineoblastomas (small blue cell tumors) and pineocytomas, are very rare.

Germ Cell Tumors

Germ cell tumors usually occur in adolescent males, arising in the midline. Germinomas exfoliate large round to polygonal cells with glycogen-rich clear cytoplasm and distinct cell borders. The nuclei are round and have characteristic large nucleoli. A dual population of tumor cells and lymphocytes is typical but not specific. Other types of germ cell tumors, such as immature teratomas, also can occur.

6.5.5 Lymphoma/Leukemia

Secondary involvement of the CNS by lymphoma is relatively common, and primary CNS lymphomas are increasing in incidence. Acute leukemias commonly involve the CNS, but CNS involvement by chronic leukemia is uncommon. Also, the patients are at higher risk for infections that can cause a reactive pleocytosis sometimes mimicking lymphoma/leukemia. Romanovsky-type stains are helpful in morphologic classification of the cells.

General Features of Lymphoma/Leukemia

Generally, the malignant cells vary in size but are usually larger than normal, small, "mature" lymphocytes. The nuclei are enlarged and often have lobulated or irregular nuclear membranes ("cleavages") or protrusions ("knobs"). Nuclear knobs are virtually never seen in normal lymphocytes. The chromatin varies from powdery fine (particularly in blasts) to coarse and hyperchromatic. Nucleoli are occasionally prominent and may have odd shapes. The amount of cytoplasm varies from very scant (eg, lymphoblasts) to abundant (eg, some large cell lymphomas). Although lymphoma/leukemia is characterized by lack of true tissue aggregates, occasionally spurious grouping and even molding of cells can be seen as an artifact of cytocentrifugation |**i6.27**|.

An important differential diagnosis is with reactive changes in inflammatory cells, which may be due to therapy, subarachnoid hemorrhage, or intercurrent infection. A mixed population of lymphocytes in which small mature forms predominate favors a benign reactive process. Plasma cells are rare in lymphoma/leukemia involving the CNS. Some benign conditions, such as multiple sclerosis, may give rise to blast-like transformed lymphocytes. In cases of doubt, a repeated examination may be helpful. A multiparameter approach, including cytochemistry, immunologic techniques, and flow cytometry, may be required for definitive diagnosis in some cases. Reactive lymphocytoses are usually predominantly T cells, while most lymphomas are of B-cell origin.

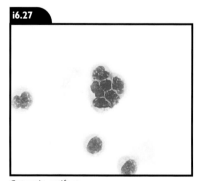

|i6.27|

Cytospin artifact

Leukemia

The diagnosis of acute leukemia, in essence, consists of the identification of blasts. Acute lymphoblastic and acute non-lymphoblastic types are discussed.

Acute lymphoblastic leukemia is the most common type of CNS leukemia in children and is also relatively common in adults. Lymphoblasts are slightly larger than normal, small, mature lymphocytes but have a higher nuclear/cytoplasmic ratio because the cytoplasm is very scant |i6.28|, |i6.29|, |i6.30|, |i6.31|. The nuclear outline varies from case to case, from smooth to convoluted. The chromatin is powdery fine; nucleoli usually are visible. Lymphoblasts never have Auer rods but may occasionally have azurophilic granules. Common acute lymphoblastic leukemia antigen may aid in detecting the presence of a few lymphoblasts. Terminal deoxynucleotidyl transferase is a highly specific marker for acute lymphoblastic leukemia.

The primary differential diagnosis is with reactive lymphocytes, which also may be enlarged and have visible nucleoli. Reactive lymphocytes have more cytoplasm and coarser chromatin than blasts. However, even normal lymphocytes may develop nuclear clefts or convolutions, probably an artifact of centrifugation. Even a minute amount of leukemic blood contamination can introduce blasts into the CSF specimen.

Acute nonlymphocytic leukemias, including acute myelogenous, acute myelomonocytic, acute monocytic, and acute undifferentiated types, as well as "blast crisis" of chronic myelogenous leukemia, also can involve the CNS. Acute myelogenous leukemia occurs in all ages but is more common in adults.

Myeloblasts appear similar to lymphoblasts in Papanicolaou stain; however, in Diff-Quik, evidence of myeloid differentiation may be appreciated, including azurophilic granules and Auer rods. The nuclei of myeloblasts tend to contain more nucleoli than lymphoblasts or monoblasts |t6.1|.

Monoblasts may resemble macrophages, with bean-shaped nuclei and prominent nucleoli. Nuclear convolutions may be particularly prominent in monoblasts. The cytoplasm is more abundant than that of lymphoblasts or myeloblasts.

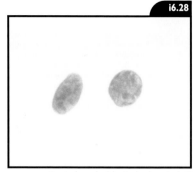

Acute lymphoblastic leukemia (oil)

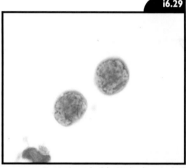

Acute lymphoblastic leukemia (oil)

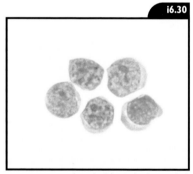

Acute lymphoblastic leukemia (oil)

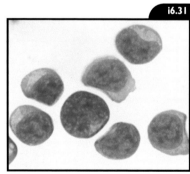

Acute lymphoblastic leukemia (DQ, oil)

t6.1 Differential Diagnosis of Blast Cells

Cell	Cytoplasm	Auer Rods	Nuclei
Lymphoblast	Scant	No	Denser chromatin
Myeloblast	Moderate	Characteristic	More nucleoli
Monoblast	Abundant	Possible	Convoluted

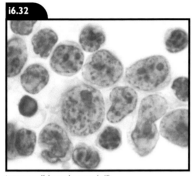

Large cell lymphoma (oil)

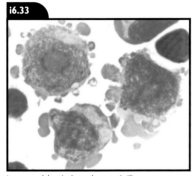

Immunoblastic lymphoma (oil)

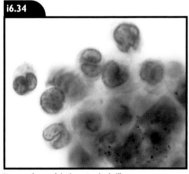

Langerhans histiocytosis (oil)

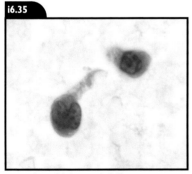

Langerhans histiocytosis (oil)

Lymphoma

In children, the most common lymphomas diagnosed in CSF are lymphoblastic and small noncleaved (Burkitt and non-Burkitt types) non-Hodgkin lymphomas. In adults, diffuse large cell lymphomas, including immunoblastic, as well as small cleaved cell non-Hodgkin lymphomas, are among the most common types. Burkitt lymphoma also is seen in patients with AIDS. Overall, the most common CNS lymphoma diagnosed by CSF cytology is usually diffuse, large, B-cell non-Hodgkin lymphoma. Follicular lymphomas and small lymphocytic non-Hodgkin lymphomas, as well as Hodgkin disease and myeloma, are rarely diagnosed in the CSF.

Lymphoblastic lymphoma sheds cells that are identical to those described for acute lymphoblastic leukemia. It is the most common type of childhood lymphoma/leukemia and has a high rate of CNS involvement.

Small noncleaved lymphoma (Burkitt, non-Burkitt) occurs in children and is being seen with increased frequency in adults with AIDS. The cells are actually medium-sized lymphoid cells with moderately abundant, deep blue cytoplasm that characteristically has tiny (lipid) vacuoles in Diff-Quik. The nuclei have fine to slightly clumped chromatin and one or more prominent nucleoli.

Large cell lymphoma is quite variable morphologically: scant to abundant cytoplasm, smooth to irregular nuclear membranes, fine to coarse chromatin, and inconspicuous to prominent nucleoli |**i6.32**|. However, it is characterized by the presence of relatively large, sometimes bizarre, noncohesive lymphoid cells. Individual tumor cells can closely resemble benign, reactive, immature lymphocytes and immunoblasts |**i6.33**|.

Small cell cleaved lymphoma is exclusively a disease of adults. There may be many atypical small cells with coarse chromatin, visible nucleoli, deep nuclear folds (ie, cleavages), and scant cytoplasm present in the CSF. Cells with bizarre twisted or irregular shapes may be encountered.

Other Lymphoreticular Diseases

Histiocytic proliferations can involve the CNS. The CNS often is affected in Langerhans histiocytoses |**i6.34**|, |**i6.35**| (histiocytosis X, Letterer-Siwe, and Hand-Schüller-Christian diseases). Malignant histiocytosis also can occur rarely. Histiocytic lesions may shed three types of cells: normal-appearing histiocytes, atypical histiocytes, and multinucleated histiocytes. The histiocytes can vary from bland to frankly malignant appearing. Evidence of phagocytosis (eg, of RBCs, WBCs, cell debris, or lipid) is a characteristic cytologic feature of (non-Langerhans) histiocytes.

Mycosis fungoides is a T-cell lymphoma that primarily affects the skin but can disseminate widely, including to the CNS. The diagnostic Sézary cells are larger than normal lymphocytes and have hyperchromatic nuclei with deeply indented, or cerebriform, nuclear membranes.

6.5.6 Meningioma

Meningioma is a benign tumor of the meninges. Consequently, although ideally situated to shed cells into the CSF, it seldom does. On rare occasions, sparse, slightly elongated cells, occasionally in whorls, containing ovoid nuclei with delicate chromatin, micronucleoli, and occasional intranuclear cytoplasmic invaginations may be seen. Psammoma bodies are frequent in the tumor. When meningeal tumors exfoliate cells, they are more likely to be malignant (meningiosarcoma).

6.6 Metastatic Malignancy

Metastatic tumors are the most common nonhematologic malignancies to be diagnosed in CSF cytology, but only about one third of metastases involving the CNS can be detected. Most are adenocarcinomas, particularly of lung and breast origin; melanoma is also relatively common. In children, small blue cell tumors, such as neuroblastoma, rhabdomyosarcoma |i6.36|, Ewing sarcoma |i6.37|, and Wilms tumor, are the most common sources of nonhematologic metastases. Although common, squamous cell carcinoma rarely sheds diagnostic cells into the CSF |i6.38|. CSF is rarely the first place a malignant diagnosis is made, because most patients have a history of malignancy. Lymphomas are discussed earlier in this chapter.

Detection of malignant cells in the CSF can be easy. Even a rare "foreign" cell can be diagnostic of malignancy |i6.39|. The cytology of metastases is usually characterized by the presence of (only) a few atypical cells in a clean background, although in some cases there may be protein precipitate, fresh or old blood, and cell debris. A normal cell count does not exclude malignancy.

The cytomorphology of metastatic malignancy in the CSF is similar to that seen in other body cavity fluids. True tissue aggregates with cellular disorder and nuclear crowding may be seen. However, in CSF, adenocarcinoma has a greater tendency to shed cells singly rather than in clusters and for the malignant cells to be smaller and less pleomorphic than in other body fluids. On the other hand, malignant cells are generally larger than any *normal* cell in the CSF. The malignant cells are often pleomorphic, with enlarged irregular nuclei, prominent nucleoli, hyperchromasia, and increased nuclear/cytoplasmic ratios.

Small cell carcinoma of lung is characterized by relatively small, cohesive cells, high nuclear/cytoplasmic ratios, nuclear molding,

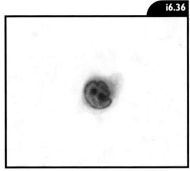
Rhabdomyosarcoma (oil)

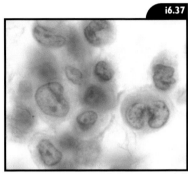
Ewing sarcoma (oil)

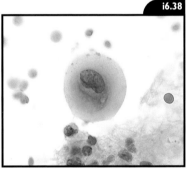
Squamous cell carcinoma

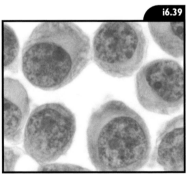
Metastatic carcinoma—foreign cells (oil)

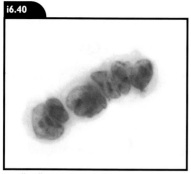

Small cell carcinoma (oil)

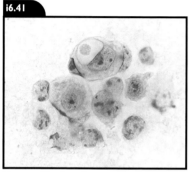

Non–small cell carcinoma

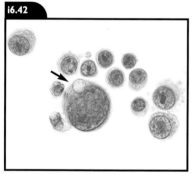

Breast carcinoma—note ICL

and cell chains |**i6.40**|. Characteristic "crush artifact" is usually not present in CSF specimens. The differential diagnosis includes neural crest tumors, eg, medulloblastoma, which together with other small blue cell tumors occur predominantly in children rather than adult cigarette smokers, and undifferentiated gliomas, which can occur at any age.

Non–small cell carcinoma of lung is characterized by pleomorphic cells with large, irregular, eccentric nuclei, irregular chromatin, prominent nucleoli, and relatively dense cytoplasm. Glandular features predominate in CNS metastases |**i6.41**|. Squamous cell carcinoma has dense cytoplasm and may form pearls but can resemble adenocarcinoma in fluid specimens. The differential diagnosis includes high-grade gliomas, which have delicate wispy cytoplasm and indistinct cell borders.

Breast carcinoma is characterized by cells that are usually single or form loose clusters; tight balls, morulae, and single-file chains of cells are rarely observed in CSF. The cells are usually larger than any normal cell in the CSF. They can range from monomorphic to pleomorphic. The cells may show round to oval nuclei, fine to coarse chromatin, prominent nucleoli, and moderate to abundant granular cytoplasm with well-defined cell borders. Intracytoplasmic lumens (ICLs) are a characteristic, but not specific, feature of breast cancer |**i6.42**|.

Gastric carcinoma is an increasingly uncommon tumor that frequently metastasizes to the CNS and may shed abundant diagnostic cells. The cells tend to be on the small side with high nuclear/cytoplasmic ratios, present singly or in small clusters, with eccentric malignant-appearing nuclei, variable nucleoli, and a moderate amount of vacuolated cytoplasm that usually contains mucin. Signet ring cells are classic but not specific.

Melanoma frequently involves the meninges and sheds diagnostic cells into the CSF |**i6.43**|. The primary tumor may be occult, or, rarely, melanoma arises in the CNS |**i6.44**|. Melanoma is characterized by large single cells with large eccentric nuclei, macronucleoli, and intranuclear cytoplasmic invaginations.

t6.2 Differential Diagnosis of CNS Tumors by Immunocytochemistry

	Keratin	S-100	HMB-45	CD45 (LCA)	GFAP
Carcinoma	+	–	–	–	–
Melanoma	–	+	+	–	–
Lymphoma/leukemia	–	–	–	+	–
Glial tumors	–	+	–	–	+
Neural crest tumors	–	+	–	–	–

CNS, central nervous system; LCA, leukocyte common antigen; GFAP, glial fibrillary acidic protein.

Double–mirror image nuclei also may be seen, as may giant tumor cells. Cytoplasmic pigment is a classic finding but not always seen and, furthermore, is not specific, since melanin can be seen in melanosis, pigmented choroid plexus neoplasms, ependymomas, nerve sheath tumors, and meningiomas.

Unknown primary tumors often derive from lung, stomach, or melanoma. Breast cancer is unlikely to be an unknown primary tumor. Although renal cell carcinoma |**i6.45**|, transitional cell carcinoma, and colorectal adenocarcinoma |**i6.46**| are common malignancies, they are unusual sources of positive CSF cytology.

Immunocytochemistry can be helpful in differential diagnosis of CNS tumors |**t6.2**|.

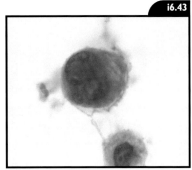

i6.43

Metastatic melanoma

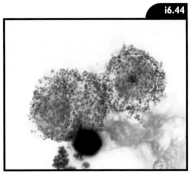

i6.44

Primary melanoma

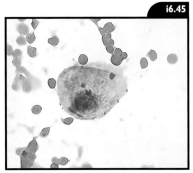

i6.45

Renal cell carcinoma

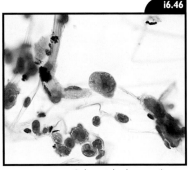

i6.46

Colorectal adenocarcinoma

CHAPTER SEVEN

Introduction to FNA Biopsy

Fine needle aspiration (FNA) biopsy goes by a number of aliases, including skinny needle, thin needle, and aspiration biopsy cytology. But, whatever name is used, fine needle aspiration is a biopsy, ie, a sample of a suspicious mass removed for diagnostic purposes. Primarily useful in diagnosing neoplasms, FNA biopsy also can be helpful in evaluating other diseases, such as infections (eg, fungal, viral, protozoal), inflammations (eg, granulomas in sarcoidosis), or infiltrations (eg, amyloidosis). The target can be a palpable superficial "lump or bump" (eg, in the thyroid, lymph node, salivary gland, or breast) or deep-seated and radiologically imaged (eg, in the lung, liver, pancreas, kidney, or retroperitoneum).

FNA biopsy is a diagnostic technique; it is usually not therapeutic (except for some cysts). It should be used only when a formal surgical tissue biopsy would be considered, because the results will affect the management of the patient. FNA biopsy is definitely not for every minor abnormality a patient may have, such as small, clinically insignificant lymph nodes. Vague inflammations or indurations are not good targets for FNA biopsy. FNA biopsy should not be used as a diagnostic shot in the dark! Occasionally, a patient without a suspicious mass is erroneously referred for FNA biopsy. In other cases, normal body structures are mistaken for abnormalities such as enlarged lymph nodes.

Fine needles, ie, 22 gauge or smaller diameter (eg, 23, 25, or 27 gauge) are used in this procedure. With fine needles, complications are rare and usually minor (See "Complications," p 132). Virtually any lesion in any organ of the body can be reached with a fine needle. For palpable targets, a syringe pistol handle facilitates performing the biopsy. For transrectal and transvaginal FNA biopsies, a needle guide (eg, Franzén) is indispensable. For deep-seated targets, long needles are placed using diagnostic imaging guidance.

7.1 **Advantages**

FNA biopsy can be performed on an outpatient basis, in the office or clinic, or at the patient's bedside. The advantages of FNA biopsy can be summed up in the acronym, SAFE. FNA biopsy is Simple, Accurate, Fast, and Economic, as well as SAFE |**f7.1**|. It has the best safety record of any method of obtaining tissue for a morphologic diagnosis. FNA biopsy is generally highly sensitive and specific, with rare false-positives. No other biopsy, including frozen section, can be processed as rapidly as an FNA

f7.1 Advantages of Fine Needle Aspiration Biopsy

FNA Biopsy is SAFE
    Simple
    Accurate
    Fast
    Economic

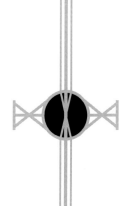

biopsy. A turnaround time of less than 1 hour is routine for an FNA biopsy service.

FNA biopsy is the most cost-effective method of obtaining a morphologic diagnosis and is far less expensive than diagnostic surgery. FNA biopsy can even be performed intraoperatively, in lieu of frozen sections. Rapid diagnosis can direct further diagnostic and therapeutic planning, which can be discussed with the patient at the initial visit. There is also the psychologic advantage of relieving anxiety or convincing the patient of the need for immediate therapy.

FNA biopsy leaves no scar. Scars are not only a cosmetic problem but can also interfere with surgery or diagnostic imaging studies such as mammography. Moreover, FNA biopsy usually does not interfere with further study of the lesion, including histopathology, flow cytometry, immunochemistry, or electron microscopy. In fact, any of these procedures, even histology (ie, cell blocks), can be performed on aspirated biopsy material. Cell blocks can be helpful when the need for numerous special studies is anticipated. Needle rinse preparations can supplement or, in certain circumstances, replace direct smears. Viable cells can be obtained, so that special studies can be performed using living material (eg, cytochemistry, tissue culture, chemosensitivity testing). Also, by using FNA biopsy, small metastases, such as in lymph nodes or skin, can be documented and then left in situ as a marker to follow the response to therapy.

There are a number of advantages specifically for the patient's convenience, too. In essence, for superficial targets, no special preparation is needed; the test is no more complicated or painful than venipuncture. Patients usually appreciate the opportunity to resolve their medical problems in an office or clinic setting rather than having to be admitted to the hospital.

7.2 Complications

Serious complications are rare, especially for superficial targets. Deep-seated organ aspiration biopsies are more likely to be associated with complications than biopsies of superficial targets. As a general rule, the incidence of complications rises exponentially with increasing diameter of the needle. As might be expected, the rate of complications tends to decrease with increasing experience with the technique.

For superficial lumps and bumps, complications are infrequent and almost always minor. Pain is usually minor and well tolerated. Bleeding can usually be controlled simply by applying local pressure, even in patients with bleeding disorders. Local infection is extremely rare, even in immunocompromised patients. An occasional patient will get light-headed (vasovagal reaction), and a rare patient will faint. (Rx = Place patient supine with legs elevated. Use smelling salts, if necessary. Monitor blood pressure. Observe patient.) A variety of other complications, including pneumothorax, have been reported but are very rare.

Deep-seated organ aspirations are somewhat more complex, and higher complication rates are seen than with superficial targets. Some complications are potentially serious and rarely even fatal.

Hematomas are somewhat more likely with deep-seated aspirations owing to the inability, in most cases, of applying direct pressure to stop bleeding. Accidental penetration of major blood vessels usually is not associated with serious bleeding when using fine needles. Rarely, however, significant hemorrhage occurs, requiring blood transfusion or even surgical intervention.

Pneumothorax is most common with transthoracic needle biopsy but also can occur during aspirations of targets near the chest (eg, breast, supraclavicular, or axillary areas or upper abdomen). A small amount of air is probably introduced into almost all patients during transthoracic aspiration biopsy, but less than one third of cases will be detectable by chest x-ray. Most pneumothoraces spontaneously resolve. A minority of cases, less than 5% to 10%, require therapy (chest tube placement or aspiration of air using a large syringe).

In the abdomen, the needle may traverse gut, but the gauge of the needle is smaller than most surgical suture needles routinely used in these organs. Thus, clinically significant bowel perforation or soiling of the peritoneum is extremely rare. On the other hand, serious infections have occurred after transrectal aspirations of active prostatitis.

Certain types or sites of lesions are associated with increased risk of complications. These include biopsies of pheochromocytoma, vascular tumors, pancreatic lesions, hepatocellular carcinoma, and infected tissues. Other rare complications of FNA biopsy, including local anaphylaxis, have been described.

By using fine needles, seeding of the needle tract with tumor is exceedingly rare; rarer still is for a tumor implant to seriously affect the patient. A needle tract can be excised during

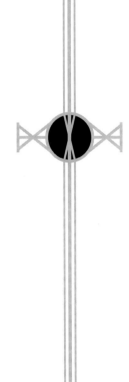

surgery; implants can be excised or radiated. In fact, seeding is so rare compared with core tissue biopsy that FNA biopsy may be favored over core biopsy for this very reason.

Although FNA biopsy can induce morphologic changes in tissue, such as hemorrhage or necrosis, such effects usually are recognized easily and rarely cause serious diagnostic problems for experienced pathologists.

Unfortunately, fatalities, or near fatalities, have been reported (eg, due to hemorrhage, pneumothorax, or air embolism), but they are extremely rare. The risks of any procedure must be kept in perspective and balanced against potential benefits, eg, major surgery may be avoided.

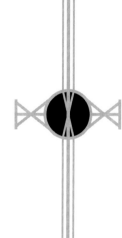

7.3 Contraindications

There are very few well-established contraindications for FNA biopsy of superficial sites. Patients who cannot suppress a cough should not undergo thyroid or transthoracic biopsy. Patients with active prostatitis should not undergo prostatic biopsy.

For deep-seated organ aspirations, coagulation parameters should be acceptable. A hemorrhagic diathesis or regular use of anticoagulants may be considered contraindications. Biopsy of a suspected vascular lesion, eg, arteriovenous malformation or angiosarcoma, risks hemorrhage—and a nondiagnostic bloody aspirate. Advanced pulmonary emphysema, especially the bullous type, severe pulmonary hypertension, severe hypoxemia uncorrected by oxygen therapy, and mechanical ventilatory assistance are generally regarded as contraindications for transthoracic needle biopsy. Suspected hydatid disease (echinococcal cyst) usually is considered a contraindication to biopsy because severe reactions or fatal anaphylaxis are possible, yet many cases have been aspirated with fine needles without untoward results. Uncooperative or excessively apprehensive patients may have to be sedated, but for transthoracic biopsy, the patients should be able to clear their own airways.

7.4 Performing, Interpreting, and Reporting the Biopsy

The first step in FNA biopsy is to obtain relevant clinical history and physical findings. The biopsy procedure should be explained to the patient, along with expected benefits, possible risks, and alternative diagnostic procedures. Informed consent should be obtained. The skin is cleaned with alcohol; iodine compounds, sterile drapes, etc, are not necessary for superficial aspirations but are used for deep sites and bone. Examining gloves should be used during the procedure.

Local anesthetic is generally not used, except for deep-seated tissues and bone. For superficial masses, the target is immobilized with one hand, and using a syringe in a pistol-type holder, the needle is introduced into the lesion. After entering the mass, suction is applied and maintained throughout the procedure (but released before withdrawing the needle). Staying within the lesion, the needle is moved, rather vigorously, in and out, several times, in a cutting motion. *This cutting motion is absolutely essential for obtaining an adequate sample!* Generally, when material is seen in the hub of the needle, the procedure is discontinued. Firm pressure is applied to the biopsy site with a sterile gauze pad, preferably by an assistant rather than the patient, to reduce bruising or hematoma formation.

No matter how expertly the biopsy is performed, if the slides are uninterpretable, the procedure is totally worthless for cytologic diagnosis. The cells must be delicately and thinly smeared, with minimal distortion, and fixed according to the requirements of the stains to be used (eg, Papanicolaou stain requires immediate fixation). Inspect the aspirate grossly. Does it appear to be adequate? (If not, repeat.) Purulent? (Culture.) Fluid? (Drain cyst, reaspirate residuum.) Necrotic? (Reaspirate periphery.) Pure blood? (Stop.)

Classic cytodiagnostic criteria (such as pleomorphism, chromatin quality, nucleoli) also apply to FNA biopsies. The exquisite cellular detail in cytologic specimens is the premier diagnostic advantage of the cytologic technique. Architectural arrangements of cells, eg, gland formation, papillae, or rosettes, are also important diagnostically. The major disadvantage of FNA biopsy, compared with tissue, is that the context of the cells, particularly invasion, cannot be assessed. However, a valuable diagnostic clue is gained by the aspiration procedure, ie, a measure of the degree of cohesion among cells, which can be an important diagnostic clue. For example, carcinomas are characterized by decreased intercellular cohesion, resulting in richly cellular aspirates composed of dyshesive atypical cells.

The results should be reported in a clinically useful and understandable format using histopathologic terms. If the diagnosis is less than certain, ie, "suspicious," a follow-up biopsy (tissue or repeat cytology) may be recommended. Do not attempt to interpret inadequate specimens.

The best results are obtained by practitioners with special interest and training in the technique of FNA biopsy. Proper use of FNA biopsy requires close communication between an experienced cytopathologist and the clinician. Major

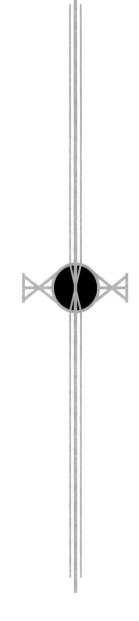

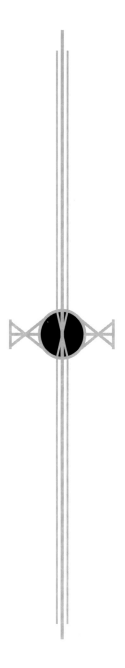

therapeutic decisions should never be based on the cytologic findings alone, but rather on the whole clinical picture, including clinical, radiologic, and pathologic data. If the cytologic findings do not correlate with the clinical suspicion, greater weight should be given to the clinical setting and further workup performed as indicated.

CHAPTER EIGHT

The Gut Course
Common Patterns and Common Problems in FNA Biopsy

If common things occur commonly, then by simply knowing what the common things *are* and what they *look like* you should, by definition, be able to diagnose most of the cases that you encounter in everyday practice. And among the common problems in daily practice is determining "Where's the primary?" when confronted with a metastasis.

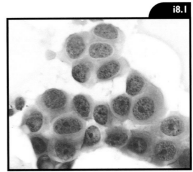

Carcinoma

8.1 Tumor Classification

At the most basic level of diagnosis, an attempt is made to classify tumors into broad categories, such as carcinoma, lymphoma, sarcoma, and melanoma |i8.1|, |i8.2|, |i8.3|, |i8.4|. Beyond this point, the number of diagnostic possibilities seems almost infinite. But in most cases at least the general category of neoplasm can be determined by cytology.

For example, carcinomas are characterized by malignant-appearing epithelial cells, which usually display at least some degree of intercellular cohesion due to the presence of desmosomes. In addition, carcinomas often form characteristic structures, such as glands or papillae, and frequently manufacture specific cellular products, such as epithelial mucin. Lymphomas, sarcomas, and melanomas typically show a more dispersed cell pattern due to absent or poorly formed intercellular connections. They also may have peculiar cytologic features (such as spindle shape) and elaborate cellular products that range from nonspecific (eg, collagen) to pathognomonic (eg, myofilaments) |t8.1|.

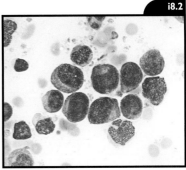

Lymphoma

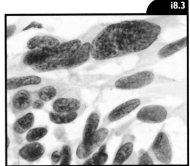

Sarcoma

8.1.1 The Unknown Primary

The initial evaluation of an unknown primary tumor can usually separate carcinomas (ie, epithelial malignancies) from the primordial group of undifferentiated tumors. Within the general category of carcinoma, three subgroups can then be recognized: (1) squamous cell carcinoma (SCC), (2) adenocarcinoma (ie, recognizably differentiated adenocarcinoma), and (3) undifferentiated carcinoma/poorly differentiated adenocarcinoma. Differentiated adenocarcinoma is the most common diagnosis in patients with unknown primary tumors, and lung and pancreas are the most common sources, followed by liver, colon/rectum, stomach, and kidney. Although adenocarcinomas of the breast, ovary, and prostate are common malignancies, they are unusual sources of unknown primary tumors because the primary site usually can be identified clinically. Similarly, SCC is a common tumor but an uncommon unknown primary. The syndrome of undifferentiated

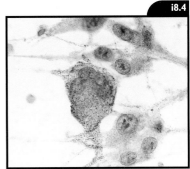

Melanoma

t8.1 Tumor Classification

Category	Cell Type	Cytodiagnostic Features	Characteristic Product
Carcinoma	Epithelial	Cohesive cells	Desmosomes
Adenocarcinoma		Glands, papillae	Mucin
Squamous cell carcinoma		Sheets, pearls	Keratin
Neuroendocrine		Rosettes	Neurosecretory granules
Lymphoma	Lymphoreticular	Single cells: round; lymphoglandular bodies	Immunoglobulin
Sarcoma	Mesenchymal	Single cells: spindle, round, or pleomorphic	Myofilaments, collagen, lipid, etc
Melanoma	Melanocyte	Single cells: D-MINs, INCIs	Melanin

D-MINs, double–mirror image nuclei; INCIs, intranuclear cytoplasmic invaginations.

carcinoma/poorly differentiated adenocarcinoma (UC/PDA) |i8.5|, |i8.6|, formerly thought to be mostly extragonadal germ cell tumors, defines a subset of patients (young adults, midline tumors, elevated serum α-fetoprotein or β–human chorionic gonadotropin levels) who may respond to therapy. Sarcomas are unusual unknown primaries (the primary site is usually obvious, although the type of tumor may not be). Melanoma is notorious for its ability to metastasize to unusual sites and mimic a wide variety of other neoplasms.

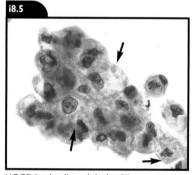

UC/PDA—hyaline globules (P)

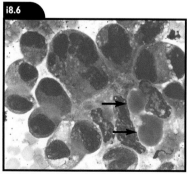

UC/PDA—hyaline globules (DQ)

8.2 The Building Blocks of Cytodiagnosis

Begin by looking at the cells. Note some of their general features. Are they all single or do they form groups (what kind of groups)? Are they squamous or glandular (see Chapter 1)? Do they have peculiar ("spindle") shapes? Is the cytoplasm particularly granular or clear? Next, look at the background. Is it clean? Mucoid or myxoid? Necrotic? Inflammatory? Etc |t8.2|.

Sometimes one building block by itself is enough to make a diagnosis (eg, malignant glandular cells → adenocarcinoma). But the power of the building blocks is enhanced by the ability to combine the blocks to build a diagnosis. For example, lung and pancreatic cancers commonly show malignant tumor cells with glandular and squamous features. Thus, a metastatic carcinoma with these dual features suggests origin in the lung or pancreas (which are two of the most common sources of unknown primary tumors).

t8.2 Building Blocks of Cytodiagnosis

Cells:

Squamous	Spindle
Glandular	Clear
Leukocytes	Granular
Giant	Neuroendocrine
Small	Melanoma

Background: Clean, mucoid/myxoid, cystic, necrotic, inflammatory, hemorrhagic, calcified, ossified, colloid, microbes, etc.

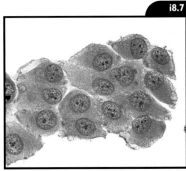

Mesothelial cells (P)

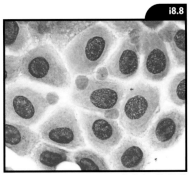

Mesothelial cells (DQ)

Histopathology is the foundation on which diagnoses are built. As an example, suppose granular cells (Hürthle onco-cytes) and leukocytes (lymphocytes) are aspirated from the thyroid. By using histopathology as a guide, these two cell types "build" a diagnosis of Hashimoto thyroiditis. On the other hand, the same kinds of cells (oncocytes and lymphocytes) aspirated from the parotid would build a diagnosis of Warthin tumor! The cytologic observations are essentially identical, but histo-pathology provides the basis to build a proper diagnosis.

8.3 Squamous Cells

Designed for protection, the squamous cell is charac-terized by its tough cytoplasm: dense cytoplasm and distinct cell boundaries are the hallmarks of squamous differentiation |t8.3|.

Mesothelial cells epitomize the features of squamous cells. Histologically, mesothelial cells form a single layer of flat cells (ie, squamous in the traditional histologic sense). In cytology, normal or reactive mesothelial cells form flat sheets that look like snakeskin leather or a mosaic of ceramic tiles |i8.7|, |i8.8|. The cells have dense cytoplasm and distinct cell boundaries. Mesothelial cells are among the most commonly misdiagnosed cells in aspira-tion cytology. They can mimic a variety of cell types, including adenocarcinoma, particularly when exhibiting reactive changes. Reactive mesothelial cells are familiar from body cavity fluids.

SCC shows the usual diagnostic features (see Chapter 1). Nonkeratinizing SCC is characterized by a fairly uniform popu-lation of malignant cells, with high nuclear/cytoplasmic ratios, chromatin that is coarse and dark but somewhat open, and conspicuous nucleoli |i8.9|, |i8.10|. The cytoplasm is dense, with well-defined cell boundaries. Keratinizing SCC is characterized by highly pleomorphic and even bizarre cells with very dark chromatin and inconspicuous nucleoli. The cytoplasm is heavily

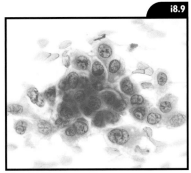

Nonkeratinizing SCC (P)

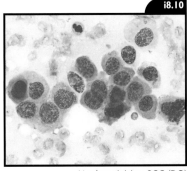

Nonkeratinizing SCC (DQ)

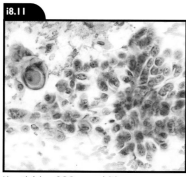

Keratinizing SCC—pearl (P)

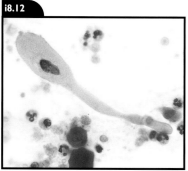

Keratinizing SCC—bizarre cell (P)

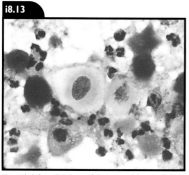

Keratinizing SCC—robin's egg blue cell (DQ)

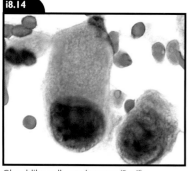

Gland-like cell—melanoma (P, oil)

t8.3 Differential Diagnosis: Squamous vs Glandular Cells

	Squamous	Glandular
Groups	Pearls	Balls
	Flat sheets	Honeycombs, palisades
	Cell-in-cell	Microacini
Cells	Polyhedral/spindle	Cuboidal/columnar
Cytoplasm	Dense	Delicate
	Orange, yellow, pink, blue	Pale blue
Nucleus	Central	Polar
Chromatin	Dense	Open
Nucleoli	Few, small	One, large

keratinized, by definition, and pearls may be seen (diagnostic of keratinization) |i8.11|, |i8.12|. Some cells have *low* nuclear/cytoplasmic ratios in keratinizing SCC.

Occasionally, very well-differentiated keratinized SCC is encountered, particularly of head and neck origin. The cells can resemble low-grade dysplasia rather than full-blown malignancy. Look for a component of less-differentiated, nonkeratinized tumor cells to help cinch the diagnosis of SCC. Atypical parakeratosis can look almost exactly like keratinizing SCC, except for the miniature size of the parakeratotic cells.

Squamous features (eg, dense cytoplasm, distinct cell boundaries, pleomorphic shapes, pearls) can be appreciated in both Papanicolaou and Diff-Quik stains. However, the Papanicolaou stain is particularly useful in the diagnosis of SCC, because keratinized squamous cells stand out, staining bright pink or orange. Keratinized cells in Diff-Quik have a glassy, "robin's egg" blue appearance |i8.13| but tend to blend into the background of other blue-staining cells.

SCC, especially the keratinizing type, often undergoes cystic degeneration, and fluid may be aspirated. This fluid can have a creamy, mucoid, or purulent appearance, mimicking pus from an abscess. Such cystic metastases are particularly common with head and neck primary tumors. Squamous cells or their keratin often elicit a foreign body granulomatous reaction.

8.4 **Glandular Cells**

Glandular cells typically have basal nuclei and apical cytoplasm (nucleocytoplasmic polarity) |i8.14|, in contrast with the "fried egg" appearance typical of squamous cells (nucleus in the middle and cytoplasm all around) |t8.3|. Glandular cells usually maintain their nucleocytoplasmic polarity, even when malignant.

Just as squamous cells are specialized for protection (manifested by keratin production), glandular cells are specialized in manufacturing (eg, mucin). Consequently, secretory product and the machinery necessary to make it are the characteristic cytologic findings in glandular cells. Thus, cells can be identified as glandular by demonstrating characteristic secretions, such as mucin, in their cytoplasm. For this, special stains, such as mucicarmine, can be helpful.

The glandular cell's cytoplasm appears delicate because it typically has a prominent Golgi apparatus and foamy secretion rather than dense filaments. Moreover, the cell boundaries of glandular cells are ill-defined. These features (polar nuclei, delicate cytoplasm, ill-defined cell borders) contrast with squamous cells (central nuclei, dense cytoplasm, distinct cell boundaries). Glandular cells characteristically have extensive rough endoplasmic reticulum in the cytoplasm, which stains basophilic in Papanicolaou stain owing to ribosomal RNA.

Malignant nuclei mirror the difference between squamous and glandular cell cytoplasm. The malignant squamous nucleus appears dense and hyperchromatic, while the glandular nucleus tends to be more delicate and open with finer chromatin. The nucleoli are typically different, too. Malignant glandular cells classically have large central ("owl's eye") nucleoli, while the nucleoli of SCC are more commonly multiple but usually not as prominent as glandular nuclei, and they may not even be visible.

Benign glandular cells typically form very orderly sheets with uniform ranks and files of cells—like endocervical cells |i8.15|. This orderly arrangement is the classic appearance of benign glandular cells from any site, including the breast, gastrointestinal (GI) tract, and prostate. (Compare with the disorder characteristic of malignant glandular cells, ie, adenocarcinoma |i8.16|.) Benign glandular cells seen from above, en face, have a regular honeycomb pattern. Seen from the side, they palisade, with the nuclei lined up in a row. In addition, glandular cells typically form three-dimensional balls of cells, or morules, recapitulating the acinar/tubular structures of glands. Or, glandular cells can form two-dimensional circles of cells, or microacinar groups, similar to rosettes |i8.17|. (See also the discussion of papillae, p 145.)

Although a columnar shape of the cells, or nucleocytoplasmic polarity, is a sensitive feature of glandular differentiation, it is not specific. A similar configuration can be seen in other tumors, including melanoma |i8.14|, carcinoid, and plasmacytic tumors. None of these other tumors form well-defined glands, although carcinoids, ie, neuroendocrine tumors, can make rosettes.

Sometimes, mucin forms a large collection in the cytoplasm that indents the nucleus, resulting in a signet ring cell |i8.18|. Signet ring adenocarcinomas most commonly arise in the stomach or breast but rarely can arise from a wide variety of

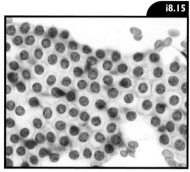
Benign glandular cells (P)

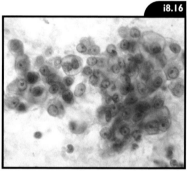
Malignant glandular cells (P)

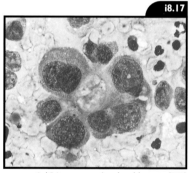
AdCA—mucus in gland lumen (DQ)

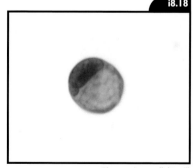
Signet ring cell (P, oil)

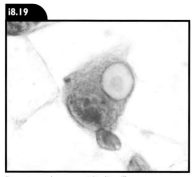

Breast carcinoma—ICL (P, oil)

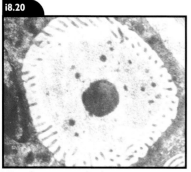

ICL—ultrastructure (EM)

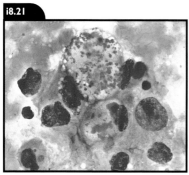

Intracellular mucin (DQ)

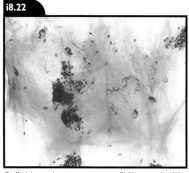

Colloid carcinoma—extracellular mucin (P)

other sites. In addition, several other kinds of cells can form collections of cytoplasmic material resulting in a signet ring appearance, including lymphoma (periodic acid–Schiff [PAS]–positive immunoglobulin), liposarcoma (lipoblasts), and melanoma, among others.

Intracytoplasmic lumens (ICLs) |i8.19| are similar to signet ring vacuoles but must be carefully differentiated from mere degenerative vacuolization. ICLs are seen as sharply punched-out holes in the cytoplasm that usually do not displace the nucleus. ICLs are outlined by a thick rim of cytoplasm (best appreciated in Papanicolaou stain) and have a dot of inspissated mucin in the center (metachromatic in Diff-Quik stain). At the ultrastructural level |i8.20|, microvilli line the ICL. It is these microvilli, which are too small to be resolved individually in the light microscope, that are responsible for the sharp dense outlines of ICLs. ICLs are associated with breast cancer but also are found in other adenocarcinomas, including stomach, lung, and ovary. In breast aspirates, ICLs are virtually diagnostic of cancer; they are rarely seen in benign breast aspirates using routine stains.

Mucin can take on a variety of morphologic appearances in fine needle aspiration (FNA) biopsies and is metachromatic in Diff-Quik stain. The inspissated metachromatic dot, as seen in ICLs, is only one appearance of mucin. Sometimes there are multiple irregular specks of mucin floating in a clear cytoplasmic space |i8.21|. Or there may be a diffuse metachromatic haze in the cytoplasm. In the proper milieu (ie, other features consistent with carcinoma), metachromatic material in the cytoplasm is presumptively mucin and points to a diagnosis of adenocarcinoma.

When islands of epithelial tumor cells are found floating in lakes of mucus, this is the pattern of colloid carcinoma (aka mucinous carcinoma) |i8.22|. The malignant cells are usually cytologically bland. This pattern suggests possible sites of origin, particularly the GI tract, but similar tumors can arise in the breast, ovary, and pancreas. Pseudomyxoma peritonei ("jelly belly") yields a similar pattern. In addition, many sarcomas and, rarely, melanoma, can have an abundant myxoid stroma, producing a pattern similar to colloid carcinoma.

Sometimes the presence of mucin is more important for tumors it *excludes* from the differential diagnosis. Three broad categories of neoplasms (lymphoma/leukemia, sarcomas, and melanoma), as well as germ cell tumors (except yolk sac tumor), "small blue cell tumors," and even certain carcinomas (eg, renal cell carcinoma, acinar/acinic carcinomas, adrenocortical carcinoma), among others, are highly unlikely in the face of intracellular mucicarmine staining. However, contrary to popular opinion, prostatic, hepatocellular, and thyroid carcinomas can sometimes be mucicarmine positive.

Of course, not every cytoplasmic inclusion is some type of mucin. Occasionally, amorphous, dense, glassy intracytoplasmic bodies—hyaline globules—may be seen. Hyaline globules occur in a wide variety of carcinomas (usually poorly differentiated), sarcomas (eg, sarcoma bodies, rhabdoid cells |i8.23|), certain lymphomas, germ cell tumors, and melanomas, as well as in benign conditions ranging from liver cirrhosis to infantile digital fibroma. Therefore, unfortunately, hyaline globules are usually a fairly nonspecific finding.

Adenoid cystic growth pattern, indicated by the presence of extracellular hyaline globules |i8.24|, is an unusual feature that can help point to a possible primary site. The mucoid or hyaline globules, which are usually composed of basement membrane–like material, are intensely metachromatic in Diff-Quik stain, staining bright magenta (like pink gum balls). Adenoid cystic growth pattern is most characteristic of a tumor of salivary gland (and related neoplasms in lacrimal, ceruminous, and sweat glands) but also can be seen in rare cancers of the breast, cervix, prostate, respiratory tract, and esophagus. The differential diagnosis of extracellular hyaline globules includes collagenous spherulosis in the breast and corpora amylacea in the prostate, neither of which is intensely metachromatic.

Another feature of glandular cells that can be useful in suggesting the site of the primary tumor is the presence of "terminal bar–like" edges on the apical cell border |i8.25|. These are microvilli with prominent glycocalyx, glycocalyceal bodies, and long anchoring rootlets that form a dense mesh and extend fairly deeply into the apical cytoplasm. As with microvilli of ICLs, these structures are too small to be resolved individually with the light microscope but impart a distinct density to the apical cell border, giving it the appearance of a terminal bar without cilia. Terminal bar–like edges are particularly characteristic of colorectal cells and their tumors but also can be seen in neoplasms of the stomach, lung (particularly bronchioloalveolar carcinoma), mucinous tumors of the ovary, and endocervical adenocarcinoma.

The manner in which gland cells arrange themselves also can be useful in suggesting a primary site. *Papillae* are defined as epithelial lined, finger-like projections with fibrovascular cores. However, for practical purposes, papillae are simply three-dimensional cell groups that are significantly longer in one dimension than in the other two. Tumors of the ovary, GI tract, lung, and thyroid are among the many that can form papillae.

Single rows of cells can help point to a primary site |i8.26|. Long single file chains of cells are particularly characteristic of breast cancer. However, other adenocarcinomas, eg, those of pancreas, stomach, and prostate, as well as other types of tumors, eg, small cell carcinoma, mesothelioma, carcinoids, and melanoma, also can form single file chains of cells.

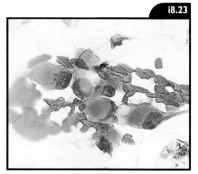

i8.23

Rhabdoid sarcoma—hyaline globules (P)

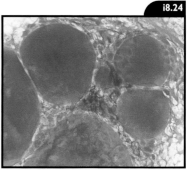

i8.24

Adenoid cystic CA—hyaline globules (DQ)

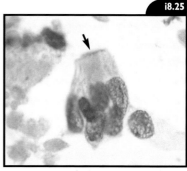

i8.25

Colonic CA—"terminal bars"

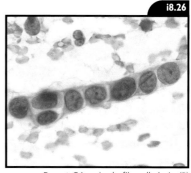

i8.26

Breast CA—single file cell chain (P)

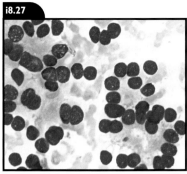

Prostate CA—microacinar complexes (DQ)

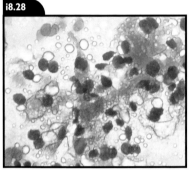

Renal carcinoma—cytoplasmic lipid (DQ)

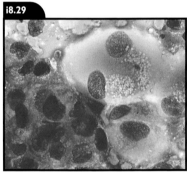

Adenosquamous CA—sharp contrast (DQ)

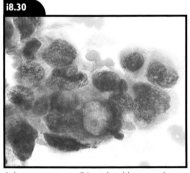

Adenosquamous CA—gland lumen, dense cytoplasm (P)

Acinar arrangement of cells is characteristic of adenocarcinoma in general. Most adenocarcinomas make microacinar groups. However, a highly repeated pattern of microacini (microacinar complexes) |i8.27| suggests origin in the prostate (common metastatic tumor of men) or thyroid (uncommon metastatic tumor). The presence of colloid or "flame cell" (see Chapter 12, p 206) change points to origin in the thyroid. On the other hand, lipid in the cytoplasm favors origin in the prostate.

When looking at a Diff-Quik–stained slide, wet and uncoverslipped, lipid appears as glistening oily droplets |i8.28|. Although the lipid dissolves in processing, it leaves clear cytoplasmic vacuoles. Cytoplasmic lipid is associated with four common adenocarcinomas: kidney, prostate, lung, and breast. However, lipid can be seen in other tumors, too, eg, sarcomas (such as liposarcoma), as well as hepatocellular carcinoma (HCC) or adrenal cortical carcinoma, among others. Occasionally, melanoma has lipid in the cytoplasm. Note that minute lipid droplets can be seen as a nonspecific degenerative change in any cell.

8.4.1 Combined Glandular and Squamous Differentiation

A common and diagnostically important combination of the building blocks is seeing glandular and squamous features in a single tumor or even in a single cell. The classic example is true adenosquamous, or mucoepidermoid, carcinoma. Remember, the essence of squamous differentiation is cellular keratin; the essence of glandular differentiation is cellular secretion.

Squamous differentiation is suggested by cytologic evidence of keratin, including dense or hyalinized cytoplasm, well-defined cell boundaries, rings of keratinization, and in the Papanicolaou stain, cytoplasmic orangeophilia. Pearls are diagnostic of keratinization and squamous differentiation. Exfoliation of cells in flat sheets and cells with central nuclei are also typical. Malignant squamous cells with bizarre shapes may be seen in keratinized cancers.

Glandular differentiation is suggested primarily by the presence of secretion, including ICLs, foamy or granular, basophilic cytoplasm, and nucleocytoplasmic polarity. Glandular origin also is suggested by three-dimensional cell balls or papillae and two-dimensional microacinar structures. Cell shape, nucleocytoplasmic polarity, and microacini are often easier to appreciate in cytology than histology. Also, Diff-Quik stains mucin metachromatically.

In practice, a sharp contrast between the hard waxy cytoplasm of squamous cells with keratin and the delicate vacuolated cytoplasm of glandular cells with secretion suggests dual differentiation |i8.29|, |i8.30|. Non–small cell lung cancer and pancreatic ductal carcinoma commonly show combined glandular and squamous features and are also common sources of unknown primary tumors. Carcinomas of the uterus (adenocarcinoma with squamous differentiation), breast (metaplastic carcinoma), and thyroid (papillary carcinoma) also show combined glandular and squamous differentiation.

Nuclear pseudoinclusions, or intranuclear cytoplasmic invaginations (INCIs) |i8.31|, are found in a wide variety of benign and malignant conditions and, although not specific, can be diagnostically useful in certain situations. For example, INCIs in a thyroid aspirate almost guarantee a malignant diagnosis (usually papillary carcinoma). INCIs are so common in melanoma that the diagnosis is doubtful in their absence. INCIs are also common in bronchioloalveolar carcinoma of the lung. INCIs in the liver can be seen in benign and malignant hepatocytes; however, their presence favors HCC over metastatic adenocarcinoma.

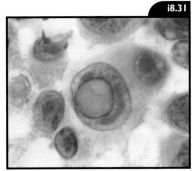

Melanoma—INCI (P)

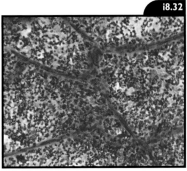

Abscess with granulation tissue (DQ)

8.5 Leukocytes

Leukocytes include neutrophils, eosinophils, lymphocytes, plasma cells, and various kinds of histiocytes (epithelioid, nonepithelioid, and giant cell).

8.5.1 Abscess

An abscess forms a mass that can mimic a neoplasm clinically. It is helpful to appreciate the gross, creamy yellow appearance of a purulent aspirate so that some can be submitted for culture. Culture often provides the most important diagnostic information in this disease.

Microscopically, an abscess is characterized by an abundance of neutrophils and, often, necrosis. Later, chronic inflammatory cells replace the neutrophils. Granulation tissue, which is, in essence, small blood vessels surrounded by histiocytes, appears |i8.32|. Myofibroblasts (spindle/stellate cells with active nuclei; see p 155) accompany the granulation tissue and help form a collagenous scar. Reactive/reparative cells can mimic malignancy, but tumors can become inflamed; therefore, look carefully for tumor cells in an abscess |i8.33|.

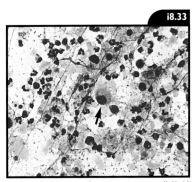

Abscess—tumor cell (DQ)

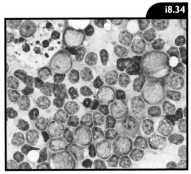

Chronic lymphadenitis (DQ)

8.5.2 Chronic Lymphadenitis

A benign, reactive lymphoid process (chronic lymphadenitis in a lymph node) looks like follicular cervicitis in the Pap smear. The lymphocytes are found in all different stages of differentiation ("range of maturation"), but small, "mature" lymphocytes predominate and plasma cells are frequently present |i8.34|. Tingible body macrophages (TBMs) usually are present.

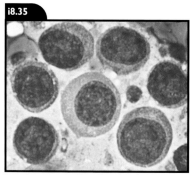

Lymphoma—single cells, LGBs (DQ)

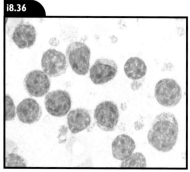

SLL (DQ)

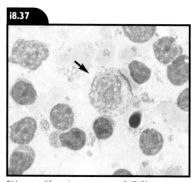

SLL—proliferation center cell (DQ)

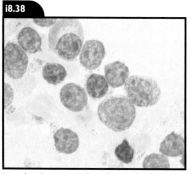

Lymphoplasmacytic lymphoma (DQ)

And, of course, foreign or malignant cells, such as metastatic carcinoma or Reed-Sternberg cells, are absent in benign disease.

8.5.3 Malignant Lymphoma

Despite their reputation for being difficult to diagnose, in some cases it is actually *easier* to determine that a tumor is a lymphoma by cytology than by histology |i8.35|. One of the most characteristic features of lymphoma in aspirates is the singly dispersed cell pattern without formation of true tissue aggregates. Clusters of cells in a lymph node aspirate are suspicious for metastases (but could be lymphohistiocytic aggregates, etc). Lymphoid cells have characteristic morphology, particularly in Diff-Quik stain. Lymphoglandular bodies (LGBs; cytoplasmic fragments) are typically present in the background of lymphoma.

8.5.4 Non-Hodgkin Lymphomas

Any lymph node aspirate that is not dominated by small, mature lymphocytes is suspicious for lymphoma. The absence of TBMs in a smear dominated by "immature" lymphocytes strongly suggests lymphoma. Note, however, that TBMs are commonly present in lymphomas, particularly high-grade non-Hodgkin lymphomas (NHLs) and Hodgkin disease. The large majority of NHLs are composed of one or two of just four types of cells: small lymphocytes, small cleaved cells, large cells, and blasts.

The Four Cells and Their Lymphomas
Small Lymphocytes: Small lymphocytic lymphoma (SLL) is composed predominantly or exclusively of small lymphocytes |i8.36|. Therefore, this lymphoma may be strikingly monomorphic. A minor component of large cells with prominent nucleoli may be present (proliferation center cells) |i8.37|, but they do not form collections (as in Richter syndrome). However, there are no cleaved cells or Reed-Sternberg cells. TBMs and mitotic figures are scarce or absent. Plasma cells and plasmacytoid lymphocytes may be seen in the lymphoplasmacytoid variant but not in ordinary small lymphocytic lymphoma |i8.38|. Clinically, the patients are usually older (> 40 years), have generalized lymphadenopathy, often have chronic lymphocytic leukemia, and may have a monoclonal gammopathy.
Small Cleaved Cells: The small cleaved cell, characteristic of small cleaved (and mixed) lymphoma, is slightly larger than the small mature lymphocyte. Its chromatin is dark and coarse but somewhat more open than the small lymphocyte, and nucleoli may be conspicuous. However, the main distinguishing feature is the presence of nuclear clefts, which are deep folds in the nuclear membranes. The classic appearance is the "coffee bean" nucleus, but the

clefts are variable, ranging from subtle notches to obvious irregularities (like popcorn) |i8.39|.

Small cleaved lymphoma is composed predominantly of small cleaved lymphocytes. A minor component of large lymphocytes usually is present. Mitotic figures, TBMs, and plasma cells are rare or absent. Clinically, the patients are usually older (> 35 years) and have diffuse lymphadenopathy. Lymphosarcoma cell leukemia may occur, but it is unusual. Mixed lymphoma is composed of roughly equal proportions of small cleaved and large cells. These follicular lymphomas are graded in the Revised European-American Lymphoid Neoplasm (REAL) classification (I, II, III) according to the proportions of small cleaved and large cells, with low-grade tumors being composed predominantly of small cleaved cells and high-grade tumors composed predominantly of large cells.

Large Cells: "Large" lymphoid cells can actually range from fairly small to giant. Large cell lymphomas are composed predominantly of large lymphocytes but may have a minor component of small cleaved lymphocytes.

There are four types of large cells: cleaved, noncleaved, immunoblastic, and "true histiocytic" |i8.40|, |i8.41|, |i8.42|. Although there may be some differences in prognosis, the treatment is similar. In particular, it makes little clinical difference whether the large cells are cleaved or not. The chromatin can vary from coarse to fine. Cleaved nuclei tend to be oblong with one or two nucleoli; noncleaved nuclei tend to be round with three to five nucleoli.

Immunoblastic lymphomas come in B- and T-cell types, and although special studies are required to reliably separate them, they have more or less characteristic morphologic features. The B-cell type usually is composed of relatively monomorphous large cells that typically have plasmacytoid cytoplasm (dark blue with a perinuclear hof in Diff-Quik stain) and single central macronucleoli. The T-cell type typically has a polymorphous population of benign and malignant cells, with a spectrum of sizes ranging from small to large. T immunoblasts most characteristically have convoluted nuclei and clear cytoplasm. This lymphoma may be associated with conspicuous numbers of epithelioid histiocytes (Lennert lymphoma).

True histiocytic lymphoma, an oxymoron, is actually composed of malignant histiocytes and, therefore, is more precisely classified as malignant histiocytosis. It is probably indistinguishable from other large cell lymphomas without special studies, but a particularly pleomorphic lymphoma with evidence of phagocytosis of RBCs suggests this diagnosis. On the other hand, the cells may be bland and resemble benign histiocytes. Lymphoglandular bodies may be scarce or absent.

Clinically, large cell lymphomas can occur at any age, including in children. Although they are aggressive tumors, they

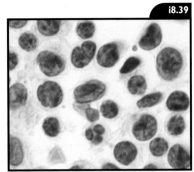

i8.39

Small cleaved lymphoma (P)

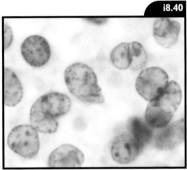

i8.40

Large cell, cleaved (P)

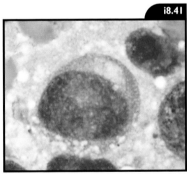

i8.41

Large cell, noncleaved (DQ)

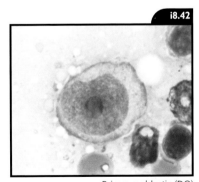

i8.42

B-immunoblastic (DQ)

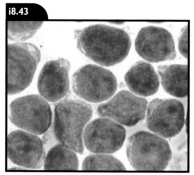

Lymphoblastic lymphoma (DQ)

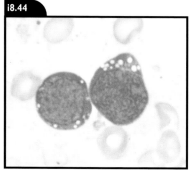

Burkitt lymphoma (DQ)

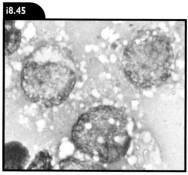

Non-Burkitt lymphoma (DQ)

are less commonly disseminated than the small cell lymphomas, discussed previously, and cure is possible. Leukemic dissemination is rare.

Blastic Cells: The blastic cells, although classified as "small, noncleaved," are actually medium-sized cells that can have smooth or convoluted nuclear membranes. An important distinguishing feature of these cells is their powdery fine to finely granular chromatin. For aficionados, there are three basic blastic lymphomas: lymphoblastic, Burkitt, and non-Burkitt |i8.43|, |i8.44|, |i8.45|. They can be subtyped according to the French-American-British (FAB) classification as FAB L1, FAB L2, and FAB L3 by nuclear and cytoplasmic as well as clinical features |t8.4|.

Lymphoblastic lymphomas also come in T- and pre–B-cell types, but they are indistinguishable morphologically. Blastic lymphomas are all very aggressive and occur mostly in children but with a second peak in old age.

Review

In benign reactive hyperplasia, there is usually a range of maturation of the lymphoid cells with a predominance of small, mature lymphocytes. Most NHLs are characterized by an excess or complete replacement of the usually very heterogeneous population of cells in the lymph node with one (or two) of the four cell types discussed previously. In fact, most NHLs are composed of various proportions of small cleaved and large cells. The percentage of large cells is an important indicator of prognosis: the more, the worse.

The presence of TBMs does not exclude lymphoma. They can be seen in any lymphoma with high mitotic rate or necrosis. However, if TBMs are rare or absent when many large cells are present, suspect lymphoma. Mitotic figures are plentiful in reactive lymph nodes and high-grade lymphomas, but are rare or absent in low-grade lymphomas. In fact, the mitotic rate is one of the best predictors of the clinical behavior of a lymphoma.

t8.4 Differential Diagnosis of Blastic Lymphomas

	Lymphoblastic	Burkitt	Non-Burkitt
Cells	*	Very uniform	More variable
Nucleoli	Invisible	2-5, smaller	1-3, larger
Cytoplasm	Scant	Dark blue	*
Site	Supradiaphragmatic	Infradiaphragmatic	Infradiaphragmatic

*Not a key distinguishing feature.

8.5.5 Hodgkin Disease

For Hodgkin disease, there is only one important cell type: the Reed-Sternberg cell. These malignant cells and their variants are often an order of magnitude larger and "uglier" than ordinary large lymphocytes and, therefore, tend to stand out conspicuously in the smear.

The classic Reed-Sternberg cell is binucleated or bilobed (but can be multinucleated or multilobated), each with an inclusion-like macronucleolus, which is often surrounded by a halo |i8.46|. There is a benign, reactive, inflammatory component consisting of a mixed population of cells, such as lymphocytes, plasma cells, and eosinophils. To be diagnostic, the Reed-Sternberg cells must be found in this benign reactive background (ie, in the proper milieu) |i8.47|. Granulomas are commonly present and provide a clue to look carefully for evidence of Hodgkin disease.

Clinically, Hodgkin disease spreads in contiguity from one nodal group to another and rarely, if ever, presents in an extranodal location (although it can disseminate later). Although four subtypes of Hodgkin disease are recognized (eg, lymphocyte predominant, lymphocyte depleted, mixed cellularity, and nodular sclerosis), age and stage are more important than subtype in therapy and prognosis.

8.5.6 Plasma Cells

Plasma cells make immunoglobulins, the antibodies, and are recognized by their typical "clock face" chromatin pattern and perinuclear hof (Golgi apparatus). Reactive plasmacytosis is typically accompanied by a mixed inflammatory infiltrate. Benign plasma cells usually appear mature. They tend to surround blood vessels. Sometimes, plasma cells contain cytoplasmic Russell bodies (inspissated immunoglobulin). In plasma cell dyscrasias, there is typically a pure population of neoplastic plasma cells, which often appear immature and form loosely cohesive sheets |i8.48|. The presence of INCIs, Dutcher bodies, is associated with malignancy, particularly Waldenström macroglobulinemia. Binucleation is common in plasma cells and their tumors. Other cells can mimic plasma cells (plasmacytoid cells), including some cases of breast cancer |i8.49|, carcinoid tumors, and melanoma. Special stains and immunocytochemistry may be useful in the differential diagnosis.

8.5.7 Epithelioid Histiocytes

Epithelioid histiocytes have elongated spindle-shaped nuclei (with fine chromatin and tiny nucleoli), which often have longitudinal folds or grooves in the nuclear membrane. They have abundant cytoplasm that is eccentrically located around the

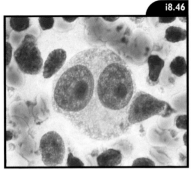
i8.46
Hodgkin disease—Reed-Sternberg cell (DQ)

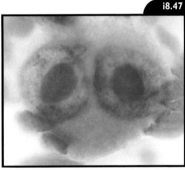
i8.47
Melanoma—Reed-Sternberg–like cell (P, oil)

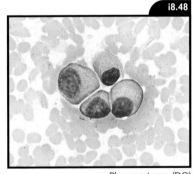
i8.48
Plasmacytoma (DQ)

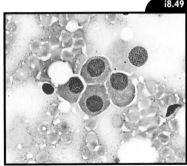
i8.49
Breast cancer—plasmacytoid cells (DQ)

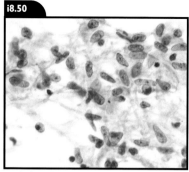

Epithelioid histiocytes (P)

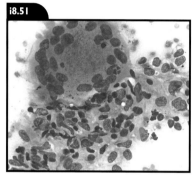

Giant cell and epithelioid histiocytes (DQ)

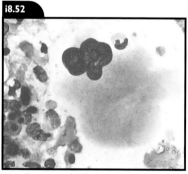

Megakaryocyte (DQ)

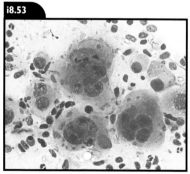

Giant cell CA—hyaline globules (DQ)

nucleus. The cytoplasm has a typical fibrillar appearance, especially in Papanicolaou stain |i8.50|, but often appears dense and homogeneous, like an epithelial cell, in Diff-Quik stain |i8.51|. Aggregates of epithelioid histiocytes are diagnostic of a granuloma. Giant cells may or may not be present.

8.6 Giant Cells

Giant cells are a characteristic feature of a granuloma but are neither necessary nor sufficient for its diagnosis. Granulomas are associated with infections (particularly tuberculosis and fungus, among many others), foreign bodies, sarcoidosis, radiation and chemotherapy, heavy metals, and necrobiotic granulomas such as rheumatoid nodules. Certain tumors are associated with granuloma formation, eg, squamous and adenosquamous carcinomas, germinomas, lymphomas (T-cell NHLs and Hodgkin disease), among others.

Tuberculosis classically causes granulomatous inflammation with caseating necrosis. Sarcoid usually produces noncaseating granulomas and may be associated with asteroid and Schaumann bodies. Special stains may be useful for identifying organisms and polarized light for identifying foreign substances. Occasionally, particularly in patients with AIDS, mycobacteria are so numerous that they can be "seen" in Diff-Quik stain as negative (unstained) images in the cytoplasm of the histiocytes or in the background of the smear.

Other benign giant cells include osteoclasts (multiple nuclei, metachromatic granules in cytoplasm) and megakaryocytes (single multilobated nuclei; may have platelets issuing from the cell periphery) |i8.52|. These cells may be sampled during FNA biopsies of bone or bone marrow. Megakaryocytes also can be seen in nonosseous cytologic specimens, eg, myelolipomas, extramedullary hematopoiesis, or myeloid metaplasia. Osteoclasts also can be seen, rarely, in stroma of malignant tumors of the pancreas, breast, liver, lung, etc.

Malignant tumor cells can become bizarre and giant |i8.53|. Giant cell carcinomas occur most commonly in the lung, pancreas, and liver, among many other sites. Giant tumor cells also are characteristic of pleomorphic sarcomas, such as malignant fibrous histiocytoma. Malignant giant cells also can be found in a variety of other tumors, eg, choriocarcinoma, neuroendocrine tumors (such as pheochromocytoma), mesothelioma, glioblastoma, giant cell tumors, anaplastic lymphomas and myelomas, Hodgkin disease, and of course, melanoma. Bizarre giant tumor cells are particularly common after radiation therapy.

8.7 **Small Cells**

Small cell tumors represent a diverse group of neoplasms, including, among others, poorly differentiated squamous or adenocarcinoma, lymphomas, neuroendocrine tumors, such as carcinoids, islet cell tumors, and small cell neuroendocrine carcinoma (particularly of the lung), small blue cell tumors of childhood, and, of course, melanoma.

The diagnosis of small cell tumors can be challenging. Dividing the tumors into three groups helps with the differential diagnosis |t8.5|. Look at the power of this simple scheme. Let's say you have a 65-year-old man with a tumor composed of small cohesive cells |i8.54|. The age practically eliminates group III, pediatric tumors; cellular cohesion eliminates group I (lymphomas); and the sex practically eliminates breast carcinoma. So, with a little bit of clinical information and only a quick glance at the cells, you have arrived at what is by far the most likely diagnosis, namely small cell carcinoma of the lung.

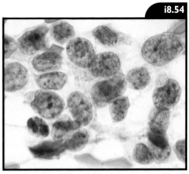
Small cell lung CA—blue bodies (P, oil)

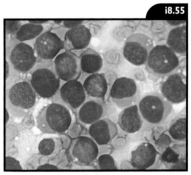
Rhabdomyosarcoma (DQ)

8.7.1 Small Blue Cell Tumors of Childhood

FNA biopsy, often used in conjunction with ancillary studies such as immunocytochemistry performed on aspirated material, is being increasingly applied to the diagnosis of pediatric small blue cell tumors |t8.6|.

Malignant lymphoma in children is usually high-grade: large (usually B) cell or blastic types (Burkitt/non-Burkitt or lymphoblastic lymphomas). (Hodgkin disease also occurs, but it is not a small blue cell tumor.) Lymphomas are characterized by a dispersed population of lymphoid cells with lymphoglandular bodies in the background. Lymphoglandular bodies are absent or rare in other small blue cell tumors. PAS stain may be positive in B-cell lymphomas due to immunoglobulin glycoproteins; also, lymphoblastic lymphomas may have PAS-positive vacuoles. Leukocyte common antigen (CD45) is characteristically expressed.

Embryonal rhabdomyosarcoma, in addition to small blue cells |i8.55|, may have spindle or strap-like cells with dense non-vacuolated cytoplasm |i8.56|, in which pathognomonic cross-striations may be identified rarely. Tumor giant cells may also be present. The cells contain PAS positive glycogen. Myxoid material may be present in the background and suggests the diagnosis (exclude Wilms tumor). Alveolar rhabdomyosarcoma can be a purely round cell tumor without spindle cells. Electron microscopy shows thick and thin myofibers. Desmin is a typical immunocytochemical marker.

Ewing sarcoma may display a dimorphic cell population of blastemic and lymphocyte-like (light and dark) cells that is highly characteristic of this tumor |i8.57|. Coarse cytoplasmic

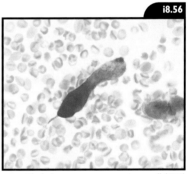
Rhabdomyosarcoma —strap cell (PAS)

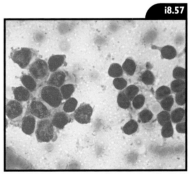
Ewing sarcoma—dimorphic cells (DQ)

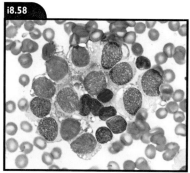
PNET (DQ)

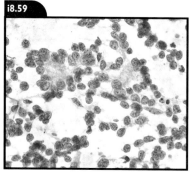
Neuroblastoma—rosettes (P)

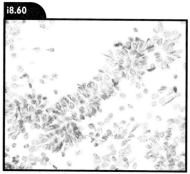
Wilms tumor—tubule (P)

t8.5 Differential Diagnosis of Small Cell Tumors

I	Lymphoma	Single cells, lymphoglandular bodies
II	Breast (adenocarcinoma) Lung (small cell carcinoma)	Adult women Older smokers
III	Ewing sarcoma/PNET Neuroblastoma Rhabdomyosarcoma Wilms tumor	Children, young adults

vacuoles, which contain glycogen—another characteristic feature—may be seen. Myogenic markers are negative, but neural markers may be positive. Ewing sarcoma is associated with a chromosomal anomaly t(11;22), which it shares with the closely related primitive neuroectodermal tumor (PNET) |**i8.58**|. Ewing sarcoma may be the poorly differentiated end of a spectrum of associated tumors (Ewing sarcoma → PNET → neuroblastoma).

Neuroblastoma is a tumor composed of monotonously uniform small blue cells |**i8.59**|. Unique to this small blue cell neoplasm is that tumor markers, such as increased catecholamines or neuron-specific enolase, can be detected in the urine or blood, respectively. Rosettes are a characteristic feature of neuroblastoma, but they are not specific and not always present. Neuropil, which is fibrillary material formed by neurites, is a unique feature of neuroblastoma among these small blue cell tumors. The cells are usually PAS-negative, although poorly differentiated neuroblastomas and primitive neuroectodermal tumors may contain PAS-positive glycogen. Neurosecretory granules may be demonstrable and are another characteristic but nonspecific feature. Ganglion cells may be seen (larger cells with more abundant cytoplasm, one or more nuclei, with vesicular chromatin and prominent nucleoli). Immunocytochemistry characteristically demonstrates neurofilaments, neuron-specific enolase, and synaptophysin.

t8.6 "Small Blue Cell Tumors" of Childhood

Tumor	Cells	Groups	PAS	Comments
Lymphoma	Monotypic	−	±	Lymphoglandular bodies, immunoglobulin
Rhabdomyosarcoma	Polymorphic	+	+	Rhabdomyoblasts and spindle cells, myxoid stroma
Ewing sarcoma	Dimorphic	+	+	Usually bone tumor; light and dark cells
Neuroblastoma	Monomorphic	+	−	Rosettes, neuropils, axons; clinical tumor markers
Wilms tumor	Triphasic	+	+	Tubules, blasts, spindle cells

Wilms tumor, or nephroblastoma, often has a biphasic or triphasic cell population, which includes stromal and epithelial cells, in addition to the small blue blastemic cells. The blastemic cells do not have prominent nucleoli, and the cytoplasm is not vacuolated, but it may be PAS-positive. Tubule formation is unique among small blue cell tumors |i8.60|. Like embryonal rhabdomyosarcoma, myxoid stroma may be present. Occasionally, anaplastic cells with considerably larger, darker nuclei and prominent nucleoli are present and correlate with an unfavorable prognosis.

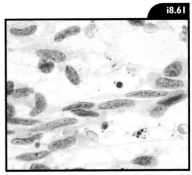

Spindle cell sarcoma (P)

8.8 Spindle Cells

Spindle cells are particularly associated with sarcomas |i8.61| but also can be found in other tumors, such as carcinomas |i8.62| and, of course, melanomas |i8.63|. Sarcomas often present as large, bulky tumors, and, therefore, the primary site is usually clinically obvious. The more likely diagnostic problem with sarcomas is trying to classify the tumor, not determine where it came from. Benign proliferations of atypical spindle cells, pseudosarcomas, can mimic malignancy: nodular fasciitis is the premier example |i8.64|. (See Chapter 9 for further discussion.)

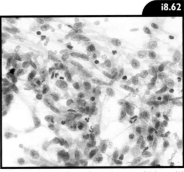

Spindle cell carcinoma, kidney (P)

One of the most notorious spindle cell carcinomas is sarcomatoid renal cell carcinoma. The metastasis can be solitary and the primary tumor occult, mimicking a primary tumor at the metastatic site. Melanoma also can do this.

Spindle SCC is, by definition, a nonkeratinizing squamous cancer, because keratinizing SCC routinely has spindly cells (tadpoles, snakes). Nasopharyngeal carcinoma, a form of SCC, also can grow in a spindle cell pattern. Other spindle cell neoplasms include mesothelioma, neuroendocrine tumors, small cell carcinoma, and thymoma.

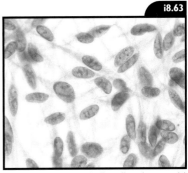

Spindle cell melanoma (P)

A biphasic combination of epithelial and spindle cells can be is seen in certain tumors, mostly carcinosarcomas, eg, in the lung, breast, and uterus (mixed mesodermal tumor). Also, synovial sarcoma, epithelioid leiomyosarcoma, and malignant schwannomas can show a combination of epithelioid and spindle cells. A variety of other tumors, ranging from benign mixed tumors (pleomorphic adenomas) of the salivary gland to melanoma, also can show this biphasic pattern.

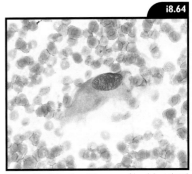

Nodular fasciitis—myofibroblast (DQ)

8.9 Clear Cells

Cells can be clear because they accumulate something transparent (eg, glycogen, lipid, mucin; also, water and electrolytes

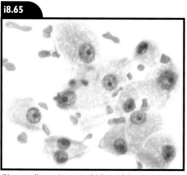

Clear cell carcinoma, kidney (P)

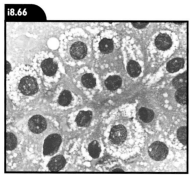

Clear cell carcinoma, kidney (DQ)

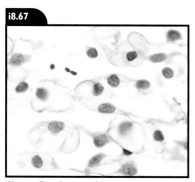

Clear cell melanoma (P)

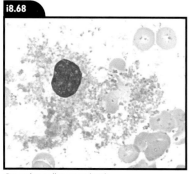

Granular cell tumor (DQ)

in hydropic degeneration), because their organelles degenerate (eg, mitochondria in oncocytes, melanosomes in balloon cell melanoma), because they have virtually no organelles (eg, clear cell lymphoma, degranulated acinic cell carcinoma), or because of artifact. All major categories of tumors, including carcinomas, sarcomas, lymphomas, germ cell tumors, and of course melanoma, can have tumors composed predominantly or exclusively of clear cells.

In cytology, clear cells are not necessarily optically clear or empty appearing, as they often are in tissue. Instead, the cytoplasm is typically abundant and very delicate but has some substance to it. In Papanicolaou stain, "clear" cytoplasm typically stains a gossamer blue |i8.65|, while in Diff-Quik stain, myriads of tiny but distinct cytoplasmic vacuoles are seen |i8.66|. Classically, the chromatin is pale and fine in Papanicolaou stain, and there is a big cherry-red nucleolus, but this classic appearance is not always present.

Most metastatic clear cell tumors, by far, come from the kidney. Bear in mind that the primary renal tumor may be small and that the metastasis can be solitary, can be found at unexpected sites, and can occur early, before the primary site is known, or years later, after the primary tumor is forgotten. Renal cell carcinoma can be composed of cells so bland that the metastasis is thought to be a *benign* clear cell tumor arising at that site.

Once a renal primary site has been carefully excluded, many other sites can give rise to benign and malignant clear cell tumors, including lung, breast, thyroid, female genital tract, liver, adrenal, salivary gland, and skin appendages. Nonepithelial clear cell tumors include clear cell sarcomas (eg, of soft parts or kidney), lipomas and liposarcoma, chordoma, epithelioid smooth muscle tumors, and fibrohistiocytic tumors, as well as clear cell lymphoma and germinoma (seminoma/dysgerminoma). And do not forget melanoma (balloon cell melanoma) |i8.67|.

8.10 Granular Cells

Granular cells can have granular cytoplasm due to the presence of numerous lysosomes (eg, granular cell tumors |i8.68|), mitochondria (oncocytic neoplasms |i8.69|, |i8.70|), or secretory granules (eg, zymogen granules—acinic/acinar carcinomas |i8.71|). Lysosomes and zymogen granules are large enough to be seen individually in the light microscope. Mitochondria give a finely granular texture to the cytoplasm. Cytoplasmic granularity also can be due to marked accumulation of smooth endoplasmic reticulum (as seen in steroid-secreting cells) or other cellular products, such as keratohyaline granules.

Granular cell tumor |i8.68| is usually benign, although it can mimic a carcinoma clinically and microscopically, particularly in the breast. The coarsely granular cytoplasm is a clue to be cautious in the diagnosis of breast cancer. Granular cell tumors probably usually arise from nerves (granular cell schwannoma), but some apparently also derive from other cells, such as smooth muscle, histiocytes, and epithelial cells.

Oncocytic neoplasms occur |i8.69|, |i8.70| in the salivary gland, kidney, thyroid, and ovary, among many other sites. In addition, oncocytic change may be seen in neuroendocrine tumors, including carcinoids (various sites of origin), islet cell tumors, medullary carcinoma, and paragangliomas. Fibrolamellar carcinoma of the liver is an oncocytic variant of HCC with a better prognosis than ordinary HCC. Also, granular renal cell carcinoma and apocrine breast carcinomas have numerous mitochondria in their cytoplasm, falling short of being oncocytic but imparting a similar granular texture.

Acinic or acinar cells are another type of granular cell |i8.71|. Their cytoplasm contains zymogen (proenzyme) granules (which may leach out, giving a foamy to clear appearance). The granules are PAS-positive, diastase resistant. Neurosecretory granules (carcinoids, paraganglioma, including pheochromocytoma) also may cause cytoplasmic granularity. Other tumors with granules or crystals, eg, alveolar soft part sarcoma, also occur. Metastatic tumor cells with the combination of a granular center and clear periphery suggest renal origin |i8.72|.

HCC and adrenocortical neoplasms have granular cytoplasm due in part to abundant endoplasmic reticulum. Glassy cell carcinoma (poorly differentiated adenosquamous carcinoma) of the cervix has a finely granular cytoplasm. Granular cell lymphomas have been described that contain intracytoplasmic azurophilic hydrolase. And, of course, melanoma characteristically has a granular cytoplasmic texture due to the presence of pigmented or nonpigmented melanosomes, which are in essence modified lysosomes. Finally, cytoplasmic granularity is a common degenerative change in cells of virtually any origin.

8.11 Neuroendocrine Cells

The neuroendocrine cell is recognized principally by its nuclear structure and cytoplasmic neurosecretory granules. Neuroendocrine cells comprise the diffuse neuroendocrine system and its tumors. Carcinoids, atypical carcinoids, and small cell carcinoma form a biologic and morphologic spectrum of closely related neuroendocrine tumors.

Typical carcinoid tumors are low-grade, very well-differentiated neoplasms that seldom metastasize. Carcinoid tumors are epithelial tumors that can arise in the appendix, small intes-

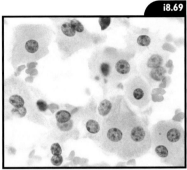
Oncocytes (P)

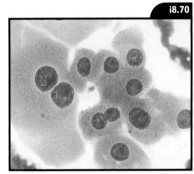
Oncocytes (DQ)

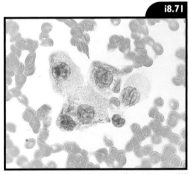
Acinic cell carcinoma (P)

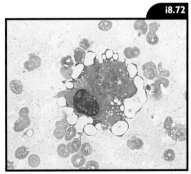
RCC—granular center, clear periphery (DQ)

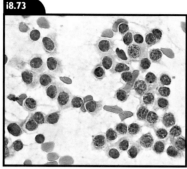

Carcinoid (P)

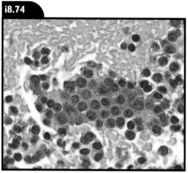

Carcinoid (DQ)

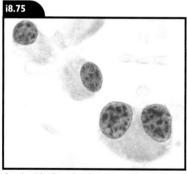

Carcinoid—lymphoplasmacytoid cells (P, oil)

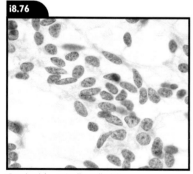

Carcinoid—spindle cells (P)

tine, Meckel diverticula, colon, stomach, and many other sites, including the lung and bile ducts. Typical carcinoids, islet cell tumors, and medullary carcinoma of the thyroid, as well as paragangliomas and pheochromocytomas (both of neural crest origin), have many similarities. Patients with inherited disorders of multiple endocrine neoplasia may have various combinations of these tumors. Classic carcinoids may secrete serotonin and, particularly when metastatic, can produce the carcinoid syndrome (flushing, diarrhea, right-sided heart valve disease, and asthma-like bronchial constriction). Other types of neuroendocrine tumors also may secrete biologically active substances and produce a variety of clinical syndromes, such as Zollinger-Ellison or Cushing syndromes.

Atypical carcinoids are of intermediate malignancy. Atypical carcinoid is more aggressive than typical carcinoid (which uncommonly metastasizes) but less aggressive than small cell carcinoma (which routinely metastasizes). Note, however, that even typical carcinoids can have atypical features, such as focal pleomorphism and atypia ("endocrine atypia"), spindle cells, and extracellular substances (eg, amyloid or bone), as well as occasional metastases.

Small cell carcinoma is considered a poorly differentiated neuroendocrine carcinoma. Other small cell tumors of neuroendocrine origin include neuroblastoma, neuroepithelioma, and primitive neuroectodermal tumors |t8.7|.

The FNA biopsy of a carcinoid-type neuroendocrine tumor obtains flat sheets, loose groups, and cords of cells |i8.73|, |i8.74|. The cells usually have a strikingly monotonous appearance and can be lymphoplasmacytoid |i8.75| or spindle-shaped |i8.76|, either pure (eg, spindle cell carcinoid of the lung) or in combination. In fact, the combination of lymphoplasmacytoid and small spindle cells in an aspirate suggests a neuroendocrine tumor. Occasional cases of otherwise typical carcinoid tumors show large, sometimes even giant or bizarre cells |i8.77|, very focally (endocrine atypia), which does not necessarily indicate the tumor will behave more aggressively. Rosettes may be seen in some cases. Necrosis is absent in typical carcinoids.

t8.7 Neuroendocrine Tumors

Carcinoid Type	Small Cell Type
Carcinoids (typical, atypical)	Small cell carcinoma
Islet cell tumors	Neuroblastoma
Medullary carcinoma, thyroid	Neuroepithelioma
Paragangliomas	Primitive neuroectodermal tumor (PNET)

The nuclei are uniform, round to oval to spindle-shaped, and have smooth nuclear borders. The chromatin often has a characteristic "salt and pepper" appearance in Papanicolaou stain (ie, moderately coarse with small parachromatin spaces). However, the chromatin can vary from fine to coarse, and other kinds of cells can have salt-and-pepper chromatin. Nucleoli are usually inconspicuous but sometimes can be prominent. Mitotic figures are absent or rare.

The cytoplasm is small to moderate in amount, pale, and finely granular. The presence of neurosecretory granules is diagnostic of neuroendocrine differentiation. Neurosecretory granules (NSGs) can sometimes be seen in Diff-Quik stain as a fine red (metachromatic) dust in the cytoplasm |i8.78|. Special studies, such as Grimelius argyrophil stain or electron microscopy, can help identify neurosecretory granules. Immunocytochemistry cannot only help to confirm the diagnosis (eg, chromogranin, synaptophysin) but also to further classify the tumor (eg, gastrinoma, insulinoma).

Atypical carcinoids are distinguished from typical carcinoids by cellular pleomorphism, mitosis, and necrosis. The cells are intermediate in appearance and behavior between typical carcinoid and small cell carcinoma |i8.79|. In essence, the more the tumor resembles small cell carcinoma, the worse the prognosis.

Small cell carcinoma shows obvious pleomorphism, marked nuclear molding, very scanty cytoplasm, irregular nuclear membranes, dark but fine chromatin, absent or inconspicuous nucleoli, numerous mitoses, and areas of crush artifact and necrosis (see |i8.54|). Three-dimensional clusters of malignant cells may be seen in small cell carcinoma, in contrast with flat sheets characteristic of typical and atypical carcinoids. Large cell neuroendocrine carcinomas have also been described |i8.80|.

8.12 Melanoma

Melanoma, last but not least, is perhaps the most notorious member of the building blocks. Although melanoma usually arises from skin, it also can arise from other, sometimes hidden sites. Moreover, it is infamous for its ability to metastasize virtually anywhere in the body, sometimes before the primary tumor is known or long after it has been forgotten. Furthermore, as has been emphasized throughout this chapter, melanoma can mimic many other tumors. Among the many features that can be seen in melanoma are high cellularity, dispersed cell pattern, epithelioid cells, giant cells, spindle cells, small cells, clear cells, granular cells, signet ring cells, eccentric nuclei, binucleation or multinucleation, prominent nucleoli, INCIs, abundant cytoplasm, cyto-

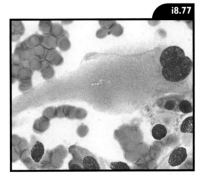
i8.77
Neuroendocrine tumor—bizarre cell (DQ)

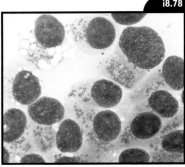
i8.78
Metachromatic NSGs (DQ, oil)

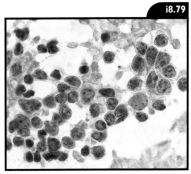
i8.79
Atypical carcinoid (P)

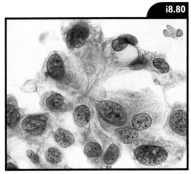
i8.80
Large cell neuroendocrine carcinoma (P)

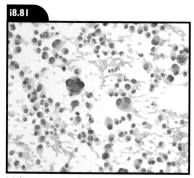

Melanoma—single cells, giant cells (P)

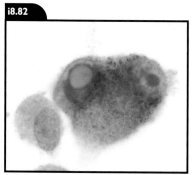

Melanoma—D-MIN, INCI, pigment (P)

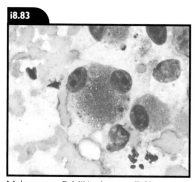

Melanoma—D-MIN, pigment (DQ)

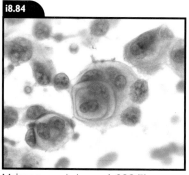

Melanoma—mimics pearl, SCC (P)

plasmic pigment, cytoplasmic vacuoles, and bloody, necrotic, or myxoid background.

The FNA biopsy usually obtains a moderately to highly cellular smear. Cases that have malignant-appearing cells containing cytoplasmic melanin pigment are easy to diagnose. However, many metastatic melanomas are not obviously pigmented, and some are completely amelanotic. Even when pigmented, only a minority of the cells may contain pigment.

The cells are usually singly dispersed, as in lymphomas or sarcomas |i8.81|, but occasionally form tissue aggregates. Also, a scattering of tumor giant cells often is present. The cells usually have an epithelioid appearance (round to polygonal to oval to columnar). Spindle cells may be present, and sometimes they predominate, mimicking a spindle cell sarcoma. Combinations of spindle and giant cells can mimic a pleomorphic sarcoma. Other patterns include clear cell, granular cell, and small cell tumors.

Binucleated cells are characteristically present in melanoma, and multinucleated cells also can be seen. Of course, binucleation is nonspecific; however, in melanoma, a few binucleated cells have a peculiar arrangement: double–mirror image nuclei (D-MINs or "demons") |i8.82|, |i8.83|. The two nuclei are widely separated and look as though they are partially extruded from the cytoplasm, giving them a "bug-eyed" appearance—hence, bug-eyed demons. Bug-eyed demons are found in most cases of melanoma and are rarely seen in other kinds of tumors (except those of neural crest origin).

The chromatin is usually finely dispersed. Macronucleoli are a characteristic nuclear feature but not always present. On careful search of an adequate specimen, INCIs almost always can be identified. Although INCIs are in no way specific for melanoma, be cautious in diagnosing melanoma in their total absence.

The cytoplasm usually has a granular quality, even in the absence of identifiable pigment. Melanin usually appears as a nonrefractile, fine (lysosome-sized), dark cytoplasmic powder (brown-black in Papanicolaou stain; blue-black in Diff-Quik stain), but sometimes it condenses into coarser granules that may resemble hemosiderin (which is golden brown and refractile in Papanicolaou stain, dark blue-green and nonrefractile in Diff-Quik stain).

Immunocytochemistry can be useful in confirming the diagnosis. The combination of positive S-100 and negative keratin supports the diagnosis. HMB-45 usually is expressed in melanoma, rarely in other tumors.

Benign pigmented cells can be found in a wide variety of body sites, and other tumors can contain melanin pigment (eg, nerve sheath tumors, occasional carcinomas). Beware of atypical macrophages containing ingested melanin pigment, which can closely mimic melanoma. Remember, melanoma can mimic practically any other tumor |i8.84|!

8.13 Background/Extracellular Material

There is a natural tendency to focus on the cells in a smear; however, there may be a great deal of information in the background. For example, colloid is very important in thyroid biopsies (the more colloid, the more likely the lesion is benign). Note that other proteinaceous fluids such as blood serum can mimic thyroid colloid almost perfectly, including "crack artifact" |8.85|. A tumor diathesis is a hallmark of malignancy. It represents a host response to the invading tumor and consists of fresh and old blood, fibrin, detritus, inflammation, and necrotic cells. Necrosis can be seen in granulomas (eg, tuberculosis), abscess, infarct, and tumors. Lymphoglandular bodies are cytoplasmic fragments of lymphoid cells and are associated with organized lymphoid tissue and malignant lymphomas. Young collagen is slightly fibrillar and metachromatic. Mucoid substances were discussed in the "Glandular Cells" section, p 144 |8.86|.

Amyloid is produced by some neuroendocrine tumors, particularly medullary carcinoma of the thyroid. Nonneoplastic amyloidosis also occurs, which can sometimes be diagnosed by FNA biopsy of abdominal fat tissue with the help of special stains (Congo red stain demonstrating apple-green birefringence) |8.87|, |8.88|. A tigroid background is characteristic of tumors with high glycogen content, particularly dysgerminoma/seminoma.

Psammoma bodies (calcospherites) are concentrically laminated, calcified structures, most characteristically surrounded by tumor cells. They stain dark red-purple in Papanicolaou stain but are clear and colorless in Diff-Quik stain. Psammoma bodies are particularly associated with papillary neoplasms, notably of the thyroid, ovary, lung, and kidney. However, psammoma bodies are seen in many tumors, benign or malignant, as well as in non-neoplastic conditions. However, in specific sites—eg, thyroid—they are highly suggestive of malignancy.

Fluid, usually poorly cellular, is obtained from cysts. Cysts are one of the most common causes of false-negative diagnoses. For example, although the great majority of aspirated cysts in the breast or the thyroid are benign (on the order of 99%), given a cystic cancer, FNA biopsy may be incapable of diagnosing half or more of the cases (owing to paucity and degeneration of diagnostic cells in cyst content). When aspirating a cyst, drain the cyst as completely as possible, then reaspirate any residual mass. Excise the cyst if it recurs more than once. The purpose of this is to exclude cystic neoplasms.

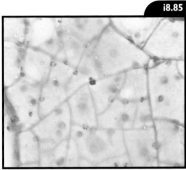

i8.85

Pseudocolloid, serum, "tissue juice" (DQ)

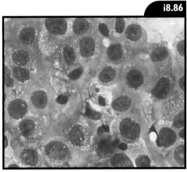

i8.86

Melanoma—myxoid stroma (DQ)

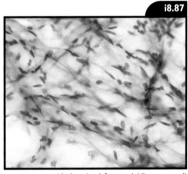

i8.87

Abdominal fat pad (Congo red)

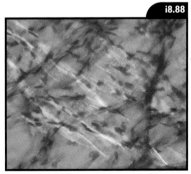

i8.88

Amyloid—apple-green birefringence

Zebras. The uncommon. Soft tissue tumors. But despite their rarity it is important to be familiar with sarcomas not only because they are likely to be encountered from time to time, but also because sarcomas can mimic benign lesions and benign lesions can mimic sarcomas. Fortunately, benign soft tissue tumors far outnumber malignant ones.

Soft tissue sarcomas are defined as nonepithelial, extraskeletal, malignant tumors, excluding tumors of the reticuloendothelial and hematopoietic systems (eg, lymphomas, leukemias, myeloma) and glia, as well as sarcomas arising in the supporting tissue of specific organs (which are considered sarcomas of the particular site). The definition includes tumors that reproduce skeletal and smooth muscle, fat, fibrous tissue, vessels, cartilage, and bone. The peripheral nervous system arises from neuroectoderm rather than mesenchyme, and, therefore, its malignant tumors are technically carcinomas rather than true sarcomas, but these tumors are generally included among sarcomas.

Sarcomas arise from primitive, multipotential, uncommitted mesenchymal cells. Because they share a common ancestor, the various mesenchymal tumors are closely related. Malignant transformation of benign soft tissue tumors is rare. One recognized exception to this general rule, however, is neurofibroma transforming into malignant schwannoma in the setting of von Recklinghausen disease. Common sarcomas are listed |t9.1|.

Most sarcomas present as painless swellings. Some, however, are associated with pain, classically: angioleiomyomas, traumatic neuroma, glomus tumor, cutaneous leiomyoma/ leiomyosarcoma, multiple painful lipomas, eccrine spiradenoma, and angiolipoma. Of course, any tumor occasionally can cause pain, depending on factors such as its location and relationship to

---

t9.1 Common Sarcomas

Adults	Children
Malignant fibrous histiocytoma	Neuroblastoma
Liposarcoma	Rhabdomyosarcoma
Rhabdomyosarcoma	Wilms tumor
Synovial sarcoma	Ewing sarcoma (bone)
Malignant schwannoma	Osteosarcoma (bone)
Fibrosarcoma	
Leiomyosarcoma	

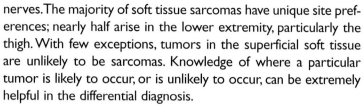

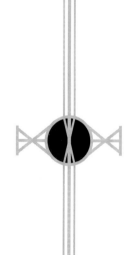

nerves. The majority of soft tissue sarcomas have unique site preferences; nearly half arise in the lower extremity, particularly the thigh. With few exceptions, tumors in the superficial soft tissue are unlikely to be sarcomas. Knowledge of where a particular tumor is likely to occur, or is unlikely to occur, can be extremely helpful in the differential diagnosis.

Older age, male sex, pain, large tumor size, and increasing depth, as well as high stage and grade of a sarcoma are factors that may adversely affect the prognosis. The grade of the tumor is particularly important and can be estimated by using fine needle aspiration (FNA) biopsy. Mitotic count and necrosis are among the best indicators of tumor grade. Of diagnostic importance, mitotic figures are generally fewer in FNA biopsy specimens (and frozen sections) than in permanent tissue sections. In addition to mitotic count and extent of necrosis, other parameters that can be evaluated in determining the grade of the tumor include cellularity, cellular pleomorphism, nuclear atypia, and degree of differentiation.

For practical purposes, a two-grade system (low and high grades) is preferred clinically for sarcomas. The behavior of some tumors can be predicted independently of grade by cytogenetic type (automatic grade). For example, rhabdomyosarcoma (especially alveolar), synovial sarcoma, osteogenic sarcoma, round cell and pleomorphic liposarcoma, angiosarcoma, Ewing sarcoma, neuroblastoma, primitive neuroectodermal tumor (PNET), and rhabdoid tumors are high-grade sarcomas, while well-differentiated and myxoid liposarcoma, epithelioid sarcoma, and dermatofibrosarcoma protuberans are low-grade.

Although many types of sarcomas are capable of metastasizing to lymph nodes, overall, less than 10% of sarcomas do so. However, certain sarcomas, such as rhabdomyosarcoma, synovial sarcoma, malignant fibrous histiocytoma (MFH), fibrosarcoma, and angiosarcoma, more frequently metastasize to lymph nodes. Although they are rare tumors, clear cell sarcoma, epithelioid sarcoma, and alveolar soft part sarcoma have a tendency to metastasize to lymph nodes. If the lymph nodes are involved, the prognosis is poor.

The precise classification of soft tissue sarcomas is among the most difficult areas of diagnostic pathology. However, the exact type of soft tissue tumor is seldom critical in the choice of therapy, including surgery. FNA biopsy may help the clinician plan therapy by pointing to the diagnosis of sarcoma and indicating its grade. When a primary diagnosis of a soft tissue tumor is made initially by FNA biopsy, the final diagnosis should probably be confirmed histologically before mutilating surgery or amputation is performed, particularly when the clinical impression does not correlate with the cytologic results.

9.1 FNA Biopsy of Soft Tissue Tumors

The FNA biopsy of soft tissue tumors obtains variably cellular smears; sarcomas tend to yield highly cellular aspirates, while benign tumors are usually less cellular. Vascular tumors result in bloody aspirates, and heavily collagenized tumors result in poorly cellular aspirates. Classic cytologic diagnostic criteria, such as pleomorphism, chromatin structure, and nucleoli, can be applied in evaluation of malignancy, but benign soft tissue tumors can yield numerous atypical, pleomorphic cells (eg, nodular fasciitis, fat necrosis), while sarcomas can be composed of deceptively bland, monomorphic cells (eg, synovial sarcoma). Clinical features and, particularly for bone tumors, the radiologic appearance may be critical in assessment of these lesions.

Hyperchromasia, atypical mitotic figures, or necrosis suggests malignancy. A highly dissociated cell pattern (ie, predominantly single cells) suggests a diagnosis of sarcoma (or lymphoma, melanoma) as opposed to carcinoma. Most sarcomas lack specific organoid structures or architectural arrangements. Therefore, as a next step in diagnosis, it can be useful to simply divide sarcomas into spindle cell, round cell, and pleomorphic types |i9.1|, |i9.2|, |i9.3|.

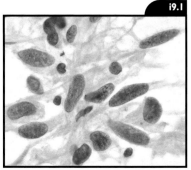
Spindle cell carcinoma

The tumors listed |t9.2| are the common varieties of soft tissue tumors and should help shape the differential diagnosis. In the spindle cell pattern, fibrosarcoma, monophasic synovial sarcoma, and malignant schwannoma can look particularly similar to each other. Synovial sarcoma is typically associated with pain, mast cells, and calcification; look carefully for evidence of a biphasic pattern. Malignant schwannoma usually arises from a large nerve or in the setting of von Recklinghausen neurofibromatosis. Fibrosarcoma usually has no giant cells, but giant cells are frequently present in MFH and other pleomorphic sarcomas. Carcinomas can grow not only in a spindle cell pattern but may also show a storiform arrangement; renal cell carcinoma is particularly likely to do this. Melanoma, too, can have a spindle cell pattern. Also, many benign lesions can show spindle cell growth, eg, fasciitis, fibrohistiocytic tumors, and nerve sheath tumors, as well as fibromatoses, including desmoid tumors (in the gray zone between benign and malignant).

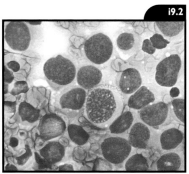
Round cell sarcoma

The round cell pattern includes "small blue cell tumors" of childhood and other small cell sarcomas; the differential diagnosis includes small cell carcinomas and lymphomas. The pleomorphic pattern is epitomized by MFH and seems to be the final common pathway of many tumors. Once a general category has been determined, look carefully for distinguishing features (eg, rhabdomyoblasts, lipoblasts, osteoid). If no specific features can be demonstrated, a pleomorphic sarcoma is "thrown into the wastebasket" of MFH.

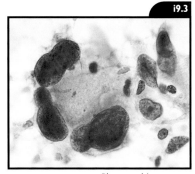
Pleomorphic sarcoma

t9.2 Differential Diagnosis of Sarcomas by Cell Shape

Cell Shape	Sarcoma	Differential Diagnosis
Spindle cell	Fibrosarcoma; rhabdomyosarcoma; leiomyosarcoma; liposarcoma; malignant schwannoma; osteosarcoma (especially fibroblastic); malignant fibrous histiocytoma; angiosarcoma; monophasic synovial sarcoma; hemangiopericytoma	Spindle cell carcinoma; melanoma; fasciitis; fibromatosis; fibrous histiocytoma; others
Round cell	Rhabdomyosarcoma (embryonal, alveolar); neuroblastoma; PNET; Ewing sarcoma; Wilms tumor; liposarcoma, round cell; angiosarcoma (poorly differentiated); synovial sarcoma (poorly differentiated); chondrosarcoma, mesenchymal; osteosarcoma, small cell type; epithelioid leiomyosarcoma; hemangiopericytoma	Small cell carcinoma; lymphoma/leukemia; melanoma; Merkel cell tumor; glomus tumor; carcinoid; paraganglioma; others
Pleomorphic	Malignant fibrous histiocytoma; liposarcoma, pleomorphic; rhabdomyosarcoma, pleomorphic; leiomyosarcoma, poorly differentiated; osteosarcoma; malignant schwannoma	Benign soft tissue tumors sometimes contain pleomorphic cells, eg, pleomorphic lipoma, benign nerve sheath tumors, fibrous histiocytoma, and leiomyoma; also, other types of malignancies can have pleomorphic cells, such as melanoma, anaplastic lymphomas, and carcinomas (eg, of lung, pancreas, and thyroid)

PNET, primitive neuroectodermal tumor.

Palisades of nuclei are prominent in nerve sheath tumors, particularly schwannomas, smooth muscle tumors, and meningiomas, but usually are not seen in fibroblastic tumors. Rosettes are suggestive of neural differentiation and are common in neuroblastoma, PNET, and other neuroendocrine carcinomas but are not specific.

The shapes of the nuclei in spindle cells can be helpful but are not specific. Neural tumors typically have wavy, bent, or twisted nuclei; smooth muscle tumors have blunt, cigar-shaped nuclei; and fibrous tumors have tapered nuclei.

Sarcoma bodies (intracellular or extracellular hyaline globules) |i9.4| are relatively common in sarcomas, eg, MFH, pleomorphic liposarcoma, and Kaposi sarcoma, but again are not specific (see Chapter 8). A myxoid background is common in sarcomas. Myxoid tumors may be fibroblastic, chondroblastic, myoblastic, or neurogenic, as well as a variety of other origins (see p 174). Myxoid sarcomas generally have a better prognosis than their nonmyxoid counterparts. Mast cells are frequently present in synovial sarcoma, neurofibroma/sarcoma, glomus tumor, hemangiopericytoma, and myxoid degeneration in lipoma, among others.

Many tumors can show calcification. However, calcification is rarely seen in certain sarcomas, such as liposarcoma and

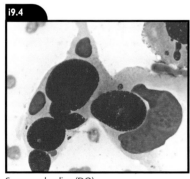
i9.4
Sarcoma bodies (DQ)

myxoid chondrosarcoma. Sometimes the pattern of calcification can be useful in distinguishing various tumors, eg, calcified hemangiomas have phleboliths with regular contours. Synovial sarcoma shows punctate calcification, which is concentrated at the periphery. Hemangiopericytoma displays so-called sweeping calcification. Ossification may follow calcification. Certain tumors are associated with osteoid or bone formation, such as osteosarcoma, synovial sarcoma, liposarcoma, MFH, and carcinosarcoma. Certain tumors are prone to cystic change, such as nerve sheath tumors, MFH, synovial sarcoma, smooth muscle tumors, and liposarcoma.

9.2 Spindle Cell Tumors

9.2.1 Nodular Fasciitis

Nodular fasciitis is a benign spindle cell tumor that can mimic malignancy. It is characterized by rapid growth but small size, and typical superficial location. It never grows in long sweeping fascicles or a herringbone pattern, but it may show a focal storiform pattern with loosely arranged bundles. The aspirate is usually rich in cells and has a myxoid background (active phase) |i9.5|, |i9.6|. The tumor cells are myofibroblasts, which are plump spindle to stellate cells, with active nuclei and prominent nucleoli but bland chromatin. Mitotic figures are frequent but not abundant, and none are atypical. Some chronic inflammation may be seen, but there is little or no hemosiderin. Variants of this tumor include proliferative fasciitis and proliferative myositis with basophilic ganglion-like giant cells (which can result in a pleomorphic cytologic picture).

9.2.2 Desmoid, Fibromatosis

Fibromatoses and desmoid tumors can occur in many sites, including the palm or sole. The tumor is poorly circumscribed; it may infiltrate muscle. The aspirate is poorly cellular; a few slender (not plump) fibroblasts without cytologic atypia may be seen. The tumor has abundant collagen (which does not aspirate well), but there usually is little or no myxoid stroma (except very early, such as fibromatosis colli in a neonate). Mitotic figures are rare or absent. There is neither significant inflammation nor necrosis.

9.2.3 Fibrosarcoma

Fibrosarcoma is a rare tumor that is often in the differential diagnosis but is seldom the final diagnosis |i9.7|, |i9.8|. It usually occurs in a superficial location but is extremely rare on the

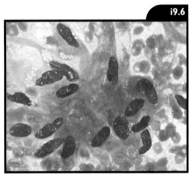
Nodular fasciitis (P)

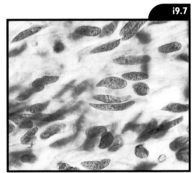
Nodular fasciitis (DQ)

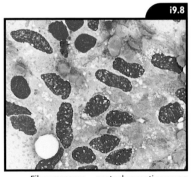
Fibrosarcoma (P)

Fibrosarcoma—metachromatic young collagen (DQ)

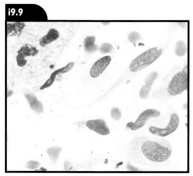

Benign fibrous histiocytoma (DQ)

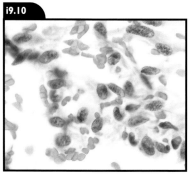

Dermatofibrosarcoma protuberans (P)

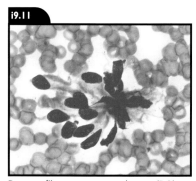

Dermatofibrosarcoma protuberans (DQ)

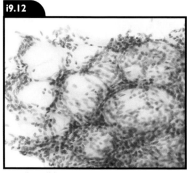

Spindle cell lipoma (P)

palm or sole (unlike fibromatosis). Fibrosarcoma is not associated with origin from nerves or with von Recklinghausen disease (unlike nerve sheath tumors). The cytology shows densely packed spindle cells, which grow in a herringbone pattern, histologically. By definition, no other specific differentiation is seen. The cells may show mild to moderate but not marked anaplasia. Mitotic figures, including atypical forms, may be observed. Necrosis may be seen. However, there are no giant cells and no bizarre tumors cells (if present, consider MFH). The periodic acid–Schiff (PAS) stain is negative. Mast cells and calcification are not present.

9.2.4 Benign Fibrous Histiocytoma

Benign fibrous histiocytoma, although not well circumscribed, typically occurs in the superficial soft tissue and rarely is deep seated. Mitotic figures can be seen, but none are atypical. The tumor is composed of spindle cell fibroblasts and rounded histiocyte-like cells that grow in a storiform but not herringbone pattern. Lipophages, siderophages, and Touton giant cells can be seen |i9.9|.

9.2.5 Dermatofibrosarcoma Protuberans

Dermatofibrosarcoma protuberans is a solitary tumor with infiltrative margins. It is composed of small, uniform, spindle cells with tapered nuclei. A prominent storiform growth pattern is characteristic, and a pinwheel configuration of the cells may be seen in cytology |i9.10|, |i9.11|. There are no giant cells, inflammatory cells, histiocytes, or xanthoma cells and no necrosis. The tumor is CD34 positive.

9.2.6 Malignant Fibrous Histiocytoma

MFH usually is a pleomorphic tumor; however, occasionally, spindle cells predominate (see "Pleomorphic Tumors," p 172).

9.2.7 Spindle Cell Lipoma

Spindle cell lipoma arises in the superficial soft tissue with characteristic location (neck, shoulder), age (45-70), sex (male), and circumscription. The tumor is composed of uniform spindle cells associated with mature collagen |i9.12|. There are neither lipoblasts nor multinucleated giant cells.

9.2.8 Liposarcoma

Liposarcoma can sometimes grow as a spindle cell neoplasm. Look for lipoblasts (see p 174). Liposarcomas are S-100 positive.

9.2.9 Leiomyoma and Leiomyosarcoma

Smooth muscle tumors, benign or malignant, usually are characterized by plump spindle cells with blunt nuclei |**i9.13**|, |**i9.14**|. The cytoplasm is dense; myofibers and perinuclear vacuoles may be appreciated. Although benign tumors (leiomyomas) are usually monomorphic with few or no mitotic figures, they can be pleomorphic or have increased mitotic figures and still behave in a benign fashion. The nuclei may form palisades, suggesting a neural tumor, but there are no neurites. Hyalinization and cystic change are possible. The cells are PAS positive and S-100 negative; muscle markers, such as muscle-specific actin, smooth muscle actin, and desmin, are positive.

9.2.10 Rhabdomyosarcoma

Rhabdomyosarcoma occasionally can be a spindle cell neoplasm. The cells are PAS positive. (See "Rhabdomyosarcoma [Embryonal, Alveolar]," p 171.)

9.2.11 Angiosarcoma

Angiosarcoma can be a spindle cell tumor. Look for neovessels and intracytoplasmic RBCs to make the diagnosis. The tumor expresses CD31, CD34, and factor VIII.

9.2.12 Monophasic Synovial Sarcoma

Synovial sarcoma, although classically a biphasic tumor, often grows predominantly and sometimes exclusively in a spindle cell pattern (monophasic synovial sarcoma) characterized by monomorphic, bland, spindle cells. Look carefully for plumper epithelioid cells, best appreciated in Diff-Quik, to suggest a biphasic pattern (see "Biphasic Tumors," p 175).

9.2.13 Benign Nerve Sheath Tumors

Benign nerve sheath tumors, including neurofibroma and schwannoma, are usually of long duration and often multiple (particularly in von Recklinghausen disease) |**i9.15**|, |**i9.16**|. Nuclear palisades are characteristic; Verocay bodies may be seen in schwannomas. The nuclei typically are wavy, bent, twisted, or squiggly. Neural differentiation, such as tactoid bodies or pacinian corpuscles, may occur and helps determine neural origin of the tumor. The tumor does not grow in a storiform or herringbone pattern. Bizarre degenerated cells may be present in benign tumors, but there are few or no mitotic figures, particularly in schwannoma. Inflammation is insignificant. The cells are S-100 positive.

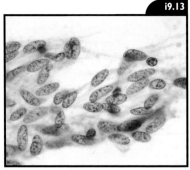

i9.13

Low-grade leiomyosarcoma (P)

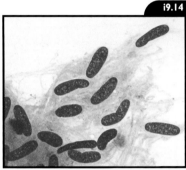

i9.14

Low-grade leiomyosarcoma (DQ)

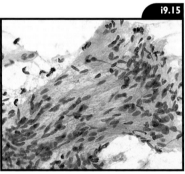

i9.15

Nerve sheath tumor, schwannoma (P)

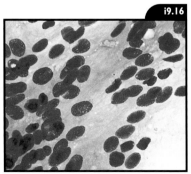

i9.16

Schwannoma—nuclear palisades (DQ)

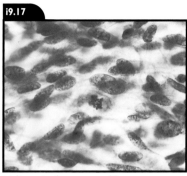

Malignant schwannoma (P)

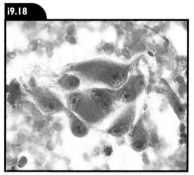

Wound healing—myofibroblasts (P)

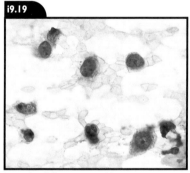

Round cell liposarcoma (P)

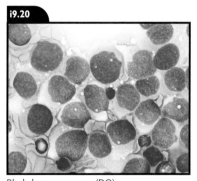

Rhabdomyosarcoma (DQ)

9.2.14 Malignant Schwannoma

Malignant schwannoma usually occurs in patients older than 35 years. The tumor is typically associated with a large nerve or occurs in the setting of von Recklinghausen disease. The patients may have projected pain. Densely cellular areas alternate with hypocellular myxoid areas |i9.17|. Variable cell types, including spindle, round, and multinucleated giant cells, may be seen. The spindle cells may form sweeping but variable fascicles, whorls, or palisades. Myxoid change, cartilage or bone formation, and even skeletal muscle (ie, triton tumor), as well as mucin-positive glands, can occur. Glycogen is absent or scant (usually PAS negative). Neural markers, such as S-100, are positive except in high-grade malignancies.

9.2.15 Osteosarcoma (Fibroblastic)

Fibroblastic osteosarcoma is a spindle cell tumor. Look for malignant osteoid to make the diagnosis (see p 173).

9.2.16 Reactive Fibrosis, Scar

Reactive fibrosis or scars are related to trauma. Scars show variable patterns but often are associated with myofibroblasts |i9.18| and granulation tissue. Stromal fragments of collagen with embedded spindle cells may be aspirated. Inflammation and hemorrhage, with hemosiderin-laden macrophages, also may be seen.

9.2.17 Other Spindle Cell Tumors

A variety of other tumors can have spindle tumor cells, including clear cell sarcoma, epithelioid sarcoma, Kaposi sarcoma, and hemangiopericytoma. Also to be considered in the differential diagnosis of spindle cell sarcomas are spindle cell carcinoma and spindle cell melanoma.

Spindle Cell Carcinoma

Carcinomas are malignant tumors characterized by epithelial differentiation. Mucin production (particularly neutral type) is typical; glycogen production also may be seen. A history of a known primary tumor is, of course, helpful. An associated dysplasia speaks for a primary lesion. Suspect spindle cell carcinoma if the spindle cell tumor is found in a visceral organ or lymph node. Epithelial markers, such as keratin, are positive.

Spindle Cell Melanoma

Melanoma also can grow in a spindle cell pattern, mimicking a sarcoma. A known history of melanoma can be extremely helpful in pointing to the correct diagnosis. Junctional change in a primary lesion is also helpful. The tumor cells are not necessarily pigmented. S-100 and HMB-45 are positive; keratin is negative. The cells may contain PAS-positive glycogen, but they do not produce mucin. Suspect this diagnosis if the spindle cell tumor is in the skin, subcutaneous tissue, or lymph node.

9.3 Round Cell Tumors

9.3.1 Round Cell Liposarcoma

Round cell liposarcoma is a "small blue cell tumor" |**i9.19**|; lipoblasts are required for the specific diagnosis of liposarcoma (see p 174). Naked nuclei are common due to fragility of the scant vacuolated cytoplasm. Look for transitions to myxoid liposarcoma to assist in the diagnosis.

9.3.2 Rhabdomyosarcoma (Embryonal, Alveolar)

Rhabdomyosarcoma is a round cell tumor |**i9.20**| in which rhabdomyoblasts are the key diagnostic cells. Rhabdomyoblasts are PAS positive. Although cross-striations are rarely identified, particularly in cytologic specimens, other features, such as thick and thin filament in electron microscopy or immunocytologic evidence of skeletal muscle differentiation, may be observed. Floret cells and multinucleated giant cells also can occur. Skeletal muscle markers, such as muscle-specific actin and desmin, are positive.

9.3.3 Neuroectodermal Tumors

Neuroendocrine neoplasms of neural crest origin, including neuroblastoma |**i9.21**| and PNET |**i9.22**|, show a cytologic pattern of uniform, small round blue cells, and may have neurites and rosettes. These tumors characteristically express neuroendocrine markers, such as neuron-specific enolase, synaptophysin, and S-100. Ewing sarcoma is a closely related, poorly differentiated tumor forming a spectrum (Ewing → PNET → neuroblastoma) that may show a characteristic dimorphic pattern |**i9.23**|.

9.3.4 Miscellaneous Round Cell Tumors

A wide variety of other soft tissue tumors can be composed of round cells, including angiosarcoma (poorly differentiated), mesenchymal chondrosarcoma (look for cartilage in small round cell background), small cell osteosarcoma (look for diagnostic osteoid) |**i9.24**|, mesenchymal chondrosarcoma (look

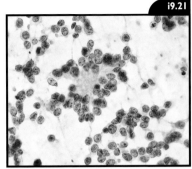
Neuroblastoma—rosette (P)

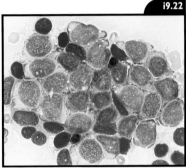
PNET (DQ)

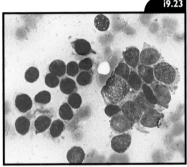
Ewing sarcoma—dimorphic cells (DQ)

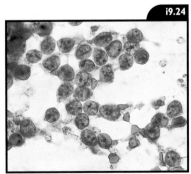
Small cell osteosarcoma (P)

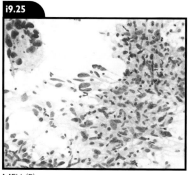

MFH (P)

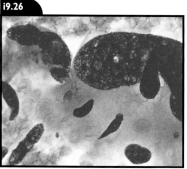

MFH (DQ)

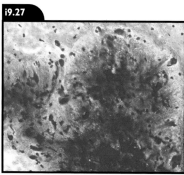

Myxoid MFH (DQ)

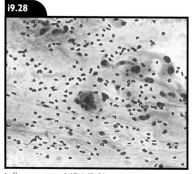

Inflammatory MFH (DQ)

for chondromyxoid stroma), epithelioid smooth muscle tumors (look for conventional spindle cell areas), and glomus tumor. Also consider carcinoid tumors, small cell carcinomas, Wilms tumor, lymphoma/leukemia, and melanoma.

9.4 Pleomorphic Tumors

9.4.1 Malignant Fibrous Histiocytoma

MFH is the classic example of a pleomorphic sarcoma. By definition, it shows no specific differentiation. MFH occurs in older patients, is usually greater than 3 cm in diameter, is deep-seated, and grows rapidly. The tumor is characterized by a strikingly malignant cytologic appearance. The cells are usually highly pleomorphic, including anaplastic tumor giant cells |i9.25|, |i9.26|. Mitotic figures, including atypical forms, are easy to find. Some cases show a myxoid stroma (myxoid MFH |i9.27|) or a conspicuous inflammatory infiltrate (inflammatory MFH |i9.28|). Also, most spindle cell sarcomas with abundant hyalinized collagen are MFH. A storiform growth pattern is typical but may not be appreciable. Hemorrhage, necrosis, and hemosiderin-laden macrophages are common. Benign-appearing Touton or osteoclastic giant cells also may be present. As stated above, there is no evidence of specific differentiation, such as lipoblasts, rhabdomyoblasts, malignant bone or cartilage, or unequivocal smooth muscle differentiation. The tumor cells are PAS negative. The tumor is typically positive for CD68, as well as for α_1-antitrypsin and α_1-antichymotrypsin.

9.4.2 Pleomorphic Liposarcoma

Pleomorphic liposarcoma is a pleomorphic sarcoma similar in appearance to MFH, except that lipoblasts are present |i9.29|. In contrast with MFH, this tumor never grows in a storiform pattern. S-100 is positive.

9.4.3 Pleomorphic Lipoma

Pleomorphic lipoma is a pleomorphic but benign tumor that contains floret cells and other multinucleated giant cells. Rare atypical mitotic figures can be present.

9.4.4 Pleomorphic Rhabdomyosarcoma

Pleomorphic rhabdomyosarcoma, formerly a common diagnosis, is now considered a rare tumor. Specific evidence of skeletal muscle differentiation must be identified to diagnose this tumor, such as rhabdomyoblasts with cross-striations (light microscope), thick and thin filaments (electron microscope), or desmin (immunocytochemistry).

9.4.5 Poorly Differentiated Leiomyosarcoma

Poorly differentiated leiomyosarcoma is a pleomorphic neoplasm that usually arises in vessels, interskeletal muscle, or the uterus |i9.30|. The cytoplasm is dense but may show prominent vacuolization (not lipoblasts). There are no benign-appearing giant cells, as can sometimes be seen in MFH. The cells may form bundles. There is little collagen production and few inflammatory cells. The cells are PAS positive. Myogenic differentiation must be demonstrated for a specific diagnosis (see p 169).

9.4.6 Atypical (Benign) Leiomyoma

Atypical leiomyoma is composed of large pleomorphic cells that are occasionally multinucleated. The nuclei are hyperchromatic, but mitotic figures are not seen. The atypia is usually not diffuse, so areas of more typical leiomyoma usually are present (see p 169).

9.4.7 Osteosarcoma

Osteosarcoma usually occurs in young patients. The malignant tumor cells are typically pleomorphic. Osteoid produced by malignant cells is diagnostic |i9.31|. Chondroid also can be seen. So-called reverse zoning is a characteristic feature seen in tissue. The tumor is infiltrative, and growth is not limited.

9.4.8 Malignant Schwannoma

Malignant schwannoma can be a pleomorphic |i9.32| or spindle cell sarcoma (see p 170).

9.4.9 Ancient Schwannoma

Ancient schwannoma, which has pleomorphic but benign tumor cells, is associated with von Recklinghausen disease. The aspiration may be painful. Spindle cells have tapered nuclei; Verocay bodies may be seen. Large, pleomorphic, hyperchromatic, often multilobulated nuclei are present, which may suggest malignancy. However, the changes are degenerative in nature: the chromatin is smudged, not crisp and distinct, and there are no mitotic figures.

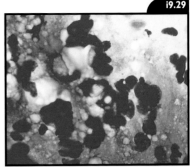

Pleomorphic liposarcoma (DQ)

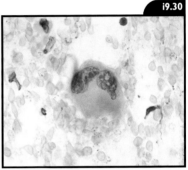

High-grade leiomyosarcoma (P)

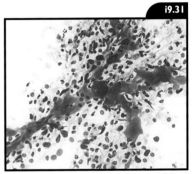

Osteosarcoma—metachromatic osteoid (DQ)

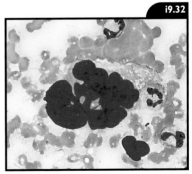

Malignant schwannoma (DQ)

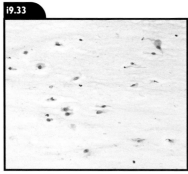

Myxoma (P)

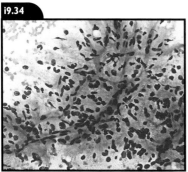

Myxoid liposarcoma (DQ)

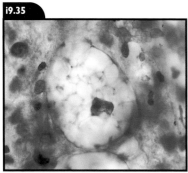

Lipoblast (P)

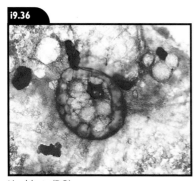

Lipoblasts (DQ)

9.4.10 Other Pleomorphic Tumors

Carcinoma

Carcinomas of the lung and pancreas, among others, can give rise to pleomorphic tumor cells. These tumors characteristically express epithelial markers, such as keratin.

Melanoma

Malignant melanoma commonly has anaplastic tumor cells. S-100 and HMB-45 are characteristically positive; keratin is negative.

9.5 Myxoid Tumors

9.5.1 Myxoma

Myxomas typically occur in deep intramuscular sites. The aspirate obtains abundant mucoid material with only a few bland to reactive appearing mesenchymal cells |i9.33|. The myxoid stroma is alcian blue positive and hyaluronidase sensitive. There are few or no blood vessels, and mitotic figures are rare or absent. By definition, there are no lipoblasts, rhabdomyoblasts, chondroblasts, or osteoblasts.

9.5.2 Myxoid Liposarcoma

Myxoid liposarcoma has abundant myxoid stroma in which vascularity is prominent, often forming a plexiform or "chicken wire fence" arrangement |i9.34|. The sarcoma is composed of bland spindle or stellate cells. Lipoblasts, in which small lipid vacuoles indent and scallop the nucleus, are diagnostic in this setting |i9.35|, |i9.36|. Mitotic figures may be present but are infrequent. There are no bizarre tumor cells (as seen in pleomorphic liposarcoma). Liposarcomas are S-100 positive.

9.5.3 Myxolipoma

Myxolipoma is a benign lipoma with myxoid stroma.

9.5.4 Rhabdomyosarcoma

Embryonal rhabdomyosarcoma (particularly the botryoid type) typically has a myxoid stroma (see p 171).

9.5.5 Myxoid MFH

MFH frequently has a myxoid stroma; when this is a dominant feature, the diagnosis of myxoid MFH can be made. Myxoid MFH has a better prognosis than ordinary MFH (see p 172).

9.5.6 Chondrosarcoma

Chondrosarcoma is a pure cartilage-producing malignant tumor. The cytology is characterized by neoplastic chondrocytes in a myxochondroid matrix, which is intensely metachromatic in Diff-Quik |i9.37|. Chondrocytes are differentiated cartilage cells within lacunar spaces.

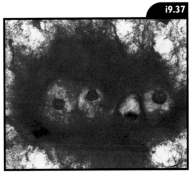

Chondrosarcoma (DQ)

9.5.7 Myxoid Chondrosarcoma

Myxoid chondrosarcoma has an abundant myxoid stroma in which malignant chondrocytes are found. The appearance of the aspirate is reminiscent of pleomorphic adenoma of the salivary gland |i9.38|. S-100 is positive, but the tumor is keratin negative in contrast with chordoma and metastatic carcinoma.

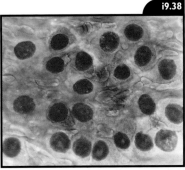

Myxoid chondrosarcoma (DQ)

9.5.8 Chordoma

Chordoma is a tumor that usually occurs in the midline at the ends of the vertebral column, particularly the lumbar-sacral area of the spine. Bone may be involved. Diagnostic physaliphorous (bubble bearing) cells may be seen |i9.39|. Vessels are sparse. The stroma is intensely metachromatic and mucicarmine positive. It characteristically surrounds individual tumor cells |i9.40|. The cells are S-100 and keratin positive (compare chondrosarcoma). The combination of keratin-positive cells and mucicarmine-positive stroma may suggest metastatic carcinoma.

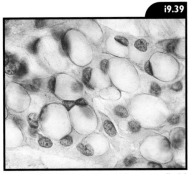

Chordoma—physaliphorous cells (P)

9.5.9 Miscellaneous Myxoid Tumors

A variety of other tumors can have a myxoid stroma, including myxoid fibrosarcoma, leiomyosarcoma, synovial sarcoma, hemangiopericytoma, malignant schwannoma, nodular fasciitis, and traumatic neuroma (with myxoid change this tumor closely resembles nodular fasciitis), as well as colloid carcinomas and, occasionally, melanoma.

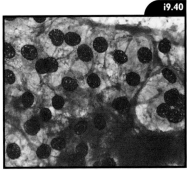

Chordoma (DQ)

9.6 **Biphasic Tumors**

9.6.1 Synovial Sarcoma

Synovial sarcoma is a classic example of a biphasic soft tissue tumor with spindle and epithelioid cells. Synovial sarcoma is a relatively common soft tissue tumor. The patients are usually adolescents or young adults (12-35 years old). The tumor typically occurs near a large joint, particularly the knee, and often is painful. The cytology shows monomorphous spindle cells with

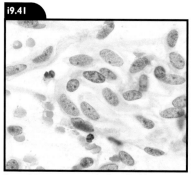

Synovial sarcoma—spindle cells (P)

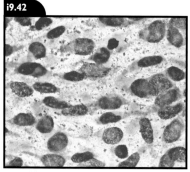

Synovial sarcoma—spindle cells (DQ)

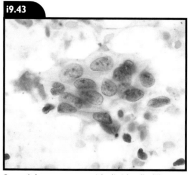

Synovial sarcoma—epithelioid cells (P)

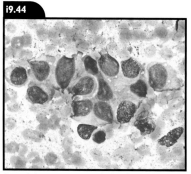

Synovial sarcoma—epithelioid cells (DQ)

highly cellular areas |i9.41|,|i9.42|. Look carefully for a biphasic pattern (plump epithelioid cells) that, when subtle, may be easier to appreciate in cytology than histology |i9.43|, |i9.44|. If well-formed glands are present (biphasic synovial sarcoma), they are PAS positive, but the stromal cells are PAS negative. Occasionally, cartilage is present (which excludes hemangiopericytoma). A mast cell infiltrate is characteristic but not specific. Mast cells have metachromatic cytoplasmic granules. The vascularity of the tumor ranges from scant to predominant (hemangiopericytomatous). Secondary changes, such as hemorrhage, hemosiderin-laden macrophages, multinucleated giant cells, chronic inflammation, or cholesterol crystals, may be seen. Keratin is positive, particularly in the epithelioid cells.

9.6.2 Epithelioid Sarcoma

Epithelioid sarcoma occurs in about the same age group as synovial sarcoma, but most occur in the hand (particularly the fingers), forearm, and elsewhere, rather than near large joints. The tumor grows in a multinodular pattern with central necrosis, mimicking granulomatous inflammation. The cells have dense cytoplasm that stains deeply eosinophilic (in Papanicolaou stain), mimicking epithelial cells. Also, like epithelial cells, the tumor cells are keratin positive. Although the tumor is classically biphasic |i9.45|, with spindle and epithelioid cells, there is not as sharp a demarcation between cell types as there is in synovial sarcoma. Also, the tumor frequently is associated with skin ulceration, unlike synovial sarcoma. In contrast with primary squamous cell carcinoma, there is no associated dysplasia. Furthermore, there are no gland-like structures, no intracellular mucin, no squamous pearls, no nesting (unlike melanoma), and no other primary tumor in epithelioid sarcoma.

9.6.3 Clear Cell Sarcoma

Clear cell sarcoma (clear cell melanoma of soft parts) usually has a distinct biphasic pattern including clear cells, typically forming nests of cells. The cells have pale nuclei with prominent nucleoli. There are few mitotic figures. The cells may contain PAS-positive glycogen, but neither lipid nor intracellular or extracellular mucin is present. The cells are keratin negative and S-100 positive.

9.6.4 Malignant Glandular Schwannoma

Malignant schwannoma with gland formation is an extremely rare biphasic tumor that occurs more often in patients with von Recklinghausen disease. The glands are of the intestinal type. Epithelioid cells can also occur |**i9.46**|. The tumor may be associated with rhabdomyosarcoma (a form of triton tumor). The tumor is S-100 positive (see p 170).

9.6.5 Epithelioid Smooth Muscle Tumor

Epithelioid smooth muscle tumors are composed of plump epithelioid tumor cells but often include a component of more typical spindle smooth muscle cells (a clue to the diagnosis), forming a biphasic pattern |**i9.47**|, |**i9.48**| (see p 169).

t9.3 Summary of Immunocytochemical Markers

Tumor	Characteristic Marker
Dermatofibrosarcoma protuberans	CD34
Malignant fibrous histiocytoma	CD68, α_1-antitrypsin, α_1-antichymotrypsin
Liposarcoma	S-100
Leiomyosarcoma	Muscle-specific actin, smooth muscle actin, desmin
Rhabdomyosarcoma	Muscle-specific actin, desmin
Angiosarcoma	CD34, CD31, factor VIII
Synovial sarcoma	Keratin (epithelioid cells)
Nerve sheath tumors	S-100 (except high-grade malignant schwannoma)
Neuroblastoma	NSE, neurofilaments, synaptophysin
Primitive neuroectodermal tumor	Vimentin, synaptophysin, NSE
Chondrosarcoma	S-100 (keratin negative)
Chordoma	S-100, keratin
Epithelioid sarcoma`	Keratin
Carcinoma	Keratin
Melanoma	S-100, HMB-45 (keratin negative)

NSE, neuron-specific enolase.

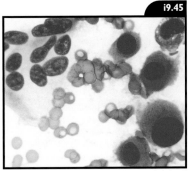

i9.45

Epithelioid sarcoma (DQ)

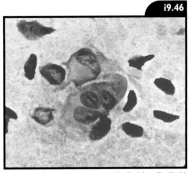

i9.46

Schwannoma—epithelioid cells (DQ)

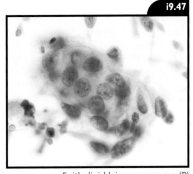

i9.47

Epithelioid leiomyosarcoma (P)

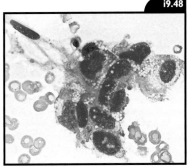

i9.48

Epithelioid leiomyosarcoma (DQ)

Head and Neck

Justifiably accepted as the initial diagnostic procedure for head and neck tumors, fine needle aspiration (FNA) biopsy is particularly useful in this region since so many disparate entities may be considered in the differential diagnosis. For example, nodules in the neck could be due to diseases involving the salivary glands, lymph nodes, thyroid, parathyroid, skin, soft tissue, or nerves. The diagnostic spectrum ranges from innocuous inflammation to life-threatening malignancy. In children, most head and neck masses are benign; however, in adults, most (nonthyroid masses) are malignant, often metastatic, frequently squamous cell carcinoma.

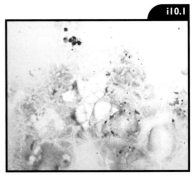

Thyroglossal duct cyst (DQ)

10.1 Cervical Cysts

The differential diagnosis of cervical cysts includes neoplasms with a cystic component and nonneoplastic cystic conditions. The two classic nonneoplastic cervical cysts are thyroglossal duct cysts and lymphoepithelial cysts. Neoplastic cervical cysts include such entities as papillary carcinoma of the thyroid and squamous cell carcinoma, which may present as cystic metastases. Cystic lesions are well-known sources of false-negative diagnoses. To reduce false negatives, drain the cyst as completely as possible, reaspirate any residual mass, and excise recurring cysts. Other cystic lesions of the head and neck region include cysts of the salivary gland, thyroid, parathyroid, and thymus, as well as dermoid/epidermoid cysts and cystic hygroma.

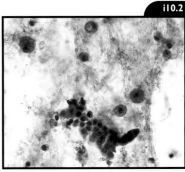

Thyroglossal duct cyst (P)

10.1.1 Thyroglossal Duct Cyst

Thyroglossal duct cysts are the classic midline cysts. They arise from embryonic remnants of the thyroglossal duct, which descends from the base of the tongue into the neck to form the thyroid gland. Although thyroglossal duct cysts can be found anywhere along this track, they are usually found in proximity—often attached—to the hyoid bone. Thyroglossal duct cysts should be distinguished from thyroid cysts, which are far more common and occur in the thyroid gland itself. Virtually any disease that affects the thyroid may (rarely) occur in a thyroglossal duct cyst, including Hashimoto thyroiditis and malignancy, most often papillary carcinoma.

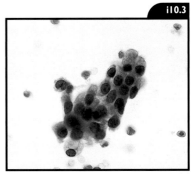

Thyroglossal duct cyst—thyroid cells (P)

The FNA biopsy of thyroglossal duct cysts obtains clear, mucinous, or "grungy" material, which usually contains few cells other than macrophages |i10.1|, |i10.2|, |i10.3|, |i10.4|. However, glandular, squamous, or ciliated respiratory-type cells may be obtained

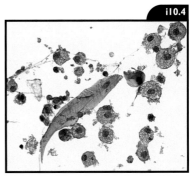

Thyroglossal duct cyst—atypical squamous cell (P)

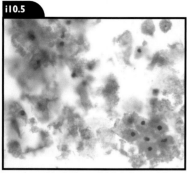

Lymphoepithelial/branchial cleft cyst (P)

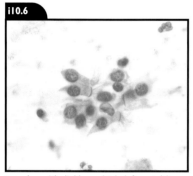

Lymphoepithelial/branchial cleft cyst (P)

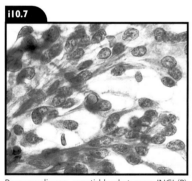

Paraganglioma, carotid body tumor, INCI (P)

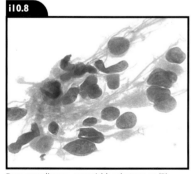

Paraganglioma, carotid body tumor (P)

from the lining of the cyst. Diagnostic thyroid tissue may occur in the wall of the cyst, but this is rarely observed in the aspirate. When present, the thyroid follicular cells often appear degenerated, with hemosiderin granules. Acute or chronic inflammation, cholesterol crystals, and reactive epithelial atypia also may be seen.

10.1.2 Branchial Cleft and Lymphoepithelial Cysts

Branchial cleft cysts and lymphoepithelial cysts are the classic lateral cysts in the neck. They can arise due to either cystic change occurring in congenital remnants of the branchial clefts, ie, branchial cleft cyst, or cystic change in salivary gland inclusions (usually parotid) trapped in cervical lymph nodes during embryologic development, ie, lymphoepithelial cyst. Similar cysts occur in the parotid gland in association with HIV infection (see page 192).

These cysts usually are found along the anterior border of the sternocleidomastoid muscle, usually near the upper middle third. They most often come to clinical attention in young patients, typically between the ages of 10 and 30 years, but can be seen at any age. Usually painless unless inflamed, they may produce a rapidly growing firm mass, suggesting malignancy in some cases.

The cysts are surrounded by dense lymphoid tissue and lined with squamous or glandular epithelium, or both (mucoepidermoid lining). The aspirate usually obtains turbid fluid, composed of proteinaceous material, mucus, foam cells, and sometimes cholesterol crystals. Epithelial cells tend to be sparse, but in some cases numerous squamous cells are present |i10.5|, which may impart a pearly or purulent gross appearance to the fluid. Glandular cells may be mucous, goblet, or ciliated (respiratory-type) |i10.6|, with bland nuclei and foamy to slightly granular cytoplasm. Inflammatory and degenerative changes are common. Lymphoid tissue, including follicular center cells and tingible body macrophages, may be aspirated. Keratin can elicit a granulomatous inflammatory response with giant cells and epithelioid histiocytes. The differential diagnosis of reactive (inflammatory) atypia occurring in a benign cyst vs a cystic metastasis of very well-differentiated carcinoma can be difficult in some cases.

10.1.3 Parathyroid Cysts

Parathyroid cysts usually occur in the lower neck but can be found anywhere from the angle of the mandible to the mediastinum. Most patients are older than 30 years, but there is a wide age range. Parathyroid cysts often are misdiagnosed clinically as a goiter or thyroid neoplasm. They are usually non-functioning.

Parathyroid cysts characteristically contain thin, clear, colorless fluid that looks like water (a clue to the diagnosis). However, some contain golden brown fluid, grossly indistinguishable from that obtained from thyroid cysts. Parathyroid cysts are usually poorly cellular, and even when cells are present, they are difficult to identify specifically as parathyroid. The fluid can be analyzed for parathormone (high) and thyroglobulin (low) to confirm the diagnosis.

10.1.4 Dermoid and Epidermoid Cysts

Dermoid and epidermoid cysts are developmental cysts that usually occur in the vicinity of the mouth, eye, or nose. Occasionally, they occur in the neck, usually near the midline, or in the submandibular triangle.

Epidermoid cysts contain only squamous epithelium. Dermoid cysts have not only skin but also skin appendages, including hair and sebaceous glands and, occasionally, respiratory-type ciliated epithelium. Sometimes cartilage can be identified. Both types of cysts are filled with a grumous cheesy material derived from keratin. Secondary inflammation may be present, including foreign body granulomas. Rarely, squamous cell carcinoma arises in these cysts, but be wary of inflammatory changes mimicking malignancy.

10.2 Head and Neck Neoplasms

10.2.1 Cervical Paraganglioma (Carotid Body Tumor, Glomus Jugulare)

Paragangliomas are neoplasms usually derived from chemoreceptor tissue of a paraganglion, such as the carotid body or glomus jugulare. Paragangliomas are composed of carcinoid-like (epithelioid) cells and spindle cells, which can range from uniform to markedly pleomorphic |i10.7|, |i10.8|, |i10.9|, |i10.10| |i10.11|. Rosettes may be seen, and "Zellballen" (rounded balls of tumor cells) are characteristic in tissue |i10.12|. The nuclei range from round to oval to spindle. Chromatin varies from "salt and pepper" to dense. Intranuclear cytoplasmic invaginations may suggest papillary thyroid carcinoma. The differential diagnosis with medullary thyroid carcinoma may be impossible based on cytologic findings alone. Pleomorphic spindle or giant cells may suggest a sarcoma. Rosettes may suggest adenocarcinoma. The cells express neuroendocrine markers, such as synaptophysin and chromogranin but not calcitonin, and are usually keratin negative.

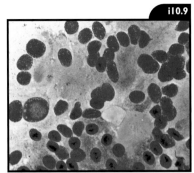
Paraganglioma, carotid body tumor (DQ)

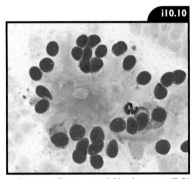
Paraganglioma, carotid body tumor (DQ)

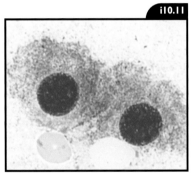
Paraganglioma, carotid body tumor (DQ, oil)

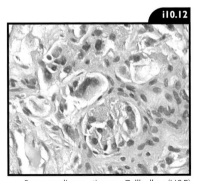
Paraganglioma, tissue—Zellballen (H&E)

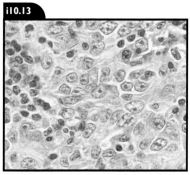

Nasopharyngeal carcinoma, tissue (H&E)

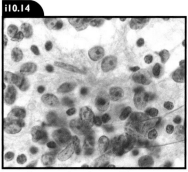

Nasopharyngeal carcinoma (P)

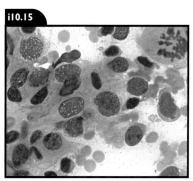

Nasopharyngeal carcinoma (DQ)

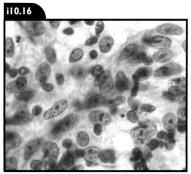

Nasopharyngeal carcinoma—spindle cells (P)

10.2.2 Nasopharyngeal Carcinoma

Nasopharyngeal carcinoma is a poorly differentiated squamous cell carcinoma. Because the tumor is usually accompanied by an intense lymphoid infiltrate, the tumor also is known as lymphoepithelioma |i10.13|. Morphologically similar tumors occur in a number of other sites, including the tonsil, salivary gland, lung, and stomach.

Nasopharyngeal carcinoma is more common in certain geographic areas and ethnic groups (southern China, North Africa, Arctic Eskimos). It is strongly associated with Epstein-Barr virus. There is a bimodal age incidence, with peaks in the teens and 50s; males are more frequently affected than females. Cervical lymphadenopathy is the most common presenting symptom. Some patients have postnasal drip, nose bleeds, impaired hearing, or otitis media. The primary lesion may be occult; even after extensive investigation, the primary tumor remains undetected in 10% to 20% of cases.

The FNA biopsy is cellular and obtains benign lymphoid tissue and cohesive sheets and crowded aggregates (Regaud pattern) or isolated (Schmincke pattern) malignant epithelial cells |i10.14|, |i10.15|. The nuclei are large and round or oval to spindle-shaped |i10.16| but usually not markedly pleomorphic. The nuclear membranes are slightly irregular, and the chromatin is somewhat hyperchromatic. Characteristically, there are one to three prominent nucleoli or macronucleoli. Mitotic figures are usually seen and naked nuclei may be conspicuous. The cytoplasm is usually scant and delicate, with ill-defined borders, producing a characteristic syncytial appearance. Variable degrees of keratinization can be seen in some cases |i10.17|. The background is composed predominantly of small, "mature" lymphocytes. Lymphocytes mixed with syncytial clusters of undifferentiated tumor cells can mimic benign lymphohistiocytic aggregates and may be overlooked. An important diagnostic clue is the presence of very large nucleoli |i10.18|. Plasma cells, macrophages, eosinophils, or giant cells can also be seen. Immunocytochemistry demonstrates keratin. The differential diagnosis includes lymphomas, germ cell tumors, and metastatic poorly differentiated carcinomas arising in other sites, eg, other head and neck tumors and lung cancer.

10.3 Parathyroid

Parathyroid glands are endocrine organs that produce parathyroid hormone (parathormone), which raises serum calcium levels. There are usually four parathyroid glands; each gland weighs 35 to 55 mg. They are usually located in the neck, near the thyroid gland, but can be found anywhere from the submandibular area to the mediastinum. The parathyroid can give rise to cysts (see p 180), hyperplasias, adenomas, and, rarely, carcinomas.

The clinical signs of hyperparathyroidism are chronic renal failure, skeletal lesions (brown tumors), and biochemical abnormalities, including elevated serum levels of calcium, alkaline phosphatase, and parathormone. Most patients with primary hyperparathyroidism have a solitary parathyroid adenoma, some have hyperplasia, and a few have multiple adenomas. Hyperplasia classically involves all four glands, while neoplasms usually involve only one gland |t10.1|.

The FNA biopsy obtains a cellular smear. The cells form thick groups, cohesive sheets, small cords, occasionally microfollicular structures, or less commonly, papillae. The cells are usually small and uniform but can be markedly pleomorphic. Hyperplastic cells tend to be more uniform and form small flat sheets |i10.19|, |i10.20|, while neoplastic cells tend to be more pleomorphic and form large, dense, crowded clusters, but, unfortunately, these distinctions are not absolute.

The nuclei are round to oval and usually smaller than RBCs, although a few larger atypical nuclei commonly are observed, and in some cases, pleomorphism can be prominent, even in benign lesions ("endocrine atypia"). The chromatin may have a typical neuroendocrine salt-and-pepper appearance, but the chromatin texture is variable. Nucleoli usually are inconspicuous but can be multiple and prominent. Naked nuclei may be numerous. The cytoplasm varies from finely vacuolar or clear (chief cells) to oncocytic (oxyphilic cells, reminiscent of Hürthle cells of the thyroid). Parathyroid cells, particularly chief cells, may contain cytoplasmic lipid. There is an inverse relationship between the amount of cytoplasmic lipid and the functional state of the cell: hyperplasia and adenomas have less cytoplasmic lipid, and the lipid droplets are smaller than those in normal or atrophic parathyroid cells. Metachromatic neurosecretory granules can sometimes be observed in the cytoplasm; their presence can be confirmed with silver stains or immunocytochemistry. The cytoplasm is usually periodic acid–Schiff positive due to glycogen content. Dense colloid-like amyloid can occur in these tumors (Congo red stain with apple-green birefringence to confirm).

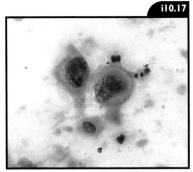
Nasopharyngeal CA—keratinized cells (P)

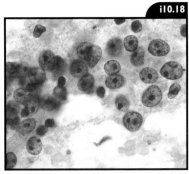
Nasopharyngeal CA—macronucleoli (P)

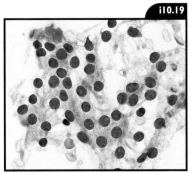
Parathyroid hyperplasia (P)

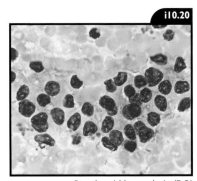
Parathyroid hyperplasia (DQ)

t10.1 Parathyroid Pathology

Favors Hyperplasia	Favors Adenoma
All four glands enlarged	One gland enlarged
Diffuse enlargement (histology)	Rim of compressed tissue (histology)
Cells more uniform	Cells more pleomorphic
Flat, orderly sheets	Dense, crowded clusters

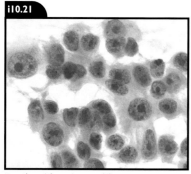

Parathyroid carcinoma (P)

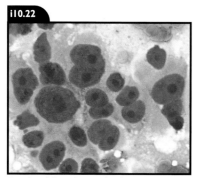

Parathyroid carcinoma (DQ)

Parathyroid carcinoma can be composed of relatively uniform cells to markedly pleomorphic cells, including bizarre giant cells and clear cells |i10.21|, |i10.22|, |i10.23|. Extreme cellularity; dyshesion; diffuse, marked, malignant anaplasia; mitotic figures, particularly abnormal forms; necrosis; and, of course, metastases favor a malignant diagnosis. Note, however, that lytic bone lesions could represent either metastases or brown tumors (osteitis fibrosa cystica) associated with hyperparathyroidism. FNA biopsy can easily distinguish between these two possibilities (epithelioid cells vs pigmented giant histiocytes, respectively).

The differential diagnosis with lesions of the thyroid can be difficult |t10.2|. To complicate matters, parathyroid adenomas coexist with thyroid neoplasms in a significant number of cases (~ 10%). Colloid and macrophages, some of which contain hemosiderin, are associated with thyroid lesions, particularly goiters. Parathyroid cells are usually smaller and have central nuclei with more finely stippled chromatin than thyroid cells, but these differences are subtle at best. Follicular thyroid neoplasms, including Hürthle cell tumors, may be particularly difficult to distinguish from parathyroid neoplasms. The presence of nuclear grooves, intranuclear cytoplasmic invaginations, squamoid cytoplasm, or true papillae favors papillary thyroid carcinoma. Other neuroendocrine neoplasms occurring in the neck (eg, medullary thyroid carcinoma and paragangliomas) may be impossible to differentiate from parathyroid neoplasia on cytologic grounds alone.

t10.2 Differentiation of Parathyroid and Thyroid Lesions

	Parathyroid	Thyroid
Hyperparathyroidism (clinical)	Often (+)	(−)
Cellularity	Usually high May form microfollicles	Variable, may be high (neoplasm) Micro → Macrofollicles
Cells	Usually smaller Monomorphic or pleomorphic	Usually larger Usually more monomorphic
Nuclei	"Salt-and-pepper" chromatin* Many naked	Moderately coarse Fewer naked
Cytoplasmic granules	Fine, red (neurosecretory granules*)	Coarse, blue (hemosiderin)
Colloid	Not present, but may have amyloid*	Often present
Background	Usually clean	Often degenerated (goiter)
Immunocytochemistry	Parathormone	Thyroglobulin

*Also seen in medullary thyroid carcinoma.

Clinical findings can be extremely helpful in the differential diagnosis and can be correlated with the cytology. High levels of parathormone in the aspirated tissue support the diagnosis of a parathyroid tumor. Immunocytochemistry, eg, to demonstrate parathormone or thyroglobulin, also can be helpful in the differential diagnosis.

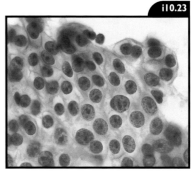

i10.23

Parathyroid carcinoma—clear cells (P)

Salivary Gland

Quick and accurate, fine needle aspiration (FNA) biopsy has gained wide clinical acceptance as a safe method to diagnose salivary gland lesions. The primary indication for FNA biopsy of a salivary gland is its enlargement. The salivary gland can harbor a wide variety of benign and malignant neoplasms, most of which are amenable to diagnosis by FNA biopsy. Diagnostic problems include cystic lesions (many salivary gland neoplasms are at least partially cystic) and interpretation of lesions with hyaline or mucinous material.

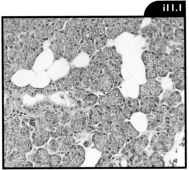

Salivary gland—normal tissue (H&E)

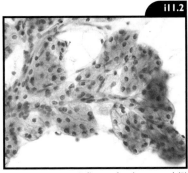

Salivary gland—normal (P)

11.1 Normal Salivary Glands

The salivary glands are exocrine secretory organs specialized for the production of saliva |i11.1|. Major salivary glands are paired and named for their site: parotid (near the ear, largest), submandibular, and sublingual. Up to 1000 minor salivary glands are widely distributed throughout the oral cavity and environs (palate, lips, tongue, and buccal mucosa). The incidence of neoplasms roughly parallels the relative size of the glands.

The parotid derives embryologically from ectoderm, arising as a bud from the oral epithelium. The developing gland is colonized by lymphocytes, which eventually form the parotid lymph nodes, part of the mucosa-associated lymphoid tissue (MALT). The submandibular and sublingual glands derive embryologically from endoderm. No lymph nodes develop within these glands.

Histologically, the salivary organs are tubuloacinar glands, arranged like bunches of grapes, set in a fibrofatty connective tissue stroma. The acini and ducts are surrounded by myoepithelial cells, which help expel the secretion when they contract. Salivary glands produce serous or mucinous secretions or both. The acini of the parotid are entirely serous. The submandibular is more serous than mucous, while the sublingual is more mucous than serous. The minor salivary glands are variably mucous and serous.

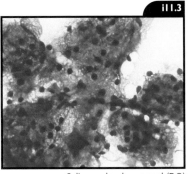

Salivary gland—normal (DQ)

11.1.2 The Cells

Acinic cells, ductal cells, myoepithelial cells, and adipose tissue may be seen. Entire lobules may be aspirated, typically accompanied by fibroadipose stromal tissue |i11.2|, |i11.3|.

Acinic Cells

Serous acinic cells are relatively large pyramidal cells |i11.4| with abundant foamy to coarsely granular cytoplasm. The granules (zymogen: proamylase, proptyalin) are lysosome-sized,

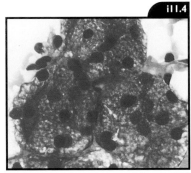

Serous acinic cells (DQ)

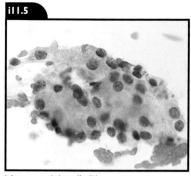

Mucous acinic cells (P)

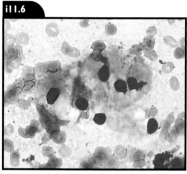

Mucous acinic cells (DQ)

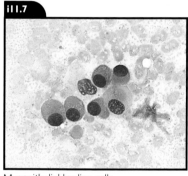

Myoepithelial hyaline cells

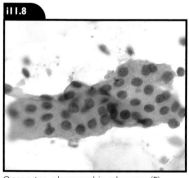

Oncocytes, pleomorphic adenoma (P)

basophilic, and refractile but often are leached from the cytoplasm, resulting in a foamy appearance. The bland nuclei are eccentric, regular, and rounded and may have a small nucleolus. Naked nuclei, which resemble lymphocytes, are common. Acinic cells typically are found in ball-like, acinic clusters.

Mucous acinic cells resemble endocervical cells but are found in acinic arrangements |i11.5|, |i11.6|. They are tall and columnar, with abundant, pale, multivacuolated, mucinous cytoplasm and eccentric bland nuclei with small nucleoli.

Ductal Cells

Ductal cells form cohesive honeycombed sheets or tubules of uniform cells with regular, round to oval, bland nuclei, reminiscent of breast duct cells. Single cells are sparse. The larger the duct, the taller the columnar cell. The cytoplasm varies from thin and pale to dense and squamoid. Mucous goblet cells also are scattered in the ducts.

Myoepithelial Cells

Myoepithelial cells are usually spindle-shaped or stellate, with delicate cytoplasm, and they have bland nuclei with smooth nuclear membranes. Plasmacytoid myoepithelial cells (hyaline cells) |i11.7| with dense epithelioid cytoplasm (due to cytoplasmic filaments) may be seen, particularly in tumors. Myoepithelial cells with clear cytoplasm also occur (see p 195).

Oncocytes

Beginning around the time a person reaches 40 years of age, oncocytes occur normally in the salivary gland ducts. Oncocytes can form nodules that may represent hyperplasia or true neoplasms (oncocytomas) and can also be a component of neoplasms such as Warthin tumor and pleomorphic adenoma |i11.8|. Oncocytes have abundant, well-defined, finely granular cytoplasm due to numerous mitochondria. The nuclei are relatively large and round and may have prominent nucleoli.

Miscellaneous

Adipose tissue is normal in the salivary gland; it increases with age and may be massive in alcoholic or malnourished patients.

Lymphoid tissue may be aspirated from intraparotid or adjacent cervical lymph nodes.

Ciliated respiratory-type glandular cells occasionally occur in salivary gland ducts.

Sebaceous cells, with abundant multivacuolated cytoplasm containing lipid, can be found normally in the parotid, as well as in various diseases; they also can be picked up from skin.

Squamous metaplasia can occur due to chronic inflammation, ischemia, radiation, or neoplasia.

Psammoma bodies are nonspecific and have been seen in normal, inflamed, irradiated, and neoplastic salivary glands.

Crystals of various kinds can be seen in salivary gland aspirates, eg, tyrosine-rich |i11.9| and collagen-rich |i11.10| crystals in pleomorphic adenomas, sulfur-rich crystals in cysts, and α-amylase crystals in sialadenitis |i11.11|.

Curschmann spirals have been identified, rarely.

11.2 Salivary Gland Diseases

Diseases of the salivary gland include sialadenosis, cysts, inflammations, and neoplasia. Salivary gland neoplasms are frequently cystic, which can cause false-negative diagnoses.

11.2.1 Sialadenosis

Sialadenosis is noninflammatory, nonneoplastic, bilateral parotid swelling. Most cases of soft, nontender, bilateral salivary gland enlargements without distinct nodules are due to sialadenosis.

Sialadenosis is usually caused by malnutrition or alcoholism. The salivary gland enlargement in sialadenosis is the result of hypertrophy of the acinic cells and acini, with fatty infiltration of the gland unassociated with inflammation or neoplasia.

The FNA biopsy can be painful. The cytology shows almost normal salivary gland cells and adipose tissue, except that the acini and acinic cells appear enlarged, as if magnified |i11.12|. The acinic cell cytoplasm is swollen and may be degranulated. By definition, there is no microscopic evidence of inflammation or neoplasia.

The clinical differential diagnosis of bilateral salivary gland enlargement includes inflammatory conditions, such as benign lymphoepithelial lesion (BLL), Sjögren syndrome, and sarcoid. Rarely, salivary gland neoplasms are bilateral, most commonly Warthin tumor.

11.2.2 Cysts

The general principle regarding aspirating cystic masses also applies to the salivary gland: drain the cyst, reaspirate any residual mass, reexamine the patient in 2 to 4 weeks to confirm resolution of the cyst, and excise if it recurs more than once. These guidelines help exclude cystic neoplasms.

Nonneoplastic Cysts

Any salivary gland, major or minor, can develop a cyst. The cysts can occur at any age. Most nonneoplastic cysts are

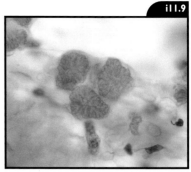
Tyrosine crystals (P)

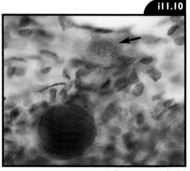
Collagen crystals (P)

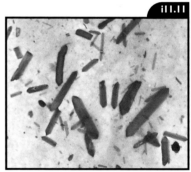
Amylase crystals (DQ)

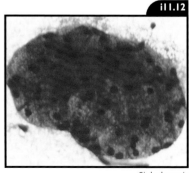
Sialadenosis

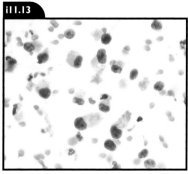

Cyst with increased cellularity, atypia (P)

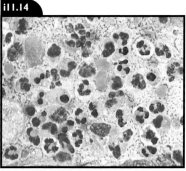

Acute sialadenitis (DQ)

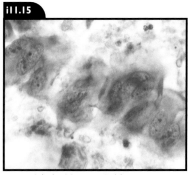

Acute sialadenitis—repair (P)

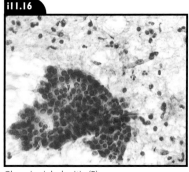

Chronic sialadenitis (P)

retention cysts (a true cyst with complete epithelial lining) or mucoceles (without lining). Retention cysts develop because of obstruction of the duct system, caused by scarring or tumors.

The FNA biopsy usually obtains clear or cloudy fluid that may be watery, like saliva, or mucoid. Cytologically, the cyst fluid contains only a few cells, mostly macrophages, sparse reactive or degenerated epithelial cells, and some inflammatory cells. Crystals may be seen occasionally.

Reactive/reparative ductal cells and squamous metaplasia can mimic low-grade mucoepidermoid carcinoma (MEC). Benign muciphages may closely resemble mucinous glandular cells of low-grade MEC. Nonneoplastic cysts are typically poorly cellular, while cystic neoplasms usually have more cells with more cytologic atypia |i11.13|.

11.2.3 Sialadenitis

The classic clinical features of sialadenitis include a history of acute or chronic recurrent pain and a swollen salivary gland without a distinct mass.

Acute Sialadenitis

Acute sialadenitis presents clinically as diffusely enlarged tender glands. The disease is usually caused by viruses (mumps, among others) or bacteria (usually *Streptococcus viridans* or *Staphylococcus aureus*). The diagnosis is usually clinically apparent, and, thus, the lesion is rarely biopsied; however, localized abscess formation may occur in bacterial sialadenitis, and these cases may be aspirated.

The FNA biopsy resembles an abscess with neutrophils, fibrin, and necrosis |i11.14|. In some cases, the probing needle encounters a stone. Organisms may be identified. Aspirated material can be submitted for culture to facilitate diagnosis. Reactive/reparative atypia can mimic tumor |i11.15|; conversely, tumors can become inflamed.

Chronic Sialadenitis

Chronic sialadenitis occurs most often in the submandibular gland, although any gland may be affected, and it can be bilateral. The most characteristic physical finding in chronic sialadenitis is a diffusely enlarged, firm gland, but occasionally a firm mass develops, mimicking a neoplasm.

The FNA biopsy is typically painful and yields a bloody smear with few cells. (In contrast, FNA biopsy of a neoplasm is usually relatively painless and yields abundant diagnostic material.)

Characteristically, ductal cells outnumber acinic cells |i11.16|, but the overall cellularity is low. There may be evidence of chronic inflammation and fibrosis (metachromatic stromal fragments containing fibroblasts) |i11.17|. Reactive atypia can closely simulate malignancy in some cases |i11.18|.

Chronic sialadenitis can be patchy, with areas of the gland being uninvolved. The diseased part of the gland may yield few cells, owing to fibrosis and atrophy, with the needle obtaining preserved healthy tissue, thereby resulting in a paradoxically normal aspirate.

The differential diagnosis of chronic sialadenitis includes aspiration of an intraparotid lymph node, BLL, Warthin tumor, and lymphoma. Metachromatic stromal fragments and ductal epithelial cells may suggest pleomorphic adenoma; however, the aspirate is scant. Mucous and squamous metaplasia with reactive atypia can mimic MEC.

Granulomatous Sialadenitis

Granulomatous sialadenitis is usually due to sarcoid (noncaseating granulomas) and occasionally tuberculosis (caseating granulomas with granular necrotic debris). Cat-scratch disease, toxoplasmosis, and various fungal diseases (suppurative granulomas) are also in the differential diagnosis.

The FNA biopsy shows aggregates of epithelioid histiocytes in which giant cells also may be found |i11.19|. Epithelioid histiocytes are characterized by fibrillar (P) to dense (DQ) cytoplasm and elongated nuclei with folded nuclear membranes, fine chromatin, and tiny nucleoli. Variable numbers of lymphocytes and degenerated epithelial cells also can be seen.

Asteroid bodies (radiating, star-like cytoplasmic inclusions), Schaumann bodies |i11.20| (concentrically laminated, calcified), and calcium oxalate crystals are rare findings but highly suggestive of sarcoidosis when present. Use special stains and culture to help identify infectious agents.

11.2.4 Benign Lymphoepithelial Lesion and Autoimmune Sialadenitis

The BLL consists, in essence, of marked lymphocytic infiltration of salivary (or lacrimal) glands. BLL is associated with autoimmune sialadenitis, but it is not specific for it.

Autoimmune Sialadenitis

Autoimmune sialadenitis usually affects middle-aged women. Autoimmune destruction of lacrimal and salivary glands results in dry eyes and dry mouth, which together constitute the sicca syndrome. The disorder can be localized to the glands (formerly known as Mikulicz disease), or it can be part of a systemic autoimmune disease, usually rheumatoid arthritis (Sjögren syndrome). Patients with Sjögren syndrome typically have hypergammaglobulinemia and antinuclear antibodies. Major and minor

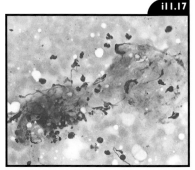
Chronic sialadenitis—stromal fragment (DQ)

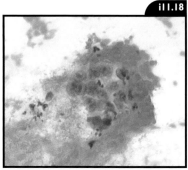
Chronic sialadenitis—reactive atypia

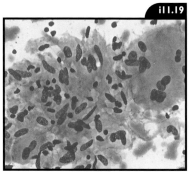
Granulomatous sialadenitis (DQ)

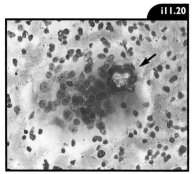
Schaumann body

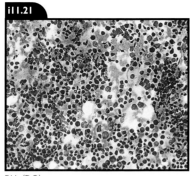

BLL (DQ)

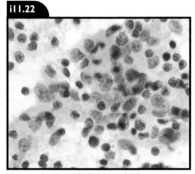

BLL—epimyoepithelial island (P)

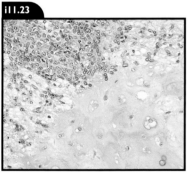

Pleomorphic adenoma, tissue (H&E)

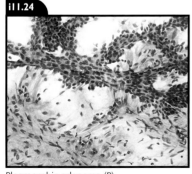

Pleomorphic adenoma (P)

salivary glands usually are involved. These patients have an increased risk of developing malignancies (lymphomas, carcinomas).

Benign Lymphoepithelial Lesion

BLL is the characteristic microscopic feature of localized and systemic forms of Sjögren syndrome. The term benign lymphoepithelial lesion is purely descriptive, and BLL can be seen in a variety of other nonmalignant lymphoproliferative reactions of the salivary gland, including granulomatous sialadenitis and HIV infection or AIDS. By definition, BLL shows salivary gland enlargement with atrophy of the parenchyma of the gland, replacement of salivary ducts by epimyoepithelial islands, and marked lymphocytic infiltration. If appropriate clinical features are present, then the patients are regarded as having Sjögren or sicca syndrome. If there are no other symptoms, the noncommittal term, benign lymphoepithelial lesion, is used.

The FNA biopsy is usually quite cellular, suggesting an aspirate of a reactive lymph node |i11.21|. It shows a range of maturation of the lymphocytes, including numerous "immature" lymphocytes or follicular center cells, with a predominance of small "mature" lymphocytes. Tingible body macrophages, lymphohistiocytic aggregates, macrophages, plasma cells, and occasionally eosinophils also are seen.

Epimyoepithelial islands are a necessary but not sufficient condition for the diagnosis of BLL, since similar groups may be seen in nonspecific chronic sialadenitis. Cytologically, the epimyoepithelial islands simply resemble small clusters of reactive or degenerative ductal cells infiltrated by lymphocytes |i11.22|. Protein precipitate or cell debris usually is present in the background.

Since either BLL or severe chronic sialadenitis may have a marked lymphoid infiltrate and epimyoepithelial islands, in practice the final diagnosis may rest on the clinical history and other laboratory findings. However, the cytologic changes in chronic sialadenitis are usually less marked than those of BLL. In intraparotid lymphadenopathy, the salivary epithelium usually appears normal. Lymphomas and Warthin tumor also could be mistaken for BLL.

11.2.5 Parotid Gland in HIV Infection

In the past, cystic lesions in the parotid were relatively rare but now are being encountered more often in HIV-positive patients. HIV-associated parotid cysts tend to be multiple and bilateral. They are true cysts, lined by epithelium that is surrounded by dense lymphocytic infiltration with or without follicular center formation.

The findings on FNA biopsy are essentially identical to those of branchial cleft and lymphoepithelial cervical cysts (see

Chapter 10). Solid lesions may show a picture reminiscent of BLL, but patients seldom have clinical features of sicca or Sjögren syndromes.

11.3 Salivary Gland Neoplasms

Salivary gland neoplasms are relatively rare; most are benign due to the overwhelming predominance of pleomorphic adenomas (benign mixed tumors). Most salivary gland neoplasms are seen in middle-aged patients, but there is a wide age range, including children. Benign tumors, except Warthin tumors, are more common in women, by a ratio of about 3:2; malignancies have a nearly equal sex distribution, except for primary squamous cell carcinoma (SCC), which occurs mostly in men.

The usual presenting complaint of patients with a benign neoplasm is a slowly growing lump in the salivary gland. Any tumor of a salivary gland that causes nerve deficit must be considered malignant until proven otherwise. Most neoplasms, by far, occur in the parotid, but there is a greater chance of finding malignancy when aspirating tumors in any of the other salivary glands. Adenoid cystic carcinoma is the most common primary malignant tumor in all salivary glands other than the parotid, where MEC overwhelmingly predominates.

11.3.1 Benign Salivary Gland Tumors

Pleomorphic Adenoma (Benign Mixed Tumor)

Pleomorphic adenomas are benign tumors (aka benign mixed tumor) but are prone to recurrence if inadequately excised (ie, simply enucleated). Multiple recurrent nodules of tumor, although benign, are difficult to completely eradicate.

Microscopically, the tumor has remarkably variable morphology, as the name implies |i11.23|. Both epithelial and mesenchymal elements must be present for diagnosis, although the mesenchymal elements are thought to be derived from myoepithelial cells.

The FNA biopsy usually obtains glistening, thick, sticky gel. Despite the highly varied morphology, the diagnosis by FNA biopsy usually is straightforward. The diagnosis is based, in essence, on the presence of epithelial cells, mesenchymal cells, and stroma in very variable proportions |i11.24|, |t11.1|. A transition from spindle stromal cells to epithelial cells is said to be particularly characteristic |i11.25|.

Fibromyxoid stroma is the most outstanding feature of pleomorphic adenoma, at least in the metachromatic Diff-Quik stain, where it stains a beautiful bright magenta |i11.26|. On the

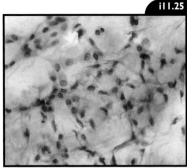
Pleomorphic adenoma (P)

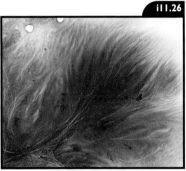
Metachromatic stroma (DQ)

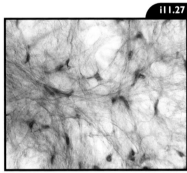
Pleomorphic adenoma—fibrillar stroma (P)

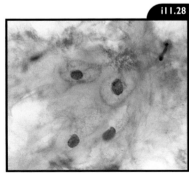
Pleomorphic adenoma—cartilage (P)

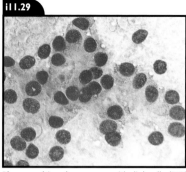

Pleomorphic adenoma—epithelial cells (DQ)

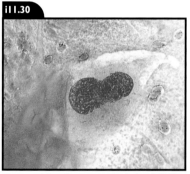

Pleomorphic adenoma—atypical cell (DQ)

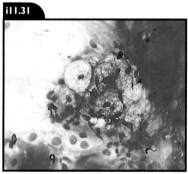

Pleomorphic adenoma—sebaceous cells (DQ)

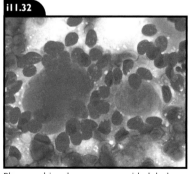

Pleomorphic adenoma—mucoid globules

t11.1 Pleomorphic Adenoma (Benign Mixed Tumor)

Epithelial cells
Mesenchymal cells } Transition is characteristic
Stroma: Metachromatic, fibrillar

other hand, the stroma practically disappears in Papanicolaou stain, being transparent and only lightly stained (usually pale blue-green or pink), or it may be mistaken for ordinary mucus. However, an important feature, which is best appreciated in Papanicolaou stain, is the characteristic fibrillar appearance of the stroma, with fine to coarse fibrils embedded in the ground substance |i11.27|. Tyrosine-rich crystals (flower-shaped) are an unusual but not specific feature |i11.9|. Mature cartilage with lacunar chondrocytes may be seen |i11.28|.

Epithelial cells may form ducts, trabeculae, glands, papillae, or cohesive sheets; single cells may be present |i11.29|. The proportion of epithelium to stroma is quite variable. The epithelial cells are usually small and uniform with pale cytoplasm and round nuclei containing bland chromatin and tiny nucleoli. Occasionally, a few scattered cells show substantial cytologic atypia, including marked nuclear enlargement and pleomorphism, membrane irregularity, hyperchromasia, and prominent nucleoli |i11.30|. The epithelial component can undergo mucinous, squamous, oncocytic |i11.8|, or sebaceous |i11.31| metaplasia.

Myoepithelial, or stromal-mesenchymal, cells are usually spindle or stellate but may be epithelioid, plasmacytoid (hyaline cells with dense cytoplasm), or clear. The cells are usually single but may form loose groups. Myoepithelial cells secrete the characteristic myxoid ground substance and other stromal elements. Spindle myoepithelial cells have delicate ill-defined cytoplasm, elongated nuclei with fine chromatin, and small nucleoli, and are characteristically embedded in the stroma.

An important potential source of diagnostic error may occur when the lumens of ducts become distended with metachromatic mucin, forming mucoid or hyaline globules |i11.32| that closely mimic the appearance of adenoid cystic carcinoma (see p 197). Squamous or mucous metaplasia could be misinterpreted as evidence of MEC. Oncocytic metaplasia can be extensive, suggesting an oncocytoma or Warthin tumor. Rarely, pleomorphic adenomas undergo malignant degeneration (see "Malignant Mixed Tumors," p 200).

Monomorphic Adenomas

Monomorphic adenomas constitute a group of tumors clinically indistinguishable from pleomorphic adenomas, including basal cell adenomas, trabecular adenomas, clear cell adenomas, and sebaceous adenomas. The fibromyxoid ground substance, characteristic of pleomorphic adenoma, is sparse or absent in these tumors, although other kinds of extracellular material may be seen. The key fact to recognize cytologically is that the lesion is benign and should not be mistaken for a malignancy such as adenoid cystic carcinoma. Clinically, evidence of nerve damage strongly suggests malignancy. Anaplastic cytologic features exclude a diagnosis of monomorphic adenoma.

Basal Cell Adenoma: The FNA biopsy of basal cell adenoma consists almost entirely of monomorphic epithelial cells in cohesive groups, cords, or irregularly branching clusters, with variable numbers of single cells. Naked nuclei may be numerous. The cells have uniform, dark, round nuclei, scant cytoplasm, and high nuclear/cytoplasmic ratios. The chromatin is granular; nucleoli are small and inconspicuous. Basosquamous whorling, akin to pearls, may be seen and, when present, excludes adenoid cystic carcinoma. Basal cell adenomas may secrete a metachromatic, hyaline, basement membrane–like material (when extensive, known as membranous type or dermal analog tumor) |i11.33|, |i11.34|, but chondromyxoid stroma is absent or very scant. Occasionally, hyaline globules, similar or identical to those of adenoid cystic carcinoma, occur.

Trabecular Adenoma: Trabecular adenoma is a subtype of basal cell adenoma that produces hyaline material (including spheres and cylinders) similar to that seen in adenoid cystic carcinoma |i11.35|, |i11.36|. Besides this hyaline material, other stroma is scant. Trabecular adenoma is composed of small, uniform, basaloid cells forming densely packed cohesive tubules, trabeculae, or papillae, with scattered single cells. Cytologically, this tumor can closely resemble adenoid cystic carcinoma, which also has hyaline globules and small basaloid cells. The hyaline globules are usually smaller and less intensely metachromatic than those in adenoid cystic carcinoma, but these are soft diagnostic criteria. There are no obviously malignant-appearing cells in trabecular adenoma. In practice, this differential diagnosis can be difficult (see "Adenoid Cystic Carcinoma," p 197).

Myoepithelioma: Myoepitheliomas are rare tumors composed almost exclusively of myoepithelial cells; they specifically lack ductal differentiation. The myoepithelial cells can be of four types: spindle, hyaline, epithelioid, or clear; they are found separately or in various combinations. Some myoepitheliomas are locally aggressive, and malignant myoepitheliomas can occur.

Spindle myoepithelial cells, naturally, have a spindle or stellate shape, with elongated oval nuclei, fine even chromatin, and inconspicuous nucleoli; the cytoplasm is thin and wispy. Hyaline myoepithelial cells have a plasmacytoid appearance with an eccentric nucleus and abundant, homogenous, dense or glassy, nongran-

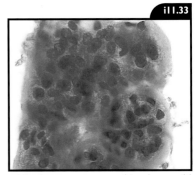

i11.33

Membranous monomorphic adenoma (P)

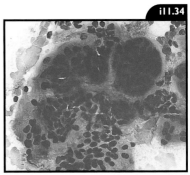

i11.34

Membranous monomorphic adenoma (DQ)

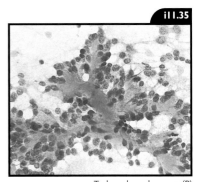

i11.35

Trabecular adenoma (P)

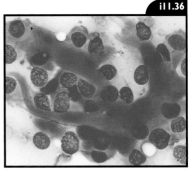

i11.36

Trabecular adenoma (DQ)

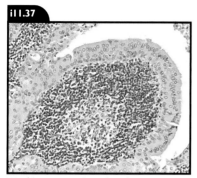

Warthin tumor—tissue (H&E)

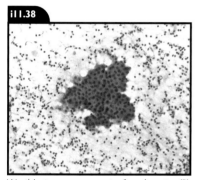

Warthin tumor—oncocytes/lymphocytes (P)

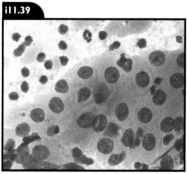

Warthin tumor—oncocytes, mast cell (DQ)

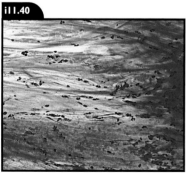

Warthin tumor—mucoid cyst content (DQ)

ular cytoplasm. Myoepithelial cells also can have an epithelioid appearance or undergo clear cell change due to the accumulation of glycogen.

Warthin Tumor

Warthin tumor, also known as papillary cystadenoma lymphomatosum and adenolymphoma, occurs almost exclusively in or around the parotid gland |t11.2|. Warthin tumor is the second most common benign salivary gland neoplasm (after pleomorphic adenoma), but it is a distant second (5% to 10% of cases). It generally occurs in patients between the ages of 40 and 70 years, and equally between the sexes. Patients usually smoke cigarettes. Warthin tumor is the most common bilateral salivary gland neoplasm and also can be multifocal.

Warthin tumor is a cystic neoplasm with papillary processes, which are lined by a double layer of oncocytes and contain a lymphoid stroma, often with follicular center formation |i11.37|. Because most Warthin tumors are predominantly cystic, they often feel soft or doughy but can be firm if the cyst is tense. Although benign, the lesion may "recur" (which actually represents a new tumor). There may be a slightly increased risk of developing malignant lymphoma.

The FNA biopsy usually obtains a variable amount of the cyst contents—an important clue to the diagnosis. The fluid typically has a greenish brown, granular, or mucoid appearance ("grungy"). The cytology consists, in essence, of oncocytes and lymphocytes, together with the contents of the cyst |i11.38|, |i11.39|, |i11.40|.

Oncocytes form orderly flat sheets and occasionally papillae with few single cells. The cells have abundant, finely granular cytoplasm (due to mitochondria, finer than lysosome-sized acinic cell granules) that typically stains bright orange in Papanicolaou stain, deep blue in Diff-Quik stain. The nuclei usually are round and uniform with granular chromatin and small nucleoli.

Lymphocytes exhibit a typical reactive pattern with a range of maturation, including follicular center cells ("immature" lymphocytes), and tingible body macrophages. Mast cells, best appreciated in Diff-Quik stain, frequently are present (but not specific). They have small, round, central nuclei and metachro-

---

t11.2 Warthin Tumor

Parotid tumor, smoking history
Cytology
   Oncocytes
   Lymphocytes
   Cyst content

---

matic cytoplasmic granules but often are seen as only a red smudge in the groups of blue oncocytes (Diff-Quik stain).

The cyst content is seen in the background of the smear, as an amorphous, granular, or ropy substance that frequently is mucoid, and is metachromatic in Diff-Quik stain. Occasionally, only cyst fluid is aspirated. Cholesterol crystals, debris, macrophages, giant cells, and granulomas, as well as corpora amylacea, may be seen in some cases. Atypical degenerated oncocytes or atypical squamous metaplasia could suggest SCC |i11.41|.

Oncocytoma and Oncocytic Carcinoma

Oncocytoma is a rare benign (and rarer still, malignant |i11.42|) neoplasm similar to Warthin tumor but composed almost exclusively of oncocytes, lacking significant numbers of lymphocytes. In contrast with Warthin tumors, oncocytomas are noncystic neoplasms that can be found in any salivary gland, not just the parotid.

11.3.2 Malignant Salivary Gland Tumors

Adenoid Cystic Carcinoma

Adenoid cystic carcinoma is the most common primary malignancy of all salivary glands except the parotid (where MEC is far more common) |i11.43|. Adenoid cystic carcinoma also occurs in a wide variety of other sites, including lacrimal and sweat glands, respiratory tract, and breast. Women are more commonly affected than men; patients are usually in their 40s or 50s.

Clinically, the tumor is characterized by slow but relentless growth, with poor long-term prognosis. Widespread perineural invasion is so characteristic that the diagnosis is doubtful in its absence. Adenoid cystic carcinoma eventually metastasizes to lung and bone.

The FNA biopsy often obtains glistening mucoid material, grossly similar to pleomorphic adenoma. Classically, the tumor grows in a cribriform or cylindromatous ("Swiss cheese") pattern but can be quite variable, including trabecular, tubular, and solid; mixtures are common. The cytology can be deceptively benign appearing. The cells are small, uniform, basaloid cells with bland nuclei, scant cytoplasm, and high nuclear/cytoplasmic ratios. They usually form cohesive clusters, cords, solid groups, cylinders, glands, or microcystic spaces, but occasionally single cells are plentiful |t11.3|.

Metachromatic basement membrane–like material, particularly in the form of extracellular hyaline globules, is highly characteristic of this tumor |i11.44|, |i11.45|. This mucoid material can be glassy (hyaline), granular, or laminated, but—in contrast with the ground substance of pleomorphic adenoma—it is not fibrillar. It stains pale blue or pink in Papanicolaou stain but is

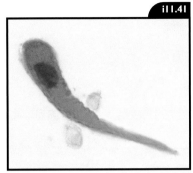

i11.41

Warthin tumor—atypical cell mimics SCC (P)

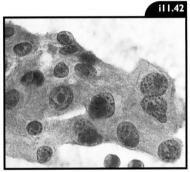

i11.42

Oncocytic carcinoma (P)

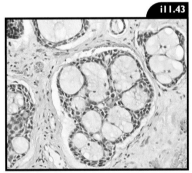

i11.43

Adenoid cystic carcinoma, tissue (H&E)

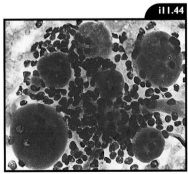

i11.44

Adenoid cystic carcinoma (DQ)

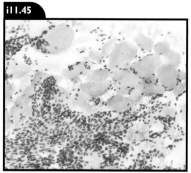

Adenoid cystic carcinoma (P)

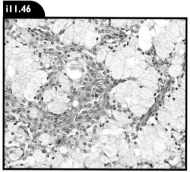

MEC, tissue (H&E)

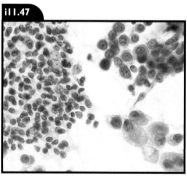

MEC—intermediate, gland, squamous cells (P)

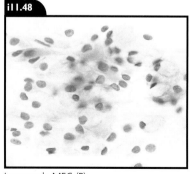

Low-grade MEC (P)

t11.3 Adenoid Cystic Carcinoma

Small uniform cells
    Bland and cohesive
Hyaline globules
    Pink "gum balls" (Diff-Quik)
    Not fibrillar

bright magenta in Diff-Quik stain, and spheres of this material look like pink "gum balls." Note well that practically identical hyaline globules can be seen in several other benign or malignant salivary gland tumors, including pleomorphic adenoma. Because of possible diagnostic problems, it is probably best to avoid making an unequivocal cytodiagnosis of adenoid cystic carcinoma, unless there is clear-cut clinical evidence of malignancy.

Poorly differentiated adenoid cystic carcinoma shows solid growth of anaplastic cells without hyaline material. The differential diagnosis includes basal cell adenomas, small cell carcinoma, and malignant lymphoma.

Mucoepidermoid Carcinoma

Overall, MEC is the most common malignant salivary gland tumor, but most by far occur in the parotid |i11.46|. Patients are usually middle-aged, but MEC is also the most common salivary gland cancer of children. The sexes are equally affected.

The tumor can be divided into low and high grades. Low-grade MEC is characterized clinically by repeated local recurrences; high-grade MEC frequently metastasizes. Low-grade tumors tend to present as soft, cystic, painless masses. High-grade tumors are usually firm and solid, and clinical symptoms (pain, skin changes, nerve paralysis) are more common.

In FNA biopsy, the key diagnostic feature of MEC is the mixture of cell types, including glandular, squamous, intermediate cells, and others |i11.47|. At a minimum, both glandular and squamous components should be present to make the diagnosis |t11.4|.

Mucous or glandular cells have abundant vacuolated cytoplasm, typically resembling goblet cells or muciphages when well-differentiated. As the grade of the tumor increases, the nuclei acquire the usual features of malignancy.

t11.4 Mucoepidermoid Carcinoma

Mixed cell types
    Glandular   ⎫
    Squamous   ⎬ Minimum diagnostic criteria
    Intermediate ⎭
Low-grade: Cystic; bland glandular cells predominate
High-grade: Solid; nonkeratinizing SCC predominates

Intermediate cells resemble normal ductal cells, ie, relatively small cells with high nuclear/cytoplasmic ratios and round uniform nuclei with vesicular chromatin and small nucleoli.

Squamous cells typically resemble parabasal-sized metaplastic (nonkeratinizing) cells. Obvious malignant nuclear features are seen in high-grade MEC. Atypical, mucin-positive, squamoid cells are highly suggestive of MEC.

Mucus is particularly characteristic of low-grade MEC. Benign muciphages often are present. Evidence of inflammation may be seen in the background, along with amorphous, granular, eosinophilic material.

Low-grade MEC is characterized cytologically by metachromatic mucoid cyst content with a predominance of fairly bland, mucous glandular cells |i11.48| and variable numbers of intermediate and squamous cells. High-grade MEC is characterized cytologically by clearly malignant-appearing glandular and squamous cells, in which the squamous component usually predominates |i11.49|, |i11.50|.

The differential diagnosis of low-grade MEC is a benign cyst: MEC shows more cells with more atypia and tends to recur. High-grade MEC may resemble nonkeratinizing SCC. Primary SCC of the salivary gland is rare; look for evidence of glandular differentiation. Marked keratinization suggests a metastasis from a head and neck primary tumor.

Acinic Cell Carcinoma

Acinic cell carcinoma is rare |i11.51|, approximately 1% of salivary gland malignancies, but it is the second most common salivary gland cancer in children, after MEC. Most occur in the parotid, usually in women, characteristically in their 40s. Acinic cell carcinoma is also the most common bilateral primary salivary gland malignancy. A striking clinical feature is the protracted course: recurrence or metastases (lymph node, lung, bone) can occur decades after first diagnosis.

In essence, the cytologic diagnosis is based on finding a pure population of acinic cells, *without* ductal cells or supporting fibrofatty stroma |i11.52|, |t11.5|.

The tumor cells, when well-differentiated, closely resemble normal serous acinic cells. Although ducts are not seen,

---

t11.5 Acinic Cell Carcinoma

Serous acinic cells
    Zymogen granules
    Diastase-resistant, PAS-positive
No ducts
No fibrofatty stroma
Chronic inflammation may be present

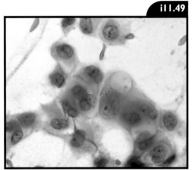
High-grade MEC—mucin vacuole (P)

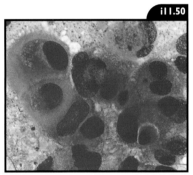
High-grade MEC (DQ)

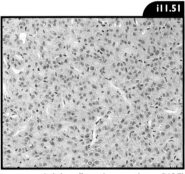
Acinic cell carcinoma, tissue (H&E)

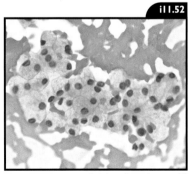
Acinic cell carcinoma (P)

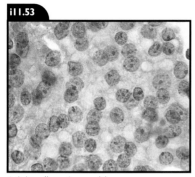

Acinic cell carcinoma (P)

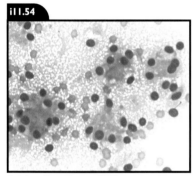

Acinic cell carcinoma (DQ)

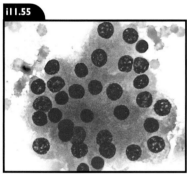

Acinic cell carcinoma (DQ)

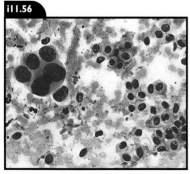

Carcinoma ex pleomorphic adenoma (DQ)

capillaries can mimic ducts. Acinic structures may be suggested, but they usually are not well-formed. Less-differentiated tumors yield crowded clusters and irregular sheets of cells and increased numbers of single cells |i11.53|. Papillae, sometimes with psammoma bodies, may be present.

The cytoplasm is abundant and, most characteristically, coarsely granular |i11.54|, |i11.55|. The granules are zymogen granules (basophilic in Papanicolaou stain, pinkish in Diff-Quik stain, diastase-resistant, PAS-positive). However, the cytoplasm frequently degranulates and appears foamy or clear. The nuclei are usually fairly bland and uniform but can show variable degrees of atypia. Naked nuclei may be numerous. The tumor frequently is associated with marked chronic inflammation.

The differential diagnosis includes oncocytoma; however, the granules of oncocytes (mitochondria) are finer, and oncocytic cytoplasm usually is not vacuolated.

Malignant Mixed Tumors

Malignant mixed tumors fall into three categories. Although relatively rare, the most common malignant mixed tumor is carcinoma ex pleomorphic adenoma (CEPA), ie, carcinoma arising out of a pleomorphic adenoma. Rarer still is the "true" malignant mixed tumor, ie, a true carcinosarcoma in which the epithelial and stromal components are both malignant. The mesenchymal component can vary but most commonly is chondrosarcoma or osteosarcoma. Rarest of all is the so-called benign metastasizing mixed tumor. This designation refers to its benign morphologic appearance, not its behavior.

Carcinoma Ex Pleomorphic Adenoma: CEPA is an epithelial malignancy arising out of a preexisting benign pleomorphic adenoma. CEPA is relatively common (~ 15% of all salivary gland cancers), but only a minority (< 10%) of all pleomorphic adenomas become malignant. Most cases occur in the parotid, more commonly after the age of 50 years. The classic clinical history is one of a slowly growing mass of long duration with recent rapid growth.

Microscopically, CEPA shows the features of a benign mixed tumor plus an epithelial malignancy |i11.56|, which usually is poorly differentiated adenocarcinoma or undifferentiated carcinoma but can be other recognized types of salivary gland cancers (eg, MEC or adenoid cystic carcinoma) or SCC. The FNA biopsy reflects the components of the tumor but is usually dominated by clearly malignant cells. Although by definition a benign component (ie, the pleomorphic adenoma) is present, it may be poorly represented in the biopsy. A particularly cellular pleomorphic adenoma with necrosis, hemorrhage, calcification, and mitoses is a warning sign of possible malignant change. Note, however, that benign pleomorphic adenomas occasionally can show considerable cytologic atypia focally.

11.3.3 Other Salivary Gland Tumors

Adenocarcinomas

This category is for the rare adenocarcinomas of the salivary gland that do not fit into other recognized diagnostic groups such as adenoid cystic carcinoma and MEC. Metastatic adenocarcinoma also must be excluded.

Mucus-producing adenocarcinoma, not otherwise specified (NOS) |i11.57|, is characterized by malignant glandular cells with abundant cytoplasm, occasionally containing small intensely metachromatic globules |i11.58|, reminiscent of similar but larger extracellular hyaline globules seen in adenoid cystic carcinoma.

Papillary adenocarcinoma shows papillary growth; psammoma bodies may be present. The cells may be mucin positive, but there are no squamous or intermediate cells or other specific features.

Salivary duct carcinoma is an extremely rare, highly malignant tumor that typically occurs in older men, usually arising in the Stensen duct of the parotid. The morphology is similar to comedocarcinoma of the breast.

Polymorphous low-grade adenocarcinoma arises exclusively in minor salivary glands and shows variable morphology. The cells are uniform myoepithelial or duct cells, growing in sheets, tight clusters, or acini with lumens. Metachromatic hyaline globules or tyrosine-rich crystals may be seen.

Epithelial-myoepithelial carcinoma is a low-grade malignancy that usually occurs in the parotid, more commonly in females. The FNA biopsy specimen shows a two-cell population (epithelial and myoepithelial). The epithelial cells resemble ductal cells and are usually located centrally in aggregates. The myoepithelial cells have clear cytoplasm and are usually located peripherally. Naked bipolar nuclei may be numerous. Hyaline material surrounds the aggregates and also may form hyaline globules similar to those in adenoid cystic carcinoma |i11.59|.

Basal cell adenocarcinoma is the low-grade malignant counterpart of basal cell adenoma that grows invasively, frequently perineurally. It may be difficult to distinguish from the more ominous solid type of adenoid cystic carcinoma.

(Primary) Squamous Cell Carcinoma

Primary SCC is rare (< 1%); metastatic SCC is far more common, especially in the parotid (intraparotid lymph node). Also, high-grade MEC must be excluded. This tumor predominantly occurs in elderly men |i11.60|.

Microscopically, the tumor shows typical features of SCC, usually keratinizing type. By definition, the tumor is mucin negative (if positive, the diagnosis is MEC).

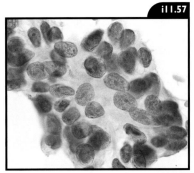

i11.57

Adenocarcinoma, NOS (P)

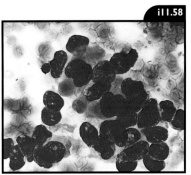

i11.58

Adenocarcinoma, NOS (DQ)

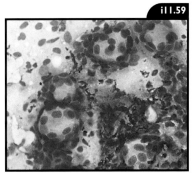

i11.59

Epithelial-myoepithelial carcinoma (DQ)

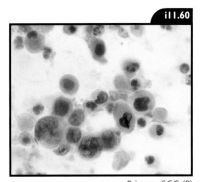

i11.60

Primary SCC (P)

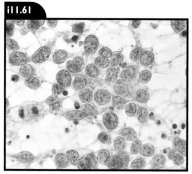

Neuroendocrine carcinoma (P)

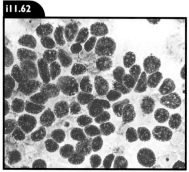

Neuroendocrine carcinoma (DQ)

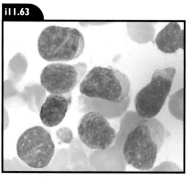

Non-Hodgkin lymphoma (DQ)

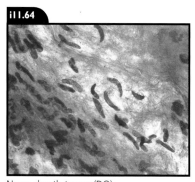

Nerve sheath tumor (DQ)

Undifferentiated Carcinoma

Undifferentiated carcinoma, aka lymphoepithelioma-like carcinoma, may be the malignant counterpart of BLL. The tumor is morphologically indistinguishable from lymphoepithelioma of the nasopharynx; both tumors are associated with Epstein-Barr virus.

Small Cell Neuroendocrine Carcinoma

Small cell carcinoma of salivary gland is a poorly differentiated neuroendocrine carcinoma that may have neurosecretory granules or express neuroendocrine markers |i11.61|, |i11.62|. The cytologic appearance is similar to small cell carcinoma of the lung; a lung primary tumor must be excluded.

Malignant Lymphoma

The lymphoid tissue of the salivary glands is a component of the mucosa-associated lymphoid tissue (MALT). Primary lymphomas of the salivary gland are relatively rare but may be increasing in frequency. They usually are associated with a history of BLL or Sjögren syndrome. They usually are non-Hodgkin lymphomas (NHLs), B-cell type, including small cleaved, mixed, and large cell types, and MALTomas.

NHLs generally are characterized by a monotypic population of neoplastic lymphoid cells as opposed to the polytypic picture seen in reactive lymphoid infiltrates |i11.63|. Tingible body macrophages can be seen in benign reactive conditions, high-grade NHLs, and Hodgkin disease but are sparse or absent in low-grade NHLs. Hodgkin disease can be diagnosed if typical Reed-Sternberg cells are recognized in the proper reactive milieu. The differential diagnosis includes BLL, which shows a reactive lymphoid infiltrate and epimyoepithelial islands. Malignant lymphoma rarely preserves epimyoepithelial islands and may infiltrate adjacent tissue.

Mesenchymal Tumors

Less than 3% of salivary gland tumors are mesenchymal neoplasms. Theoretically, virtually any benign or malignant soft tissue tumor could arise in the salivary gland.

Hemangioma is the most common salivary gland tumor presenting in infants younger than 1 year, usually in girls and usually parotid. The FNA biopsy is bloody and frequently nondiagnostic. Occasionally, rare clusters of small oval to spindle endothelial cells with moderate cytoplasm and bland oval nuclei are obtained. Lymphangiomas also can occur in this region.

Lipoma of the salivary gland also occurs and may result in formation of a suspicious mass. The FNA biopsy yields fibroadipose tissue, which may have admixed acinic-ductal fragments.

Nerve sheath tumors, including neurofibromas and schwannomas |i11.64|, arising in the facial nerve occasionally produce a mass in the salivary gland. Schwannoma is characterized by spindle cells embedded in acellular ground substance, mimicking the stroma of pleomorphic adenoma. The aspirate typically shows organoid Verocay bodies, with nuclear palisading, but lacks an epithelial component. Note that palisading nuclei can be seen, focally, in pleomorphic adenomas.

Metastasis

Metastases to the salivary gland are not rare. Most are head and neck SCCs or melanomas |i11.65| metastatic to intra-parotid lymph nodes. Clinical history provides an important clue to the diagnosis. Metastatic SCC can be difficult to differentiate from primary SCC (very rare) or high-grade MEC (relatively common). Marked keratinization is common in metastatic head and neck SCC but not in MEC; mucin positivity is seen in MEC but not SCC. Because it can grow in papillary, glandular, or solid formations with clear, granular, or spindle cells, metastatic renal cell carcinoma (RCC) |i11.66| can closely mimic several primary salivary gland tumors, particularly MEC, acinic cell carcinoma, oncocytoma (or Warthin tumor), and clear cell tumors.

11.4 Salivary Gland Masses in Children

Inflammation, the most common salivary gland disease of childhood, can be viral or bacterial. Salivary gland neoplasia is rare in childhood. However, the most common salivary gland tumor in children (particularly in those younger than 1 year old) is hemangioma (probably a hamartoma) |i11.67|, |i11.68|, followed by pleomorphic adenoma (which becomes more common in older children); all other benign salivary gland tumors are particularly rare. MEC is the most common malignant salivary gland tumor in children; rhabdomyosarcoma is the most common primary sarcoma |t11.6|.

t11.6 Salivary Gland Masses in Children

Most are inflammatory
Hemangioma: Most common tumor (? hamartoma)
Pleomorphic adenoma: Most common neoplasm
Mucoepidermoid carcinoma: Most common carcinoma
Rhabdomyosarcoma: Most common sarcoma

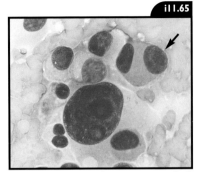
Metastatic melanoma—D-MIN (DQ)

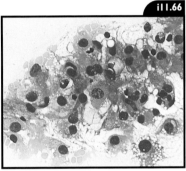
Metastatic RCC (DQ)

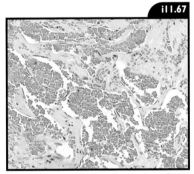
Hemangioma, tissue (H&E)

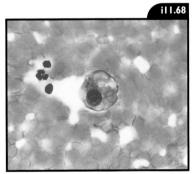
Hemangioma (DQ)

Thyroid

A thyroid nodule is the classic clinical finding in thyroid cancer. But virtually any disease of the thyroid can present as a nodule, and it is usually not possible to distinguish between benign and malignant thyroid nodules by any noninvasive procedure. To compound the diagnostic dilemma, there are millions of benign nodules (~ 5% of adults have goiters, clinically) but relatively few cancers (17,000 cases, 1200 deaths, annually), most of which are low grade.

Risk factors for thyroid cancer include male sex, youth or old age, radiation exposure, and iodine deficiency. Although solitary nodules usually are considered more suspicious clinically, thyroid cancer probably occurs in a multinodular gland as often as in a solitary nodule. A hard, fixed nodule is more worrisome than a soft or cystic nodule. Although most cancers are "cold" on radioiodine scan, in practice, most thyroid nodules are cold and most cold nodules are benign. However, cancer virtually never occurs in a "hot" nodule. Failure of a nodule to suppress under hormone therapy, and particularly growth of a nodule while under suppression, increases the risk of cancer |t12.1|.

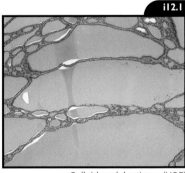

i12.1

Colloid nodule, tissue (H&E)

12.1 Fine Needle Aspiration Biopsy: The Best Test

Fine needle aspiration (FNA) biopsy is the best test short of surgery for evaluation of a thyroid nodule |i12.1|, |i12.2|. In general, about 1 in 20 patients with a benign FNA biopsy diagnosis has a malignancy (5% false-negative rate), while about 1 in 100 patients with a malignant FNA biopsy diagnosis does not (1% false-positive). With experience, less than 5% to 10% of thyroid aspirates are unsatisfactory. The principal reason for false-negative biopsies is inadequate sampling, ie, unsatisfactory aspirates. As a

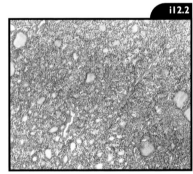

i12.2

Follicular nodule, tissue (H&E)

t12.1 Risk of Thyroid Cancer

	Increased Risk*	Decreased Risk
History	History of radiation therapy Youth, old age, male	Family history of goiter Middle age, female
Physical examination	Firm, solitary nodule	Soft, cystic, multinodular
Radioiodine scan	Cold	Hot
Hormone suppression	Fails to regress	Regresses

*When these factors are used to select patients for surgery, at most 25% will be found to have thyroid cancer.

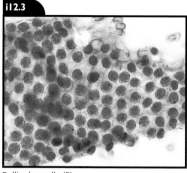

Follicular cells (P)

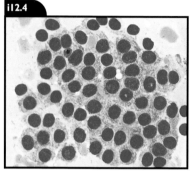

Follicular cells (DQ)

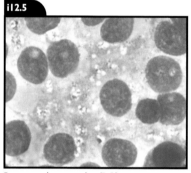

Paravacuolar granules (DQ)

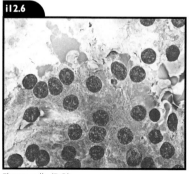

Flame cells (DQ)

rule of thumb, if the quality of the smear is such that you would even think about counting the number of cells to determine adequacy, the specimen is probably inadequate! Because of the known false-negative rate of FNA biopsy, even patients with benign diagnoses must be carefully followed up, eg, by another biopsy in 6 to 12 months, provided the lesion is not clinically suspicious. If the FNA biopsy is consistently benign, observation may be safely continued. Some practical diagnostic advice: thyroid aspirates are benign until proven otherwise.

12.2 The Normal Thyroid Gland

The functional unit of the thyroid is the follicle, which is composed of a central ball of colloid surrounded by an outer skin of follicular epithelium. These two elements of the follicle, follicular cells and colloid, play a fundamental role in FNA biopsy diagnosis.

12.2.1 The Cells

Follicular Cells

Follicular cells are normally uniform and form orderly honeycomb sheets; single cells are sparse |i12.3|, |i12.4|. Intact follicles also may be aspirated. The nucleus is round, usually about the size of a lymphocyte, with smooth nuclear membranes. The chromatin usually is distinctly granular and moderately hyperchromatic. However, nuclear size and chromatin texture vary with the functional state of the cell. Nucleoli normally are inconspicuous to invisible.

The cytoplasm normally is pale and delicate in Papanicolaou stain and light purple in Diff-Quik stain. The more active the cell, the more abundant the cytoplasm. Degenerated follicular cells, or foam cells, resemble histiocytes. Paravacuolar granules are tiny hemosiderin or lipofuscin deposits (dark blue in Diff-Quik stain, golden brown in Papanicolaou stain) surrounded by a small, clear, cytoplasmic vacuole |i12.5|. They are a nonspecific finding associated with degeneration. Occasionally, repair/regeneration occurs, reminiscent of that seen in the Pap smear (see p 213).

Flame Cells

Flame cells (aka flare cells) are follicular cells with cytoplasmic vacuoles containing metachromatic material (pink in Diff-Quik stain) |i12.6|. Because these metachromatic vacuoles tend to occur at the margins of small groups of cells, they also are known as marginal vacuoles. Flame cell change indicates that the individual cells are hyperfunctioning. Flame cells are numerous in toxic goiters but also can be seen focally in nontoxic goiters, Hashimoto thyroiditis, and even neoplasms.

Hürthle Cells

Hürthle cells are oncocytes, characterized by abundant, dense, finely granular cytoplasm (due to mitochondria) staining orange to blue in Papanicolaou |i12.7|, purplish in Diff-Quik stain |i12.8|. The nuclei usually are enlarged; binucleation and multinucleation are common. Prominent nucleoli can be seen. Although associated with Hashimoto thyroiditis, Hürthle cells can be seen in many other thyroid conditions ranging from goiters to neoplasms.

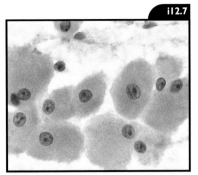
Hürthle cells (P)

Miscellaneous Cells

Ciliated cells usually indicate that the trachea was entered. This is particularly common with nodules in the isthmus of thyroid. Fragments of intensely metachromatic fibrocartilage, as well as air, also are usually aspirated. Skeletal muscle, from the platysma or sternocleidomastoid, can mimic colloid (look for cross-striations and nuclei). Skin, adipose tissue, blood vessels, and, rarely, hematopoietic elements (eg, from marrow containing cartilaginous structures of the larynx or upper trachea) can all be seen in "thyroid" aspirates.

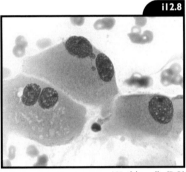
Hürthle cells (DQ)

12.2.2 Colloid

Colloid has a central role in the FNA biopsy diagnosis of several common thyroid diseases, particularly follicular lesions (goiter and follicular neoplasms). Grossly, colloid often looks like honey but can vary from semisolid to liquid. Microscopically, colloid has a wide variety of morphologies, but in essence there are two basic forms: watery (diffuse) and dense (solid).

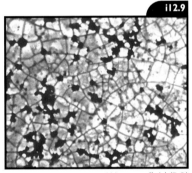
Watery colloid (DQ)

Watery Colloid

Thin watery colloid is usually better visualized in Diff-Quik stain |i12.9| than in Papanicolaou stain |i12.10|. In Diff-Quik stain, diffuse watery colloid has a tendency to crack in a geometric pattern ("crack artifact"), resulting in stained glass–like "panes" of purple colloid. Sometimes, the panes wash off the slide, leaving a spider web–like or chicken wire appearance (corresponding to the frames of the panes). Thick, honey-like colloid has a tendency to bunch up, especially in wet-fixed, Papanicolaou-stained slides, and looks like wrinkled, colored, plastic wrap. Blood serum can mimic watery colloid microscopically; therefore, be cautious diagnosing colloid in the absence of follicular cells (|i8.85|, p 161).

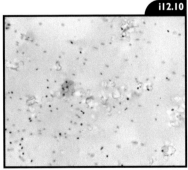
Watery colloid (P)

Dense Colloid

Dense, inspissated colloid usually looks like irregular or rounded "chips" of translucent homogeneous material that stains

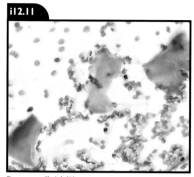

Dense colloid (P)

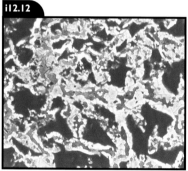

Dense colloid (DQ)

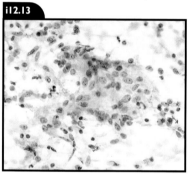

Granulomatous thyroiditis (P)

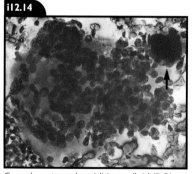

Granulomatous thyroiditis—colloid (DQ)

shades of blue or pink in Papanicolaou stain |i12.11| and deep purple in Diff-Quik stain |i12.12|. In contrast with watery colloid, dense colloid is usually easy to appreciate with either the Papanicolaou or the Diff-Quik stain. Occasionally, especially in older patients, the dense colloid may be granular and can resemble necrotic debris.

12.3 Diseases of the Thyroid

12.3.1 Inflammation

Acute Thyroiditis

Acute thyroiditis is rare. Patients, often immunosuppressed, present with fever and a pain in the neck. Most cases are bacterial in origin, eg, *Staphylococcus aureus*, *Streptococcus pyogenes*, or *Streptococcus pneumoniae*. The clinical diagnosis usually is obvious, and the disease responds to appropriate antibiotic therapy. It is, therefore, unlikely to be aspirated. However, occasionally, acute thyroiditis presents as a focal nodular lesion (ie, an abscess); an inflamed tumor may be considered in the differential diagnosis (particularly anaplastic carcinoma).

The FNA biopsy obtains yellow-green pus, which when recognized grossly, can be cultured for definitive diagnosis. Microscopically, numerous neutrophils and histiocytes are characteristic. In addition, granulation tissue, necrosis, and debris may be present. Atypical reparative cells also can be seen. Bacteria (usually gram-positive cocci) or, rarely, other organisms (fungus, viral changes) may be identified. Look carefully for tumor cells.

Granulomatous (de Quervain or Subacute) Thyroiditis

Granulomatous (aka de Quervain or subacute) thyroiditis is a postviral syndrome that usually presents clinically after a recent viral illness, such as a "cold." Granulomatous thyroiditis is a classic cause of painful thyroid. Patients are typically young women, who usually have chills, fever, and fatigue. Although relatively common clinically, granulomatous thyroiditis is rarely aspirated because the diagnosis usually is clinically apparent; there usually is no distinct suspicious nodule; and the disease is self-limiting, typically resolving within a few weeks. In some cases, however, subacute thyroiditis may be painless and form a nodule; these patients are more likely to undergo FNA biopsy.

The aspirate may be somewhat scanty because the biopsy may not be well tolerated due to pain, and the granulomas are "tacked down" by reticulin fibrosis. Microscopically, giant cells and noncaseating granulomas (ie, nodular aggregates of epithelioid histiocytes without necrosis) are present |i12.13|. Very large giant cells surrounding and engulfing colloid are particularly character-istic |i12.14|. Chronic inflammation may be seen, but Hürthle cells are unusual. Follicular epithelium is sparse and degenerated.

When epithelioid giant cells are found in a thyroid aspi-rate, papillary carcinoma must be considered. The differential diag-nosis also includes systemic granulomatous disease (eg, sarcoid), specific infections (eg, tuberculosis |i12.15|, fungal), Hashimoto thyroiditis, and "palpation thyroiditis."

Hashimoto Thyroiditis

Hashimoto thyroiditis is the archetypal example of an autoimmune disease |i12.16|. The classic patient is a middle-aged white woman who has a diffuse goiter and signs of hypothy-roidism. Autoantibodies (antithyroglobulin and antimicrosomal or antiperoxidase) usually are elevated in the serum and help confirm the diagnosis.

The thyroid gland typically shows diffuse moderate enlargement (two to four times normal) and is firm and non-tender. With time, the gland may become bosselated, or "pebbly" (akin to micronodular liver cirrhosis), due to fibrosis. (In contrast, multinodular goiter typically results in a macronodular pattern.)

The diagnosis of Hashimoto thyroiditis usually is clinically apparent. However, some patients present with nonclassic findings (eg, male, hyperthyroid, dominant nodule, low antibody titers). Such atypical cases are more likely to be selected for FNA biopsy.

The cytologic diagnosis of Hashimoto thyroiditis is usually straightforward, consisting in essence of *lymphocytes* and *oncocytes* (Hürthle cells). The autoimmune process, represented by a chronic inflammatory reaction, results in destruction of the thyroid follicles. There is a lymphoplasmacytic infiltrate, complete with follicular center formation. In addition, lymphoid tangles (crushed lymphocytes), lymphohistiocytic aggregates, tingible body macrophages (TBMs), and lymphoglandular bodies may be present. Giant cells, macrophages, and occasionally granulomas can be seen.

Hürthle cells are present in most cases |i12.17|, |i12.18|. The Hürthle cells sometimes can be quite atypical in appearance. Degenerated nononcocytic follicular epithelium also is usually present. Microfollicular structures may be seen. Colloid usually is scant, except in unusual cases in which the disease occurs in a preexisting goiter. Flame cells can be present, especially during the thyrotoxic phase.

Lymphocytes range from scant (in nonneoplastic Hürthle cell nodules, mimicking neoplasm) to abundant (in the florid lymphoid phase, mimicking lymph node) |i12.19|, |i12.20|, |i12.21|. Lymphocytes infiltrating aggregates of Hürthle cells is particularly characteristic of Hashimoto disease. Also, plasma cells, which in contrast with lymphocytes do not normally flow in

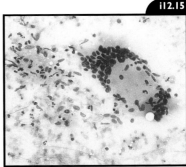

Tuberculous thyroiditis—Langhans cell (DQ)

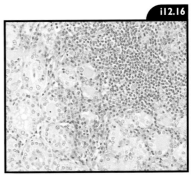

Hashimoto thyroiditis, tissue (H&E)

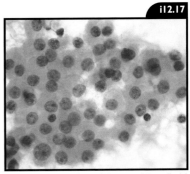

Hashimoto thyroiditis—Hürthle cells (P)

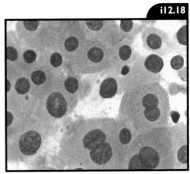

Hashimoto thyroiditis—Hürthle cells (DQ)

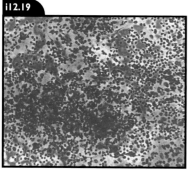

Hashimoto thyroiditis—lymphoid phase (DQ)

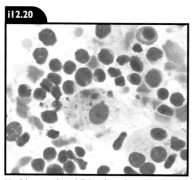

Hashimoto thyroiditis—lymphs, TBM (DQ)

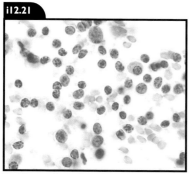

Hashimoto thyroiditis—lymphs, plasma cell (P)

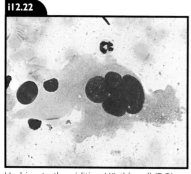

Hashimoto thyroiditis—Hürthle cell (DQ)

the blood, provide a good clue to chronic inflammation. Patients with Hashimoto thyroiditis are at increased risk of developing malignant lymphoma and possibly carcinoma. Beware of atypical Hürthle cells mimicking malignancy |i12.22|.

12.4 Follicular Lesions

In the following discussion, the term *follicular lesion* includes nodules of nonneoplastic goiters and follicular adenomas and carcinomas, as well as the follicular variant of papillary thyroid carcinoma (PTC); *goiter* refers to an enlarged thyroid gland resulting from benign nonneoplastic hyperplasia and colloid storage; and *follicular neoplasm* includes follicular adenomas and carcinomas. In essence, all follicular lesions, whether neoplastic or nonneoplastic, consist of more or less encapsulated nodules of thyroid follicles. Consequently, the distinction among them sometimes can be difficult or impossible, even in the resected specimen.

12.4.1 Goiter

There are many causes of goiter, but in an individual patient, the cause usually is unknown. The overall function of the gland usually is normal (euthyroid goiter), although its function also can be low (hypothyroid goiter) or high (hyperthyroid or toxic goiter). As a goiter develops, the thyroid gland enlarges diffusely: this is simple goiter. With time, some areas of the gland undergo involution, while others undergo further hyperplasia. The continued cycle of degeneration and regeneration causes the gland not only to enlarge but also to become nodular; this is multinodular goiter. Goitrous nodules usually are multiple, although one nodule may be dominant. Microscopically, multinodular goiters can be subclassified as colloid or adenomatous (cellular), depending on whether the colloid storage or the glands, respectively, predominate.

12.4.2 Follicular Neoplasms

Follicular Adenoma

Follicular adenoma is defined as a benign neoplasm, usually single, that fulfills the following criteria: (1) complete encapsulation, (2) different composition inside than outside, and (3) no evidence of invasion (capsular or vascular) or metastases |i12.23|. The follicles in adenoma tend to be more uniform than in goiter. From case to case they range from macro to micro; the neoplastic cells can be follicular, Hürthle, or atypical. Mitoses are rare or absent. There is usually no degeneration |t12.2|.

A putative adenoma occurring in a background of any significant damage to the thyroid gland ("nodularity") is far more likely to be a nodule of a goiter than a true neoplasm, particularly if the interior of the lesion is histologically variable or shows evidence of degeneration. Whether truly neoplastic or not, adenomas are benign, by definition, and are not precursors of cancer.

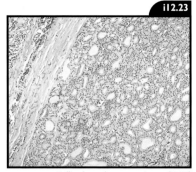
Follicular adenoma, tissue (H&E)

Follicular Carcinoma

Follicular carcinoma has a predilection for middle-aged women. It is associated with iodine deficiency and therefore recently has become quite rare. Follicular carcinomas are of two major types: widely invasive and microinvasive. Microinvasive follicular carcinomas (so-called encapsulated carcinomas) have a capsule and are similar to follicular adenomas, but microscopically they exhibit evidence of capsular or vascular invasion |i12.24|. Encapsulated follicular carcinomas have a much better prognosis than widely invasive tumors, with 10-year survival rates as high as 95% (vs < 50%).

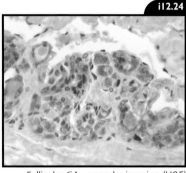
Follicular CA—vascular invasion (H&E)

Atypical adenomas are follicular neoplasms that exhibit cytologic atypia and mitotic figures but lack evidence of invasion or metastasis. They are likely to be considered malignant on FNA biopsy.

12.4.3 FNA Biopsy of Follicular Lesions

The diagnosis of follicular lesions is not an exact science. Basically, FNA biopsy can assign diagnostic probabilities but often cannot provide a precise diagnosis. In theory, the bigger the follicle, the more likely the lesion is benign; the smaller the follicle, the more likely the lesion is neoplastic (benign or malignant). Thus, macrofollicles are low risk and microfollicles are higher risk for a follicular neoplasm. FNA biopsy can predict follicle size by assessing the ratio of colloid to cells. In practice, the more colloid, the more likely the lesion is benign; the more cells, the more likely the lesion is neoplastic. Now, a simple graph can be constructed |f12.1|.

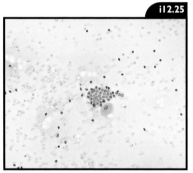
Colloid nodule (P)

The graph forms the basis for a simple approach to the cytologic diagnosis of follicular lesions that proceeds through three

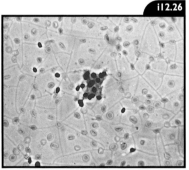
Colloid nodule (DQ)

t12.2 Follicular Adenoma vs Goiter

Follicular Adenoma	Goiter
Single nodule	Multiple nodules
Complete encapsulation	Variable encapsulation
Uniform follicles	Variable follicles
Different inside from outside	Same or different
Preservation	Degeneration/Regeneration
No invasion; no metastasis	No invasion; no metastasis

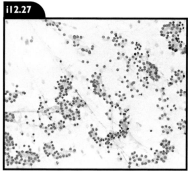

Follicular nodule (P)

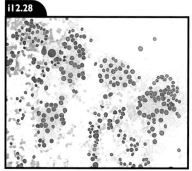

Follicular nodule (DQ)

diagnostic stages. First, assess the amount of colloid and cells, which assigns the biopsies into three risk zones (I, II, III) and roughly separates goiters from neoplasms. Then, look at the architecture (honeycomb vs microfollicles) and background, refining the distinction between goiters and neoplasms. Finally, the cytology (cellular atypia, nuclear membranes, etc) helps classify benign or malignant neoplasms, including the follicular variant of PTC.

First: Colloid vs Cells

At low scanning power, assess colloid and cells. Assign the follicular lesion to one of the following three zones:

Zone I: Colloid dominates the smear and cells are few; the pattern of a colloid nodule |i12.25|, |i12.26|.

Zone II: Many cells but colloid conspicuously present; the pattern of a cellular nodule.

Zone III: Almost entirely cells with little or no colloid; the pattern of a follicular nodule (suspicious for follicular neoplasm, but many are cellular nodules of goiter) |i12.27|, |i12.28|.

Zones I, II, and III correspond to low, intermediate, and high risk of a neoplasm. However, the corresponding risk of cancer is very low, low, and moderate.

f12.1 Diagnosis of Follicular Lesions

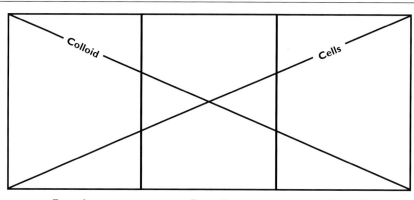

	Zone I	Zone II	Zone III
Cytologic diagnosis	Colloid nodule (most common, by far)	Cellular nodule	Follicular nodule
More diagnostic clues	Multiple nodules; honeycomb pattern; favors goiter	See zones I and III	Solitary nodule; microfollicular pattern; favors neoplasm
Risk of neoplasm	Low (~ 10%)	Moderate (~ 20%)	High (~ 40%)
Risk of cancer*	Very low	Low	Moderate

*Because it has become rare, the risk of follicular carcinoma in *any* zone is low. However, nuclear grooves or intranuclear cytoplasmic invaginations suggest papillary thyroid carcinoma, regardless of zone.

Zone I: Colloid Nodule. Zone I, the most common pattern by far, has little practical risk of being follicular carcinoma (~ 1%), and at least 90% of cases will correspond to nodular (colloid) goiter. A few patients will have colloid adenomas, but such colloid adenomas are virtually never malignant. A rare patient may have macrofollicular variant of papillary carcinoma (see p 215).

Zone II: Cellular Nodule. Zone II biopsies represent a gray area between the more diagnostic patterns of zones I and III. Patients with zone II biopsies have an intermediate risk of neoplasm (~ 20%) and a low risk of cancer.

Zone III: Follicular Nodule. Zone III biopsies carry a higher risk of being a follicular neoplasm (~ 40%) but at most a moderate risk of being follicular carcinoma. Clinical factors, such as extremes of age; new, solitary, dominant, or growing nodule; and history of radiation, increase the risk of malignancy, while lack of additional risk factors and bland cytology reduce the risk. The risk of follicular carcinoma in *any* of the three zones is low because follicular carcinoma has become rare. However, follicular variant of papillary carcinoma must be excluded (see p 215).

Almost all primary follicular carcinomas have a micro-follicular architecture, ie, fetal, embryonal, trabecular, or solid (or Hürthle cell pattern; see p 220), that usually translates into a zone III biopsy. However, only a minority of follicular carcinomas show obvious cytologic features of malignancy. Cellular nodules of goiters are common causes, and dyshormonogenetic goiters rare causes, of nonneoplastic zone III aspirates.

Second: Architecture and Background

Certain features favor goiter over neoplasm. Degenerative and regenerative changes are so common in multinodular goiter that they are virtually part of the definition. In contrast, these changes are unusual in follicular neoplasms. Thus, evidence of hemorrhage |i12.29|, fibrosis (including stromal fragments and perifollicular fibrosis |i12.30|), cystic degeneration, foam cells, macrophages, cholesterol crystals, stromal calcification (not psammoma bodies), repair |i12.31|, and focal pleomorphism favors goiter over neoplasm.

Characteristically, there is a wide range of follicle size in a goiter, from small to very large, but medium to large size follicles usually predominate. Microfollicles, if present, usually simply represent part of the size spectrum in goiters. Sheets of cells remain very orderly and regularly spaced ("honeycombed") |i12.32| and seldom show overlap or crowding of nuclei. The honeycomb pattern is usually maintained in goiters but lost in neoplasia. The individual cells usually are quite uniform, although an occasional cell may be more pleomorphic ("endocrine atypia"). The nuclei usually are about the size of a lymphocyte or slightly larger. As in normal thyroid cells, the chromatin is granular and uniform, and nucleoli usually are incon-

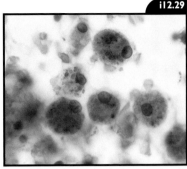
i12.29
Goiter—hemorrhagic degeneration (P)

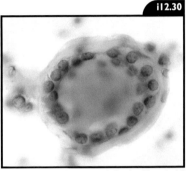
i12.30
Goiter—perifollicular fibrosis (P)

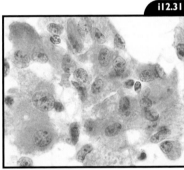
i12.31
Goiter—repair/regeneration (P)

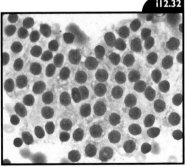
i12.32
Goiter—honeycomb sheet (DQ)

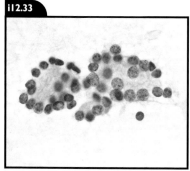

Follicular neoplasm (P)

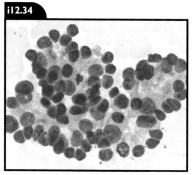

Follicular neoplasm (DQ)

spicuous. The presence of different types of cells (eg, follicular, Hürthle, flame, foam) also favors a diagnosis of goiter over neoplasm. Evidence of repair/regeneration, similar to that seen in the Pap smear, is common in goiters but rare in neoplasms.

Certain features favor a diagnosis of neoplasm over goiter. High cellularity and scant colloid occur in most follicular neoplasms but also can occur in adenomatous (cellular) nodules of goiters. A prominent microfollicular pattern is characteristic of follicular neoplasms |i12.33|, |i12.34| and is seen in most cases, but it also occurs in some goiters. Microfollicular lesions are more likely to be neoplastic. The combination of high cellularity and a microfollicular pattern is suggestive of a follicular neoplasm. The nuclei of follicular neoplasms may—or may not—be diffusely enlarged but usually remain uniform. The chromatin may—or may not—be coarse, and although nucleoli can be seen, they are infrequent. In practice, however, atypical follicular epithelium usually correlates with nonneoplastic goiter. Follicular neoplasms composed of normal or large-sized follicles are difficult to recognize as neoplastic (because they result in zone I pattern) but are unlikely to be malignant |t12.3|.

Third: Cytology

It often is not possible to distinguish between follicular adenomas and follicular carcinomas by cytology alone. This is because many well-differentiated follicular carcinomas look cytologically benign, and, conversely, a few benign but atypical adenomas look cytologically malignant.

Cytologic features suggestive of carcinoma include high cellularity, markedly crowded, irregular microfollicles, numerous single cells, large, pleomorphic nuclei (three to four times normal size), abnormal (coarse, dark, irregular) chromatin, prominent or multiple nucleoli, and atypical mitotic figures. In essence, if there

t12.3 Differential Diagnosis of Goiter and Follicular Neoplasm

	Goiter	Follicular Neoplasm
Colloid	Usually abundant	Usually scant
Cellularity	Usually low	Usually high
Cell types	Multiple	Single
Nuclei	About the size of a lymphocyte	May be enlarged
Nucleoli	Inconspicuous	Variable
Follicles		
Size	Variable	Uniform
Microfollicles	Less common	More common
Honeycomb	Maintained	Lost
Degeneration	Common	Uncommon
Clinical nodules	Multiple	Solitary

is marked architectural disorganization or marked cytologic atypia, suspect follicular carcinoma |i12.35|, |i12.36|.

Finally, if the nuclear membranes are markedly irregular or deeply "grooved" (most cells, most fields) or if there are *any* intranuclear cytoplasmic invaginations (INCIs), the most likely diagnosis is PTC, regardless of which of the three zones the aspirate falls into. The nuclei of PTC are more oval than round, the chromatin is powdery fine and pale, and micronucleoli are present and tend to be marginated. In contrast, follicular nuclei are round with moderately granular chromatin and smooth nuclear membranes; nucleoli usually are inconspicuous. Other characteristic features of PTC, including papillae, squamoid cytoplasm, and psammoma bodies, also may be present. (For further discussion, see next section.)

12.5 Malignancy (Other Than Follicular Carcinoma)

12.5.1 Papillary Thyroid Carcinoma

PTC accounts for at least three quarters of all thyroid malignancies. PTC is more common in females and has a peak incidence in the 20s through the 40s, although no age is exempt. PTC usually has an excellent prognosis, particularly in young patients, but may be more aggressive in older age and in men. Regional cervical lymph node metastases are common and may be the presenting sign. Distant blood-borne metastases (lung, bone, etc) are much less common in PTC than in follicular carcinoma. A few cases recur, and recurrence may be late. Cystic change is common in PTC and uncommon in most other thyroid cancers. Multicentricity (intrathyroidal metastasis) occurs in at least 20% of cases (substantially higher on careful search), even when the disease is clinically unilateral. Partial or complete encapsulation is common in PTC. Microscopically, PTC can be predominantly papillary (classic pattern) |i12.37|, mixed papillary-follicular (most cases), or predominantly follicular (follicular variant). Occult PTCs (≤ 1 cm) are common but rarely metastasize.

The FNA biopsy usually obtains abundant diagnostic material, except in the cases that are predominantly cystic. Numerous large monolayered sheets of cells are a common and typical finding. The malignant cells are larger than normal and may be crowded, losing their normal honeycomb spacing. Follicular structures also are commonly present and may be the predominant or exclusive growth pattern in some cases (follicular variant of PTC). An occasional case has a predominance of single cells, an unfavorable prognostic sign.

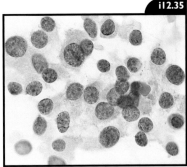
i12.35

Follicular carcinoma (P)

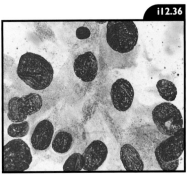
i12.36

Follicular carcinoma (DQ)

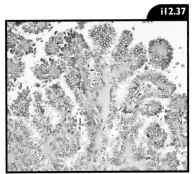
i12.37

Papillary carcinoma, tissue (H&E)

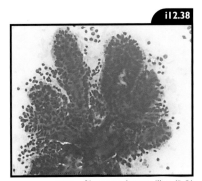
i12.38

PTC—fibrovascular papillae (DQ)

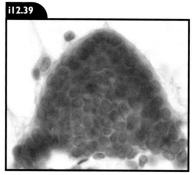

PTC—"cap" (P)

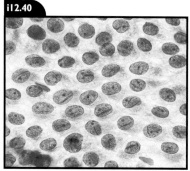

PTC—nuclear grooves (P)

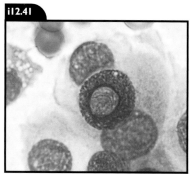

PTC—INCI (DQ)

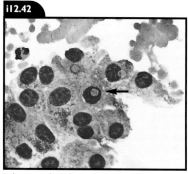

False pseudoinclusion—RBC (DQ)

Papillary structures are an important diagnostic feature of PTC and are found in up to 90% of cases on FNA biopsy. Three types of papillae may be seen. The first is classic three-dimensional branching papillae with fibrovascular cores |i12.38|. These papillae are highly characteristic of PTC but are found in only a minority of cases. The second type of papillary structure seen in PTC is avascular, three-dimensional, rounded dome-shaped structures that may represent the tips of papillae ("caps") |i12.39|. These caps are the most frequently present type of papillary structure seen in aspirates of PTC. Finally, two-dimensional flat sheets of cells arranged in finger-like projections also can be seen.

Although papillae are highly characteristic of PTC, they are not necessary for the diagnosis (and are absent in the pure follicular variant). The diagnosis of PTC also can be based on certain nuclear features, including nuclear grooving and INCIs.

Nuclear grooving, or irregularity of the nuclear membrane, is present in at least 90% of cases of PTC. At a minimum, the nuclear outline should have a deep longitudinal fold, like a coffee bean |i12.40|, but can be as irregular and lobulated as a piece of popcorn. To be diagnostically useful, grooved nuclei must be present diffusely in the smear (most cells, most fields), because nuclear grooves can be found focally in many thyroid conditions, including goiter, thyroiditis, adenomas, and other carcinomas. Nuclear grooves are more easily appreciated in cytology than histology, particularly in Papanicolaou stain.

INCIs, also known as nuclear pseudoinclusions, are one of the most important diagnostic features of PTC |i12.41|. On careful search of an adequate specimen, they are present in at least 90% of cases. Note that INCIs are completely different from the ground-glass "Orphan Annie eye" nuclei seen in permanent tissue sections, although in the proper milieu, INCIs have similar diagnostic significance. INCIs can be easily appreciated in histology or cytology, Papanicolaou or Diff-Quik stain.

Because a variety of artifacts can mimic INCIs, great care must be taken to identify them accurately. INCIs have a homogeneous center, which stains more like the cytoplasm than like the rest of the nucleus. INCIs are completely contained within the nucleus. Any bubble that goes through the nuclear membrane cannot be an INCI. Further, since the INCIs are surrounded by nuclear membrane, they have a very sharp margin, which is outlined by a rim of condensed chromatin. INCIs are not traversed by strands of chromatin, and if a nucleolus is visualized within the space, it is not an INCI. More than one INCI can be seen in a nucleus, but to be diagnostic, an INCI should occupy a significant part of a given nucleus. An RBC overlying the nucleus can closely mimic an INCI |i12.42|.

INCIs are exceptionally rare in benign thyroid disease but can be seen in other thyroid malignancies, particularly medullary carcinoma. INCIs also occur in a wide variety of other kinds of head and neck tumors, including parathyroid adenomas, paragangliomas, and metastases (eg, melanoma, renal cell carcinoma). But, in the proper milieu, INCIs are practically diagnostic of PTC.

The chromatin of PTC usually is powdery fine and pale. This is in contrast with the chromatin of ordinary follicular cells (seen in normal thyroid, goiters, or follicular neoplasms), which usually is distinctly granular and moderately hyperchromatic. One to three small but conspicuous nucleoli, which tend to be marginated near the nuclear membrane, also are characteristic of PTC.

There are several other characteristic cytologic features of PTC. These include squamoid cytoplasm (dense cytoplasm, distinct cell boundaries, similar to squamous metaplasia) |i12.43|, septate cytoplasmic vacuoles (tiny well-defined vacuoles, not foam cells), giant cells (particularly those with an epithelioid cytoplasm, often with peculiar shapes—an important clue to look carefully for evidence of PTC |i12.44|), and psammoma bodies (present in only one third of cases but rare in other benign or malignant thyroid disease) |i12.45|. Colloid usually is scanty but can range from sparse to abundant. A particular form of altered dense colloid, so-called bubble gum or sticky colloid, is diagnostically important but found only in a minority of cases. This peculiar "gummy" colloid stains pink in Diff-Quik |i12.46| and pink-purple or blue-green in Papanicolaou. Occasional cases are predominantly cystic; the smears are dominated by macrophages and debris with a paucity of diagnostic cells, which can result in a false-negative diagnosis.

In Summary

There is practically an embarrassment of riches when it comes to diagnostic features of PTC. The following diagnostic features are among the most commonly present in PTC (ie, most sensitive) and most commonly absent in other diseases (ie, most specific):

Architecture: Papillae, especially "caps"
Nuclei: Irregular membranes
     Grooved nuclei (most cells, most fields)
     Intranuclear cytoplasmic invaginations
Cytoplasm: Dense and squamoid (some cells)

If all of these features are present, PTC can be diagnosed with a high degree of confidence. In fact, if even one feature is present, PTC is a likely diagnosis.

12.5.2 Medullary Thyroid Carcinoma

Medullary thyroid carcinoma (MTC) is a neuroendocrine (carcinoid type) tumor arising from or mimicking the parafollicular or "C" (for calcitonin) cell. The neoplasm characteristically secretes calcitonin, causing elevated serum calcitonin levels,

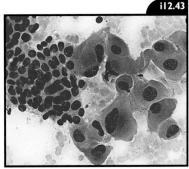

PTC—squamoid cytoplasm (DQ)

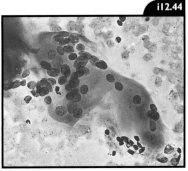

PTC—epithelioid giant cell (DQ)

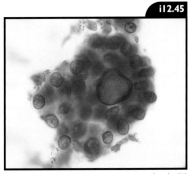

PTC—psammoma body (P)

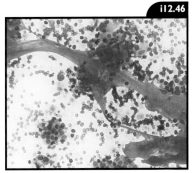

PTC—gummy colloid (DQ)

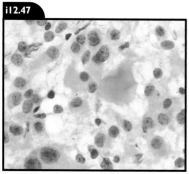

Medullary carcinoma—cells, amyloid (P)

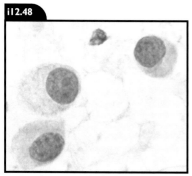

MTC—plasmacytoid cells (P, oil)

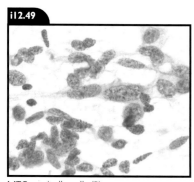

MTC—spindle cells (P)

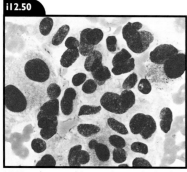

MTC—pleomorphism, red granules (DQ)

which can be used as a tumor marker for MTC. The combination of elevated serum calcitonin plus a thyroid nodule is virtually pathognomonic of MTC.

Familial and sporadic forms of MTC occur. Sporadic cases are much more common (~ 80% of cases) and usually present as a solitary nodule. Familial cases, often part of multiple endocrine neoplasia syndromes, are usually multifocal and bilateral and present in younger patients. The tumor is typically located in the mid to upper pole of the thyroid, is often well-circumscribed, and sometimes is even encapsulated, although microscopic evidence of invasion is commonly present. MTC has a characteristic coarse calcification pattern that can be detected radiologically. Metastasis occurs most commonly to regional lymph nodes, followed by distant metastases (lung, liver, bone).

The FNA biopsy characteristically obtains carcinoid-like neuroendocrine cells and amyloid in variable proportions |i12.47|. The cells can be predominantly dispersed or form loose clusters. There are three common cell types, which vary in proportion from case to case: lymphoplasmacytoid |i12.48|, spindle |i12.49|, and granular ("Hürthloid"). A characteristic finding in neuroendocrine carcinoid-type tumors, including MTC, is the combination of lymphoplasmacytoid and small spindle cells. The tumor cells are usually mildly pleomorphic, although individual cases can range from very monomorphic (typical of carcinoids in general) to markedly pleomorphic with bizarre tumor cells |i12.50|. In some cases, spindle cells predominate.

The most characteristic feature of the stroma is amyloid, which is very variable in amount and not seen in all cases. Amyloid resembles dense colloid. Although it is variably metachromatic (in Diff-Quik stain) |i12.51|, special stains (eg, Congo red with diagnostic apple green birefringence |i12.52|) are needed to confirm its presence.

The nuclei of MTC cells typically have "salt-and-pepper" chromatin. While not present in every case, this characteristic chromatin pattern suggests the diagnosis of a neuroendocrine tumor. Scattered binucleated or multinucleated cells are relatively common. Nucleoli usually are not prominent. INCIs, identical to those seen in PTC, can be found in many cases. Mitotic figures are sometimes identified.

The cytoplasm is well-defined and fibrillar or finely granular. Dendritic cytoplasmic processes—spindle or stellate cells—are a characteristic feature of MTC. In Diff-Quik stain, a dusting of fine red (metachromatic) granules may be seen in the cytoplasm of some cells, which corresponds to neurosecretory granules. Silver stains, such as Grimelius, usually are positive, but nowadays, immunocytochemical demonstration of calcitonin is more often used to confirm the cytologic diagnosis. Thyroglobulin is usually negative but may be focally positive in some cases. Psammoma bodies occur in a few cases.

The morphologic appearance of MTC can mimic a variety of other thyroid neoplasms, including follicular neoplasms, PTC, anaplastic carcinoma, Hürthle cell neoplasms, lymphoma, and sarcoma. Variants of MTC include oncocytic, spindle cell, clear cell, small cell, and giant cell types. The presence of plasmacytoid and spindle cells, salt-and-pepper chromatin, red cytoplasmic granules, and amyloid, as well as an increased serum calcitonin level or a positive family history, supports the diagnosis of MTC.

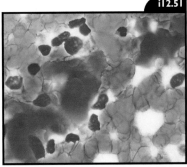

MTC—metachromatic amyloid (DQ)

12.5.3 Giant and Spindle Cell (Anaplastic) Carcinoma

Giant and spindle cell (anaplastic) carcinoma is a highly aggressive but rare thyroid neoplasm. It is more common in women than men (3:1) and usually occurs in elderly patients (60s-80s). Although capable of metastasis, giant and spindle cell carcinoma usually strangles the patient by local infiltration of vital structures in the neck. The tumor does not respond well to surgery or radiation, and most patients die within a year of diagnosis, unless the disease is caught early.

Giant and spindle cell carcinoma is thought to arise, at least in some cases, from "dedifferentiation" of a preexisting thyroid tumor (which also may be sampled in the aspirate). Rapid increase in the size of a long-standing thyroid nodule in an elderly patient is a classic history.

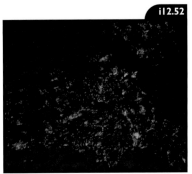

MTC—amyloid, apple green birefringence

Cytologically, the diagnosis of malignancy usually is obvious |i12.53|, |i12.54|. The smears usually are quite cellular and contain highly malignant-appearing cells. The cells are extremely variable in size and shape, often bizarre; many are spindle or giant, hence the name. The nuclei have obvious malignant features, such as highly irregular membranes, abnormal, coarse, dark, irregular chromatin, and macronucleoli. Mitotic figures, including abnormal forms, may be numerous. INCIs can be present. The cytoplasm can range from pale and vacuolated (clear) to granular (Hürthle-like) to dense (squamoid). Neutrophils may be present in the cytoplasm in some cases. Hyaline globules may be seen. Inflammation, necrosis, and a malignant diathesis are typical of the background. Immunocytochemically, most cases are thyroglobulin negative, and some are keratin negative.

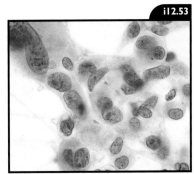

Giant and spindle cell carcinoma (P)

MTC is perhaps the most common differential diagnostic problem |t12.4|, since it can grow in a similar giant and spindle cell pattern. The differential diagnosis also includes primary spindle cell or pleomorphic sarcomas, which are extremely rare in the thyroid. Metastatic anaplastic carcinomas, eg, from lung or pancreas, also must be excluded. When a poorly differentiated tumor is encountered in a thyroid aspirate, consider giant and spindle cell carcinoma and exclude metastasis.

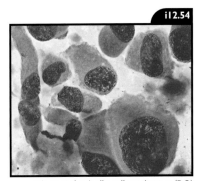

Giant and spindle cell carcinoma (DQ)

t12.4 The "Big Four" Thyroid Cancers

	Papillary	Follicular	Medullary	Anaplastic
Clinical features				
Associations	Radiation	Iodine deficiency	Familial (20%)	Long-standing goiter
Peak age (y)	25-30	40-55	30-50*	> 60
Incidence (%)	75-85	< 5[†]	5-10	5-10
Metastasis	Cervical lymph nodes	Blood, distant	Nodal and distant	Local infiltration
Mortality (%)	10	25-33[‡]	50	> 90
Cytologic features				
Cells	Monotonous	Monotonous	Spindle or plasmacytoid	Anaplastic spindle or giant
Nuclei	Monotonous	Monotonous	Variable	Pleomorphic
Membrane	Grooved	Smooth	Smooth	Highly irregular
INCIs	> 90% of cases	None	50% of cases	Can occur
Chromatin	Powdery, pale	Granular	Salt and pepper	Very abnormal
Nucleoli	Small, marginated	Can occur	Small	Macro
Cytoplasm	Squamoid	Delicate	Red granules	Variable
Papillae	Characteristic	Absent	Rare	Absent
Follicles	Common	Characteristic	Rare	Absent
Other	Psammoma bodies	Colloid (scant)	Amyloid	Neutrophils

INCIs, intranuclear cytoplasmic invaginations.
*Younger in familial type.
[†]Formerly 15%-20%.
[‡]Widely invasive type; microinvasive < 5%.

12.5.4 Hürthle Cell Tumors: Nonneoplastic Nodules and Neoplasms

Hürthle cell tumors are controversial lesions that have a reputation for unpredictable behavior. There are several reasons for this. First, not every Hürthle cell tumor is a Hürthle cell neoplasm. Nonneoplastic proliferations of Hürthle cells, forming nodules, are relatively common in goiters and Hashimoto thyroiditis. Furthermore, some have regarded "Hürthle cell neoplasm" as a specific diagnosis. In fact, oncocytic metaplasia (ie, Hürthle cell change) can occur in any of the usual types of thyroid neoplasms, including follicular adenomas and carcinomas, PTC, anaplastic carcinoma, and, rarely, MTC. Naturally, if benign and malignant neoplasms as well as nonneoplastic nodules are all placed into a single diagnostic category, the behavior will be unpredictable. Unfortunately, it sometimes can be difficult to accurately sort out all these possibilities, even in the resected specimen.

Certain clinical features help to differentiate nonneoplastic Hürthle cell nodules (in Hashimoto thyroiditis or goiters) from Hürthle cell neoplasms. A Hürthle cell nodule in a goiter is usually part of a multinodular gland and a Hürthle cell nodule in Hashimoto thyroiditis usually presents in a diffusely abnormal gland, while a true neoplasm is classically a solitary nodule in an otherwise normal gland. Moreover, Hashimoto thyroiditis is associated with hypothyroidism and antithyroid antibodies, in contrast to goiters and neoplasms. Use caution in diagnosing a Hürthle cell neoplasm in the presence of clinical, laboratory, or cytologic evidence of Hashimoto thyroiditis.

Cytologic factors that favor a nonneoplastic nodule include cohesive honeycombed sheets, a spectrum of morphology (ranging from typical follicular cells to Hürthle cells), degeneration, colloid (in goiters), and lymphoplasmacytic infiltrate (in Hashimoto thyroiditis). Neoplasms tend to show a dissociated single cell pattern or disorganized three-dimensional groups and microfollicles with a pure population of Hürthle cells. Neoplastic Hürthle cells often have more uniform nuclei than nonneoplastic nodules, with prominent or macronucleoli in most cells. Nuclear size and the degree of anisokaryosis are not completely reliable in distinguishing between benign and malignant Hürthle cell neoplasms. Features favoring Hürthle cell carcinoma include marked pleomorphism, numerous microfollicles, crowded sheets with ill-defined cell borders, smaller cells with high nuclear/cytoplasmic ratios, abnormal chromatin, multiple or macronucleoli, INCIs, and psammoma bodies |i12.55|, |i12.56|.

12.5.5 Clear Cell Neoplasms

Clear cell neoplasms are a subtype of all major variants of thyroid neoplasms. The clear cell change can be focal or diffuse. The clarity of the cytoplasm usually is due to greatly dilated mitochondria in Hürthle cells but can be due to accumulation of substances, such as glycogen, thyroglobulin, or lipid. Although clear cells can be seen in benign lesions of the thyroid (eg, goiter, Graves disease, Hashimoto thyroiditis, or follicular adenomas), they occur more commonly in thyroid malignancy. Also, consider metastasis from renal cell carcinoma.

12.5.6 Insular Carcinoma

Insular carcinoma |i12.57|, |i12.58|, despite its deceptively bland cytologic appearance, is considered a poorly differentiated thyroid cancer, intermediate in behavior between the differentiated thyroid malignancies (ie, papillary and follicular carcinomas)

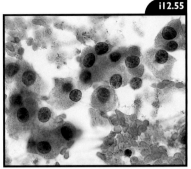

i12.55

Hürthle cell carcinoma (P)

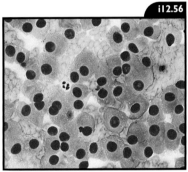

i12.56

Hürthle cell carcinoma (DQ)

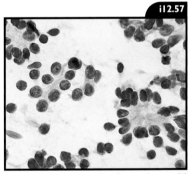

i12.57

Insular carcinoma (P)

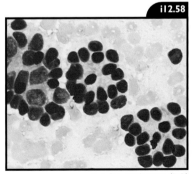

i12.58

Insular carcinoma (DQ)

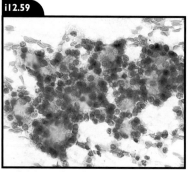

Hyalinizing trabecular neoplasm (P)

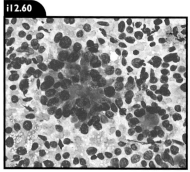

Hyalinizing trabecular neoplasm (DQ)

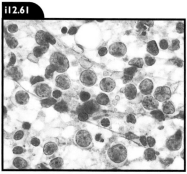

Non-Hodgkin lymphoma, large cell type (P)

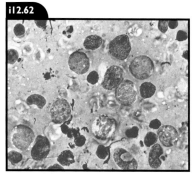

Non-Hodgkin lymphoma, large cell type (DQ)

and anaplastic giant and spindle cell carcinoma. Insular carcinoma grows in solid nests and islands—hence the name—reminiscent of carcinoid tumors. Small loose clusters, trabeculae, and follicles, as well as single cells, may be seen, but papillae are not. The cells are small, monomorphic, and bland appearing with scant pale cytoplasm and high nuclear/cytoplasmic ratios. The nuclei are round with smooth membranes, although focally the nuclei may be grooved (but not to the extent seen in PTC). INCIs have been reported. Nucleoli range from inconspicuous to prominent. Some nuclear crowding can occur. Intracytoplasmic vacuoles containing thyroglobulin may be a characteristic finding. Necrosis often is present in the background, but colloid is scant. The cells express thyroglobulin, and stains are negative for neurosecretory granules.

12.5.7 Hyalinizing Trabecular Adenoma

Hyalinizing trabecular adenoma, also known as paraganglioma-like adenoma of the thyroid, is a rare, usually benign neoplasm of the thyroid. It has a marked predilection for women. The cytologic diagnosis is difficult; the tumor often is mistaken for PTC or MTC. The tumor may be more closely related to PTC than previously appreciated.

The cells tend to be spindle shaped. The nuclei often are enlarged slightly and atypical appearing with pale chromatin, INCIs, and nuclear grooves, similar to PTC. Psammoma bodies may occur. A clue to the diagnosis is the presence of metachromatic stromal (basement membrane–like) material found as irregular deposits between cells |i12.59|, |i12.60|. This material could be mistaken for colloid (but is metachromatic) or amyloid (but is Congo red negative). Metachromatic (red) cytoplasmic neurosecretory granules are not present. Hyalinizing trabecular adenoma expresses thyroglobulin but not calcitonin, which is similar to PTC but the opposite of MTC (calcitonin, positive; thyroglobulin, negative).

12.5.8 Hematopoietic Neoplasms

Malignant lymphoma rarely arises in the thyroid, accounting for only about 2% of all primary thyroid cancers (but the incidence may be increasing); secondary involvement is more common. The typical patient is an older woman (60-65 years old). There is a strong association with Hashimoto thyroiditis, a possible clue to the diagnosis. Sudden enlargement of a long-standing diffuse goiter suggests the diagnosis clinically. Patients also may complain of pain.

The course is unpredictable, but it can be aggressive. However, when confined to the thyroid, the disease often is curable. The majority of cases are non-Hodgkin lymphomas, predominantly large B-cell type |i12.61|, |i12.62|. There may be a relationship with neoplasms of mucosa-associated lymphoid tissue (MALTomas). Other hematologic malignancies, including Hodgkin disease, plasmacytoma, and Langerhans histiocytosis, also can involve the thyroid |i12.63|, |i12.64|. Ancillary studies, such as immunologic markers, flow cytometry, and gene rearrangement, can be performed on aspirated material.

The details of the cytologic diagnosis depend on the type of lymphoma, but in general the tumor is composed of dispersed monotypic lymphoid cells with lymphoglandular bodies in the background. Remnants of Hashimoto thyroiditis may be present in some cases, including Hürthle cells and degenerated follicular epithelium.

The florid lymphoid phase of Hashimoto thyroiditis may simulate a lymphoma owing to the presence of an abundance of "immature" follicular center cells. Characteristic of a benign infiltrate, small "mature" lymphocytes predominate, and tingible body macrophages and plasma cells are present.

Sarcomas

Primary sarcomas of the thyroid are extremely rare. Most thyroid "sarcomas" are actually anaplastic (giant and spindle cell) carcinomas, which can mimic pleomorphic or spindle cell sarcomas and can have a metaplastic stroma. Anaplastic carcinoma may be negative for both thyroglobulin and keratin, mimicking a sarcoma. Liposarcoma, leiomyosarcoma, and angiosarcoma are among the primary sarcomas that can occur in the thyroid.

12.5.9 Other Rare Tumors

Primary squamous cell carcinoma in the thyroid gland is very rare (~ 1% of cases). Far more commonly, squamous cell carcinoma in the thyroid is secondary to another source (eg, head and neck, esophageal, or lung cancer). Squamous differentiation can be seen in PTC, giant and spindle cell carcinoma, MTC, and mucoepidermoid carcinoma.

Mucoepidermoid carcinoma (MEC) is a very rare, low-grade cancer with both malignant squamous cells |i12.65| and mucin-positive glandular cells |i12.66|, similar to mucoepidermoid carcinoma in other body sites. Mucoepidermoid features (squamoid cytoplasm, malignant glandular cells) are commonly seen in ordinary PTC.

Small cell carcinoma of the thyroid is vanishingly rare, although there is a small cell variant of MTC. Most putative cases of small cell carcinoma actually represent malignant lymphoma or metastasis of small cell carcinoma of the lung.

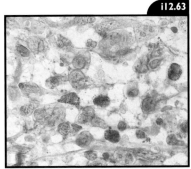
Langerhans histiocytosis (P)

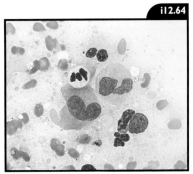
Langerhans histiocytosis (DQ)

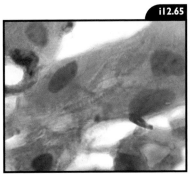
MEC—intercellular bridges (P)

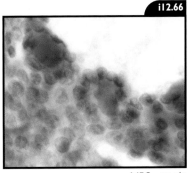
MEC—mucin

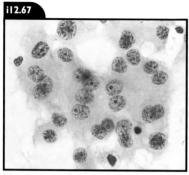

Metastatic renal cell carcinoma (P)

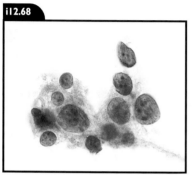

Therapeutic effect—methimazole (P)

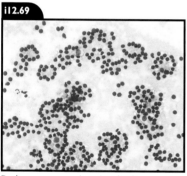

Dyshormonogenetic goiter (DQ)

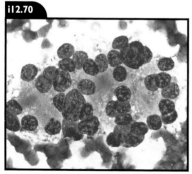

Dyshormonogenetic goiter (DQ)

12.5.10 Metastatic Carcinoma

Metastases to the thyroid are not rare but were formerly diagnosed only rarely during life. However, with the increasing use of FNA biopsy, the antemortem diagnosis of metastatic tumors in the thyroid has become more common. The most common sources of metastases are carcinomas of the kidney, colon, lung, and breast, and melanoma.

For thyroid tumors that do not fit one of the common patterns of primary thyroid carcinoma or are poorly differentiated, consider a metastasis. Metastases of kidney and breast carcinomas can be almost indistinguishable from follicular neoplasms or PTC on cytologic grounds. Single file chains of cells or intracytoplasmic lumens suggest breast origin. Renal cell carcinoma can mimic Hürthle cell or clear cell neoplasms |i12.67|. Small cell carcinoma usually is metastatic from the lung. Giant and spindle cell carcinoma can be mimicked by tumors from the lung or pancreas or metastatic sarcomas. Most cases of squamous cell carcinoma in the thyroid represent direct extension from an esophageal or laryngeal primary site.

Benign thyroid lesions and most differentiated thyroid cancers express thyroglobulin, while metastases of nonthyroidal origin do not. Note, however, that MTC and giant and spindle cell thyroid carcinomas also are frequently negative for thyroglobulin.

12.6 Therapeutic Effects

Radiation, especially radioactive iodine, can cause marked cytologic atypia, including cellular crowding, nuclear enlargement, irregular nuclear outlines, INCIs, hyperchromasia, prominent nucleoli, and high nuclear/cytoplasmic ratios, mimicking malignancy. However, the abnormal cells tend to be randomly distributed, and mitotic figures are rare. Also, radiation may be associated with an increased risk of developing thyroid cancer, especially PTC. Antithyroid therapy, eg, methimazole, thioimidazole, or thiouracil, can also cause marked cytologic atypia |i12.68|.

12.7 Dyshormonogenetic Goiter

Congenital hypothyroidism, due to autosomal recessively inherited enzyme defects in thyroid hormone synthesis, is associated with the formation of a goiter. Microscopically, the follicles are poorly formed, colloid is scant, and the epithelium is hyperplastic and may be atypical and mitotically active due to thyroid-stimulating hormone. An FNA biopsy is essentially indistinguishable from that of a follicular neoplasm (high cellularity, numerous micro-follicles, and scant colloid) |i12.69|, |i12.70|, and because of cellular atypia, which is common, carcinoma may be favored. These changes mimic malignancy, but actual malignant change is rare.

12.8 **Pregnancy**

During pregnancy, iodine is lost in the urine; the thyroid gland compensates by becoming hyperplastic, causing it to enlarge. During pregnancy, an aspirate of a thyroid nodule may be very cellular, with thin watery colloid and flame cells |i12.71|. Papillary hyperplasia may suggest PTC, a disease that predominates in women of childbearing age. Look for the usual features of PTC, eg, irregular nuclear membranes, INCIs, and squamoid cytoplasm, before making this diagnosis.

12.9 **Cysts**

Cystic thyroid nodules are common. Aspiration of a thyroid cyst is a "good news, bad news" proposition for the patient. The good news is that only about 1% of aspirated thyroid cysts are malignant (most are PTC). The bad news is that only about half of cystic malignancies can be diagnosed by aspiration cytology. A diagnosis of a cyst (or cyst content) |i12.72| does not completely exclude malignancy, and patients with thyroid cysts should be carefully followed up. When aspirating a cyst, drain it as completely as possible and reaspirate any residual mass. If the cyst recurs, it can be drained again, but if it recurs again, it probably should be excised (for two reasons: first, to "catch" missed cancers and second, because it is impractical to come in every few weeks to have a cyst drained).

12.10 **Hot Nodules and Graves Disease**

In most cases, the FNA biopsy of a hot nodule shows a colloid-predominant smear pattern that indicates a benign lesion. Sometimes, however, the aspirate may suggest a follicular neoplasm owing to the presence of marked cellularity, microfolli-cles, and nuclear pleomorphism |i12.73|. Flame cells may be numerous |i12.74|. Papillary hyperplasia may suggest PTC (look for usual diagnostic features, such as INCIs). Although hot nodules may be neoplastic, they are unlikely to be malignant.

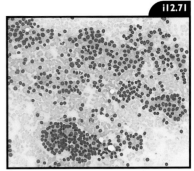
Pregnancy hyperplasia (P)

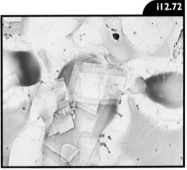
Cyst content—cholesterol crystals (DQ)

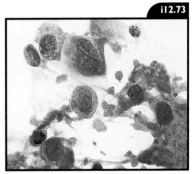
Graves disease (P)

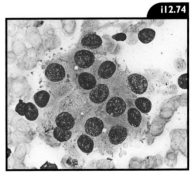
Graves disease (DQ)

CHAPTER THIRTEEN

7 ⋈ Lymph nodes are small bean-shaped organs with highly organized anatomic and functional compartments |f13.1|. Lymph arrives in the lymph node via afferent lymphatics and, after filtering through the cortex, paracortex, and medulla, leaves by the efferent lymphatics on its way to the blood. Particulate matter is removed by macrophages (histiocytes) that also have an important role in antigen concentration and processing for lymphocytes. Lymph nodes are sites of lymphocyte proliferation (lymphocytopoiesis) and antibody production |i13.1|.

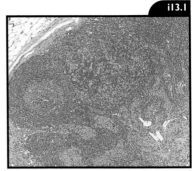

Lymph node, tissue (H&E)

The cortex, or outer cortex, of the lymph node contains the lymphoid follicles, which are B-cell areas. B cells produce immunoglobulin (Ig) and are responsible for humoral antibody-mediated immunity, such as is seen in response to bacterial infection. B cells are characterized by the presence of Ig heavy chains, and each cell has a single (monoclonal) light chain on the cell surface membrane. Follicular hyperplasia and follicular center cell (FCC) lymphomas are associated with the cortical zone of the lymph node.

The paracortex, or inner cortex, is located in the inter-follicular area, between the cortex and medulla, and is a T-cell area. T cells are responsible for cell-mediated immunity, including graft rejection and delayed hypersensitivity, as well as response to viruses and certain drugs. Cell-mediated (T-cell) response is characterized by paracortical hyperplasia with proliferation of T immunoblasts. The paracortex also is associated with T-cell lymphomas.

The medulla of the lymph node is composed of cords and sinuses. The medullary cords are plasma cell areas. When humoral immunity is stimulated, the medullary cords become expanded by reactive plasmacytosis. The medullary cords also are associated with lymphoplasmacytoid lymphoma and plasmacytoma. The medullary sinuses are primarily histiocyte areas, but they also contain small B lymphocytes. The phagocytic (macrophage) response, sinus histiocytosis, may be seen, eg, in lymph nodes draining infection or cancer. The sinuses also are associated with anaplastic (CD30/Ki-1) lymphoma and malignant histiocytosis.

13.1 **The Cells**

Diff-Quik stain is particularly useful in identifying lymphoreticular and hematopoietic cells and their tumors. However, the Papanicolaou stain also is useful, particularly for the evaluation of nuclear features, such as membrane irregularities ("cleaves"), chromatin, and nucleoli.

f13.1 Lymphoid Morphology and Immunophenotypes

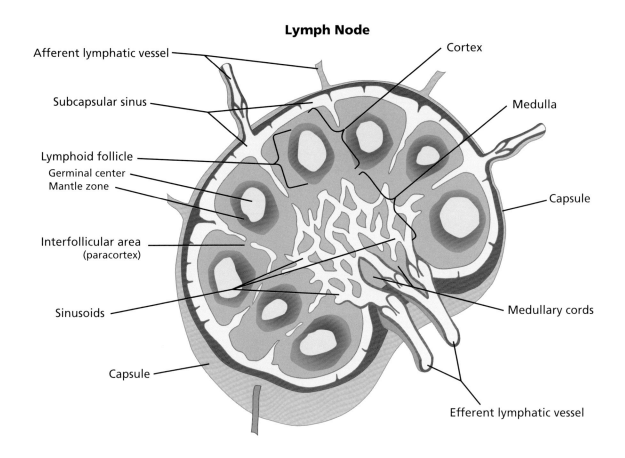

Lymph Node

Afferent lymphatic vessel

Cortex

Subcapsular sinus

Medulla

Lymphoid follicle
Germinal center
Mantle zone

Capsule

Interfollicular area
(paracortex)

Sinusoids

Medullary cords

Capsule

Efferent lymphatic vessel

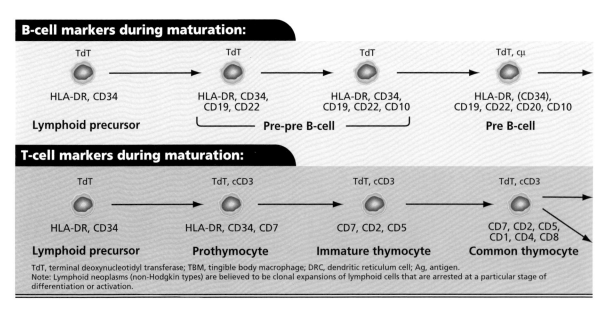

B-cell markers during maturation:

TdT

HLA-DR, CD34

Lymphoid precursor

TdT

HLA-DR, CD34,
CD19, CD22

TdT

HLA-DR, CD34,
CD19, CD22, CD10

Pre-pre B-cell

TdT, cμ

HLA-DR, (CD34),
CD19, CD22, CD20, CD10

Pre B-cell

T-cell markers during maturation:

TdT

HLA-DR, CD34

Lymphoid precursor

TdT, cCD3

HLA-DR, CD34, CD7

Prothymocyte

TdT, cCD3

CD7, CD2, CD5

Immature thymocyte

TdT, cCD3

CD7, CD2, CD5,
CD1, CD4, CD8

Common thymocyte

TdT, terminal deoxynucleotidyl transferase; TBM, tingible body macrophage; DRC, dendritic reticulum cell; Ag, antigen.
Note: Lymphoid neoplasms (non-Hodgkin types) are believed to be clonal expansions of lymphoid cells that are arrested at a particular stage of differentiation or activation.

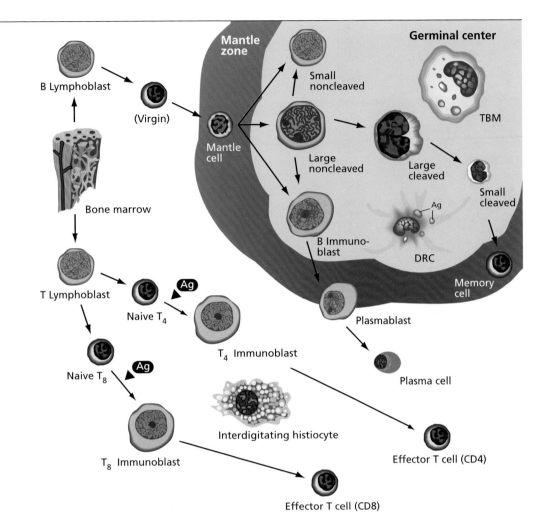

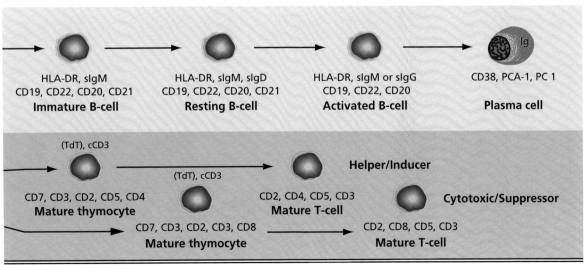

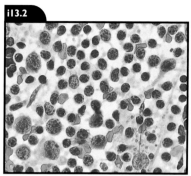

Small lymphocytes, FCCs, TBM (P)

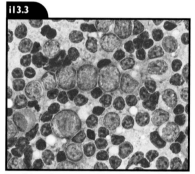

Small lymphocytes, FCCs, plasma cell (DQ)

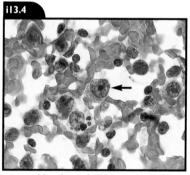

Immunoblast (arrow), mononucleosis (P)

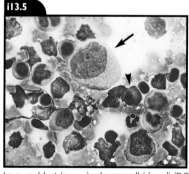

Immunoblast (arrow), plasma cell (-head) (DQ)

13.1.1 Lymphocytes

Small Lymphocytes

Small, "mature" lymphocytes are the lymphoid cells of the primary follicle, mantle zone, and medullary cords |i13.2|. Small lymphocytes normally compose the large majority (up to 90%) of the cells in a lymph node. They are larger in Diff-Quik stain and smaller in Papanicolaou stain, but average about 8 μm. The nucleus is round, has a smooth membrane, and is surrounded by a thin rim of pale cytoplasm. The chromatin is very coarse, or blocky, and stains dark. Nucleoli are invisible or inconspicuous.

Follicular Center Cells

FCCs, so-called immature lymphocytes, are found in the follicular centers, and normally compose the minority (~ 5%-15%) of the cells |i13.3|. FCCs can be small or large, and the nuclei can be relatively smooth (noncleaved) or irregular with deep folds (cleaved). The chromatin is variable but usually is at least somewhat more open than the chromatin of small lymphocytes. (Equivalent Kiel classification terms are given in parentheses.)

Small and Large Cleaved Cells (Centrocytes): Cleaved cells have scant cytoplasm and cleaved to angulated nuclei with coarse chromatin and inconspicuous marginal nucleoli. Large cleaved nuclei are larger than a histiocyte nucleus and tend to be elongated.

Large Noncleaved Cells (Centroblasts): The nuclei are round, larger than histiocyte nuclei, have relatively smooth or slightly irregular (ie, noncleaved) membranes, one to three prominent, often marginated nucleoli, and a rim of basophilic cytoplasm.

Small Noncleaved Cells (Lymphoblasts): The nuclei are round and medium sized, ie, about the size of a histiocyte nucleus, with inconspicuous or invisible nucleoli, fine chromatin, and very scant cytoplasm.

Immunoblasts

Immunoblasts are large lymphocytes of B- or T-cell origin |i13.4|, |i13.5|. B immunoblasts are characterized by large round nuclei, prominent central macronucleoli, and abundant plasmacytoid cytoplasm (in Diff-Quik stain, dark blue with perinuclear hof). T immunoblasts are characterized by very irregular (convoluted) nuclear membranes, two or more marginated nucleoli, and variable cytoplasm. In practice, it may be difficult to distinguish B- and T-cell immunoblasts from one another, as well as from large, noncleaved, follicular center lymphocytes or even Reed-Sternberg cells.

13.1.2 Histiocytes (Macrophages)

Histiocytes occur singly or in loose aggregates. The nuclei are round to oval or, most characteristically, bean-shaped.

They have a bland chromatin pattern, similar to monocytes ("salt and pepper" in Papanicolaou stain; "raked sand" in Diff-Quik stain). Single or multiple nucleoli may be seen but usually are small and inconspicuous. The cytoplasm is abundant and pale, foamy or granular, and usually has poorly defined outlines. Phagocytosed debris, eg, hemosiderin, carbon, or melanin, may be seen. Histiocytes proliferate in a wide variety of conditions, including nonspecific histiocytic reactions (to infections, malignancy, etc), granulomas, storage diseases, and neoplastic histiocytoses. In sinus histiocytosis with massive lymphadenopathy (Rosai-Dorfman disease), emperipolesis of lymphocytes is a characteristic but nonspecific finding |i13.6|, |i13.7|. Crescentic histiocytes with debris in the cytoplasm are characteristic of Kikuchi lymphadenitis |i13.8|. LE cells may be seen in lupus lymphadenitis.

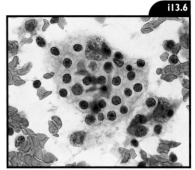

Rosai-Dorfman disease—emperipolesis (P)

Tingible Body Macrophages

Tingible body macrophages (TBMs) are specialized histiocytes, associated with follicular centers, containing debris (the tingible, or stainable, bodies) from necrobiotic cells |i13.9|. Although TBMs are associated with benign disease, particularly follicular hyperplasia, they also are seen in high-grade lymphomas (with high mitotic rate and cell turnover), Hodgkin disease (HD), and metastatic carcinoma. However, an aspirate in which "immature" lymphocytes are numerous and TBMs are sparse or absent is suspicious for lymphoma.

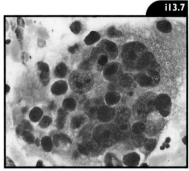

Rosai-Dorfman disease—nuclear atypia (DQ)

Lymphohistiocytic Aggregates

Lymphohistiocytic aggregates are associated with follicular center formation, including follicular hyperplasia and follicular lymphomas, and are rare in diffuse lymphomas. Lymphohistiocytic aggregates are large aggregates of histiocytes, intimately admixed with lymphocytes, that form loose flat sheets or cohesive three-dimensional clusters |i13.10|, |i13.11|. The cytoplasm is abundant, pale, and delicate and barely stands out against the background of the slide. Metastatic carcinoma and granulomas have denser (epithelioid) cytoplasm and characteristic nuclei (see p 233).

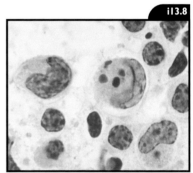

Kikuchi—crescentic histiocytes (P)

13.1.3 Lymphoglandular Bodies

Lymphoglandular bodies (LGBs) are detached fragments of lymphocyte cytoplasm. They are associated with benign or malignant lymphoid processes. LGBs also can be seen in carcinoma metastatic to lymph node, and occasionally a few similar structures are seen in "small blue cell" tumors. Conversely, LGBs sometimes are missing in lymphoma, eg, T-cell, anaplastic, and "true histiocytic" types. Nevertheless, the absence of LGBs makes a diagnosis of lymphoma unlikely.

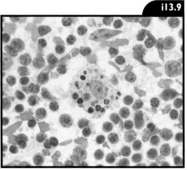

TBM (P)

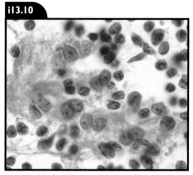

Lymphohistiocytic aggregate (P)

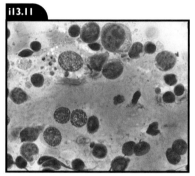

Lymphohistiocytic aggregate (DQ)

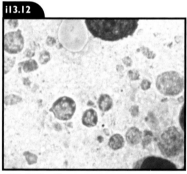

LGBs (DQ, oil)

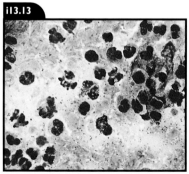

Acute lymphadenitis—bacteria (DQ)

LGBs are round globules, which vary from about 2 µm to 8 µm in diameter, and usually have a uniform, pale gray-blue appearance but can be vacuolated |i13.12|. LGBs express leukocyte common antigen (CD45). LGBs could be confused with platelets, which have metachromatic granules and tend to clump, or with necrotic debris, which is irregular in shape, nonuniform in staining, and associated with nuclear fragments.

13.1.4 Other Cells

A variety of other cell types, including mast cells, neutrophils, plasma cells, giant cells, eosinophils, and basophils, can be seen in lymph node aspirates.

13.2 Nonneoplastic Diseases of the Lymph Node

13.2.1 Acute Lymphadenitis

Acute lymphadenitis usually is clinically apparent. The local area is red, warm, and tender. The usual cause of acute lymphadenitis is infection (especially *Staphylococcus* or *Streptococcus*). Culture and sensitivity provide the most useful diagnostic information. Besides infection, cell debris or foreign matter also can cause acute lymphadenitis.

The fine needle aspiration (FNA) biopsy usually shows the characteristics of an abscess, including numerous neutrophils and other inflammatory cells |i13.13|. Bacteria may be easier to appreciate in Diff-Quik stain than in Papanicolaou stain, but a Gram stain can be helpful. Necrosis is common. With organization, capillaries proliferate, accompanied by histiocytes (ie, granulation tissue). Occasionally, reactive cells can appear quite atypical and mimic malignancy.

13.2.2 "Chronic Lymphadenitis" (Reactive Hyperplasia)

Chronic lymphadenitis is a general diagnostic term that encompasses follicular hyperplasia, paracortical hyperplasia, sinus histiocytosis, and mixed reactions. Chronic lymphadenitis is one of the most common processes encountered in FNA biopsy of lymph nodes.

Chronic lymphadenitis can occur at any age. There is often a history of infection in the region drained by the lymph node. The process usually involves only a single lymph node or a single group of nodes, without hepatomegaly or splenomegaly. The nodes usually are no more than moderately enlarged (< 3 cm) and are nontender. Chronic lymphadenitis is particularly common in the inguinal, axillary, and cervical lymph nodes, because these nodes drain large areas of the body.

The FNA biopsy of chronic lymphadenitis is typically highly cellular. The aspirate is dominated by small "mature" lymphocytes, but there usually are lymphocytes in various stages of maturation (small and large, cleaved and noncleaved FCCs, and immunoblasts) |i13.14|, |i13.15|. This combination of mature and immature lymphocytes results in a highly characteristic "range of maturation" associated with a benign reactive process.

Histiocytes, including TBMs, are typically present. Lymphohistiocytic aggregates also are common. Mitoses may be frequent. Plasma cells and plasmacytoid lymphocytes, neutrophils, and eosinophils may be seen. In essence, there is a good mixture of cell types, but small mature lymphocytes predominate, and TBMs usually are present. In response to viral infections, drug reactions, and the like, a proliferation of immunoblasts with prominent nucleoli, sometimes mimicking Reed-Sternberg cells or variants, may be seen.

13.2.3 Granulomatous Lymphadenitis

Granulomatous lymphadenitis is characterized by nodular collections of epithelioid histiocytes; multinucleated giant cells need not be present |i13.16|, |i13.17|. Necrosis (caseating or gummatous granulomas) or acute inflammation (suppurative granuloma) may be seen.

Epithelioid histiocytes have elongated, spindle- or carrot-shaped nuclei with fine pale chromatin and tiny but distinct nucleoli. The nuclear membrane characteristically has a longitudinal fold or groove (best seen in Papanicolaou stain). In Diff-Quik stain, the cytoplasm is abundant, somewhat dense ("epithelioid"), and eccentrically located around the nucleus. In Papanicolaou stain, the cytoplasm often has a fibrillar character. Granulomas may aspirate poorly, since they are anchored in the tissue by reticulin fibrosis.

A wide variety of diseases can be associated with granulomas, including various infections, such as tuberculosis (associated with caseating necrosis and acid-fast bacilli), cat-scratch disease (suppurative granulomas), and toxoplasmosis ("baby" granulomas without giant cells); sarcoid (noncaseating granulomas); and foreign bodies. The presence of granulomas does not exclude malignancy; eg, HD, T-cell non-Hodgkin lymphomas (NHLs), and some carcinomas, particularly those with squamous differentiation, may be associated with granulomatous inflammation.

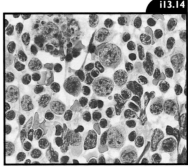
i13.14
Chronic lymphadenitis (P)

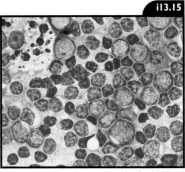
i13.15
Chronic lymphadenitis (DQ)

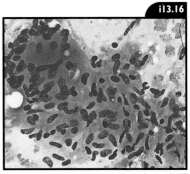
i13.16
Granuloma (DQ)

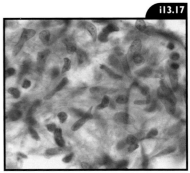
i13.17
Granuloma—epithelioid histiocytes (P)

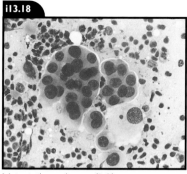

Metastatic carcinoma (DQ)

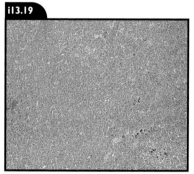

Diffuse lymphoma, tissue (H&E)

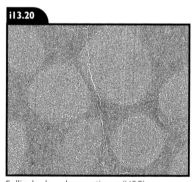

Follicular lymphoma, tissue (H&E)

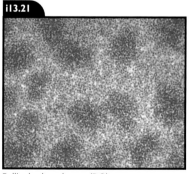

Follicular lymphoma (DQ)

13.3 Metastatic Malignancy

One of the premier uses of FNA biopsy of the lymph node is diagnosis of metastatic malignancy: the diagnosis usually is easy, accurate, and safe. As a general rule, the key to diagnosis of metastatic tumor is the presence of "foreign" cells in a lymph node. Metastatic carcinoma, which is the most common source of lymph node metastasis, usually forms cohesive clusters of malignant cells |i13.18|. Metastatic melanoma and sarcomas are less likely to form cohesive groups (and lymphoma typically yields a dispersed cell pattern). Note that LGBs can be present in lymph node metastases of any tumor type. Lymph node inclusions and "pick ups" from skin are possible benign sources of foreign cells in lymph node aspirates. (Metastases are discussed in Chapter 8.)

13.4 Malignant Lymphomas

13.4.1 Classification of Lymphoid Neoplasms

Malignant lymphomas are broadly grouped into two categories: Hodgkin disease and, for lack of a better term, non-Hodgkin lymphomas. The Revised European-American Lymphoma (REAL) classification |t13.1| and one by the World Health Organization |t13.2| are the most recent of a long line of diagnostic schemas for lymphomas. NHLs, HD, plasma cell tumors, and even some leukemias are included in these classifications.

13.4.2 Biology of Non-Hodgkin Lymphomas

Monoclonality usually indicates malignancy. Although polyclonality favors a benign process, it also can be seen in HD, T-cell lymphomas, or focal nodal involvement by B-cell lymphomas. Monoclonality of B cells can be determined by identification of a single immunoglobulin light chain (κ or λ), Ig heavy chain, or non-Ig B-cell antigens. Although no immunologic marker of clonality analogous to Ig light chains is currently available for T cells, the demonstration of a dominant or abnormal T-cell phenotype in morphologically atypical lymphoid cells suggests T-cell malignancy. Cytogenetic analysis can be useful, eg, by demonstrating the t(11;14) translocation in mantle cell lymphoma and small B-cell lymphoma/chronic lymphocytic leukemia (CLL); t(14;18) in FCC lymphoma; t(8;14) in small noncleaved lymphoma, or t(2;5) in anaplastic large cell lymphomas.

Follicles (aka nodules) are the neoplastic counterpart of the normal lymph node's germinal centers |i13.19|, |i13.20|. Follicular lymphoma is generally associated with a better prognosis than diffuse lymphoma of the same cell type. Follicular lymphomas are always of B-cell origin. They are graded in the REAL classification by the proportion of small and large cells |t13.1|. Certain lymphomas, such as small lymphocytic, lymphoblastic, Burkitt, and T-cell lymphomas, never grow in a follicular pattern. FNA biopsy cannot reliably diagnose follicle formation, although rarely, vague dense aggregates of lymphoma cells suggest follicular differentiation |i13.21|. Also, follicular center fragments are more commonly present in follicular lymphomas. Immunophenotyping is important in the diagnosis and classification of lymphomas |t13.3|, |t13.4|. For example, CD10 positivity suggests follicular lymphoma but is negative in 30% to 40% of cases.

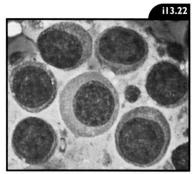

Malignant lymphoma (DQ, oil)

13.4.3 FNA Biopsy of Malignant Lymphoma: General Features

The aspiration of lymphoma usually yields a highly cellular specimen characterized by a dispersed cell pattern, with LGBs in the background |i13.22|, |t13.5|. These features can actually make the diagnosis of lymphoma easier in cytology than histology in some cases (especially large cell types). Sclerotic lymphomas yield a poorly cellular specimen. A poorly cellular aspirate from a large lymph node or a patient with generalized lymphadenopathy is suspicious for lymphoma.

Lymphomas are classically "monotypic" (ie, the cells look alike in the way that siblings do) or show a limited range of maturation, while benign processes classically display a full range of maturation in which small mature lymphocytes predominate. Cell size, or more precisely, nuclear size, is judged in relation to a histiocyte nucleus. Small cell lymphomas and mixed lymphomas are usually more difficult to diagnose by cytology, and medium and large cell lymphomas are usually easier. Suspicious cytologic findings include numerous large cells with few or no TBMs, presence of bizarre cells, or absence of plasmacytoid cells.

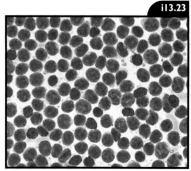

SLL (DQ)

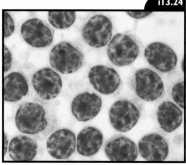

SLL (Pap, oil)

13.4.4 Small Lymphocytic Lymphoma

Small lymphocytic lymphoma (SLL) typically occurs in older patients, more commonly men, and is rare before 40 years of age |i13.23|, |i13.24|, |i13.25|. Patients usually present with generalized lymphadenopathy and often have mild to moderate hepatosplenomegaly. The bone marrow usually is involved, and most patients have leukemia (CLL) or an absolute lymphocytosis. Conversely, all patients with CLL have SLL in their lymph nodes. CLL and SLL are probably different expressions of the same disease. Some patients have a monoclonal gammopathy (hypergammaglobulinemia). Although

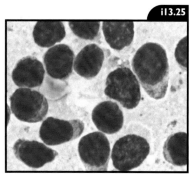

SLL (DQ, oil)

t13.1 Revised European-American Lymphoma (REAL) Classification

B-Cell Neoplasms

I.   Precursor B-cell neoplasm: Precursor B-lymphoblastic leukemia/lymphoma
II. Peripheral B-cell neoplasms
   1. B-cell chronic lymphocytic leukemia/prolymphocytic leukemia/small lymphocytic lymphoma
   2. Lymphoplasmacytoid lymphoma/immunocytoma
   3. Mantle cell lymphoma
   4. Follicle center lymphoma, follicular
      Provisional cytologic grades: I (small cell), II (mixed small and large cell), III (large cell)
      Provisional subtype: Diffuse, predominantly small cell type
   5. Marginal zone B-cell lymphoma
      Extranodal (MALT-type ± monocytoid B cells)
      Provisional subtype: Nodal (± monocytoid B cells)
   6. Provisional entity: Splenic marginal zone lymphoma (± villous lymphocytes)
   7. Hairy cell leukemia
   8. Plasmacytoma/plasma cell myeloma
   9. Diffuse large B-cell lymphoma*
      Subtype: Primary mediastinal (thymic) B-cell lymphoma
   10. Burkitt lymphoma
   11. Provisional entity: High-grade B-cell lymphoma, Burkitt-like*

T-Cell and Putative NK-Cell Neoplasms

I.   Precursor T-cell neoplasm: Precursor T-lymphoblastic lymphoma/leukemia
II. Peripheral T-cell and NK-cell neoplasms
   1. T-cell chronic lymphocytic leukemia/prolymphocytic leukemia
   2. Large granular lymphocyte leukemia (LGL)
   3. Mycosis fungoides/Sézary syndrome
   4. Peripheral T-cell lymphomas, unspecified*
      Provisional cytologic categories: medium-sized cell, mixed medium and large cell, large cell,
         lymphoepithelioid cell
      Provisional subtype: Hepatosplenic γδ T-cell lymphoma
      Provisional subtype: Subcutaneous panniculitic T-cell lymphoma
   5. Angioimmunoblastic T-cell lymphoma (AILD)
   6. Angiocentric lymphoma
   7. Intestinal T-cell lymphoma (± enteropathy associated)
   8. Adult T-cell lymphoma/leukemia (ATL/L)
   9. Anaplastic large cell lymphoma (ALCL), CD30+, T- and null-cell types
   10. Provisional entity: Anaplastic large cell lymphoma, Hodgkin-like

Hodgkin Disease

I.   Lymphocyte predominance
II. Nodular sclerosis
III. Mixed cellularity
IV. Lymphocyte depletion
VI. Provisional entity: Lymphocyte-rich classical HD

*These categories probably include more than one disease entity.

t13.2 Proposed World Health Organization (WHO) Classification for Neoplastic Diseases of the Lymphoid Tissues (February 1998)

B-Cell Neoplasms

Precursor B-cell lymphoblastic leukemia/lymphoma*
Mature B-cell neoplasms
    B-cell chronic lymphocytic leukemia/small lymphocytic lymphoma
    B-cell prolymphocytic leukemia
    Lymphoplasmacytic lymphoma *(lymphoplasmacytoid lymphoma)*†
    Mantle cell lymphoma
    Follicular lymphoma‡ *(follicle center lymphoma)*
    Marginal zone B-cell lymphoma of mucosa-associated lymphoid tissue (MALT) type
    Nodal marginal zone lymphoma with or without monocytoid B cells
    Splenic marginal zone B-cell lymphoma
    Hairy cell leukemia
    Diffuse large B-cell lymphoma‡
        Subtypes: mediastinal (thymic), intravascular, primary effusion lymphoma
    Burkitt lymphoma
    Plasmacytoma
    Plasma cell myeloma

T-Cell Neoplasms

Precursor T-cell lymphoblastic leukemia/lymphoma*
Mature T-cell and NK-cell neoplasms
    T-cell prolymphocytic leukemia
    T-cell large granular lymphocytic leukemia
    NK-cell leukemia
    Extranodal NK/T-cell lymphoma, nasal type *(angiocentric lymphoma)*
    Mycosis fungoides‡
    Sézary syndrome
    Angioimmunoblastic T-cell lymphoma
    Peripheral T-cell lymphoma (unspecified)‡
    Adult T-cell leukemia/lymphoma (HTLV1†)‡
    Systemic anaplastic large cell lymphoma (T- and null-cell types)‡
    Primary cutaneous anaplastic large cell lymphoma‡
    Subcutaneous panniculitis-like T-cell lymphoma
    Enteropathy-type intestinal T-cell lymphoma
    Hepatosplenic $\gamma\delta$ T-cell lymphoma

Hodgkin Lymphoma (Hodgkin Disease)

Nodular lymphocyte predominance Hodgkin lymphoma
Classic Hodgkin lymphoma
    Hodgkin lymphoma, nodular sclerosis (grades I and II)
    Classic Hodgkin lymphoma, lymphocyte-rich
    Hodgkin lymphoma, mixed cellularity
    Hodgkin lymphoma, lymphocytic depletion (includes some *"Hodgkin-like anaplastic large cell lymphoma"*)

---

* The classification of acute lymphoid leukemias will expand on the classification of the precursor B-cell and T-cell malignant neoplasms, incorporating immunophenotypic and genetic features.

† Terms shown in italics have been altered in the WHO classification. The italicized version represents the term as it was used in the Revised European-American Classification of Lymphoid Neoplasms (REAL). Where no italicized term appears, the REAL and WHO terms are essentially equivalent.

‡ Morphologic and/or clinical variants of these diseases are not listed, for the purpose of clarity and presentation.

t13.3 Immunophenotypes of Small Cell Lymphomas

	SLL	FCC	SLL, L-P	Marginal	Mantle	T Cell*
Ig	+	Usually +	+	+	+	–
Heavy	IgM, ± IgD	IgM, IgG	IgM	IgM, IgD, IgA	IgM, IgD	–
κ/λ	2:1	2:1	2:1	2:1	1:1	NA
CD20	+	+	+	+	+	–
CD43	Usually +	–	Often +	Often +	Often +	+
CD5	Usually +	–	Usually –	Usually –	Usually +	Usually +
CD10	Usually –	Often +	Usually –	Usually –	Usually –	–
CD23	Usually +	Usually –	Usually –	Usually –	Usually –	–

SLL, small lymphocytic lymphoma; FCC, follicular center cell lymphoma; L-P, lymphoplasmacytic; Ig, immunoglobulin; NA, not applicable.
*Usually CD4+, CD8– (helper); occasionally CD4–, CD8+ (suppressor/cytotoxic).

t13.4 Selected Major Leukocyte Antigens

Antibody	Predominant Expression
CD2	T cells and T-cell lymphomas
CD3	T cells and many T-cell lymphomas
CD4	Histiocytes and their neoplasms, T helper cells, many T-cell lymphomas
CD5	T cells and T-cell lymphomas, many B-cell SLL/CLL, mantle cell lymphoma
CD7	Most T cells and T-cell lymphomas, some myeloid leukemias
CD8	T cytotoxic/suppressor cells, some T-cell lymphomas
CD10 (CALLA)	Precursor B cells and B-cell lymphoblastic lymphomas, many FCC lymphomas
CD15 (Leu M1)	Myeloid cells, Hodgkin disease, some non-Hodgkin lymphomas
CD19	B cells and B-cell lymphomas
CD20	B cells and B-cell lymphomas, nodular L&H lymphocyte predominant Hodgkin disease
CD23	Mantle zone B cells and mantle zone lymphoma, most B-cell SLL/CLL
CD30 (Ki-1)	Activated lymphoid cells, Hodgkin disease, anaplastic large cell lymphoma
CD43	T cells and T-cell lymphomas, myeloid cells and neoplasms, mast cells and neoplasms
CD45 (LCA)	Hematolymphoid cells (not plasma cells)

SLL/CLL, small lymphocytic lymphoma/chronic lymphocytic leukemia; FCC, follicular center cell.

t13.5 Non-Hodgkin Lymphomas

Small lymphocytic lymphoma
Small cleaved lymphoma
Mixed lymphoma
Large cell
    Cleaved, noncleaved
    Immunoblastic (B, T)
    "True histiocytic"
Lymphoblastic
Burkitt types
Other, miscellaneous

incurable, the lymphoma usually follows an indolent course. In some patients, however, the disease transforms to large cell lymphoma (Richter syndrome).

The aspirate usually is highly cellular and has a monotonous appearance |i13.23|. The large majority (> 80%) of the cells resemble ordinary small mature lymphocytes |i13.24|, |i13.25|, although they are often slightly larger than normal, and the chromatin is not quite as condensed. The nuclear membranes are smooth. In some cases, the chromatin is "clotted" (cellules grumelées, or cells with little clots) and resembles the "clock-face" chromatin of plasma cells |i13.26|. Nucleoli are invisible or small and inconspicuous. The cytoplasm is pale and scant, and there is a very high nuclear/cytoplasmic ratio. Plasmacytoid cytoplasmic features are inconspicuous or absent, by definition.

Large "proliferation center cells" are present in some cases |i13.27|, |i13.28|. However, FCCs (particularly cleaved lymphocytes), immunoblasts, TBMs, lymphohistiocytic aggregates, and mitotic figures are absent or rare, although a few ordinary histiocytes may be seen. The characteristic immunophenotype is CD5+, CD19+, CD20+, CD23+.

Lymphoplasmacytic lymphoma is morphologically and clinically similar to SLL, except for the additional presence of plasmacytoid lymphocytes and mature plasma cells |i13.29| and the more common occurrence of a monoclonal gammopathy, particularly IgM (Waldenström macroglobulinemia). Dutcher (intranuclear) bodies are common and Russell (cytoplasmic) bodies occur. The characteristic immunophenotype is CD19+, CD20+, CD5–, CD10–, CD23–.

13.4.5 Small Cleaved Lymphoma

Small cleaved lymphoma usually occurs in mid to old age and is rare before 35 years of age. Patients have generalized moderate to marked lymphadenopathy. Hepatosplenomegaly and bone marrow involvement may occur. The disease is virtually incurable but follows a protracted course unless it transforms to large cell lymphoma. About 10% develop a leukemic phase, which is associated with a poor prognosis. In most cases (> 75%), the lymphoma shows a follicular growth pattern histologically. Small cleaved lymphoma is the most common follicular lymphoma. The diffuse form may actually be a different disease (mantle cell lymphoma).

The aspirate usually is cellular, but occasional cases undergo sclerosis, resulting in a poorly cellular aspirate. The large majority of the malignant cells (> 80%) are small to medium lymphocytes. The most characteristic cytologic feature is the deeply folded, or cleaved, nucleus. The "coffee bean" nuclear shape is classic but not common; many cells have very abnormally shaped

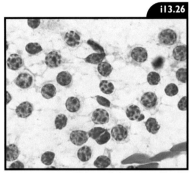
SLL—cellules grumelées (P)

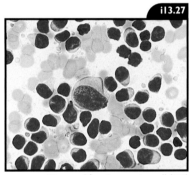
SLL—proliferation center cell (DQ)

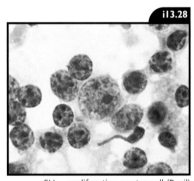
SLL—proliferation center cell (P, oil)

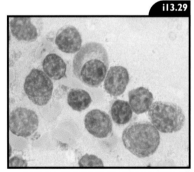
Lymphoplasmacytic lymphoma (DQ, oil)

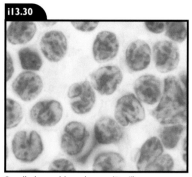

Small cleaved lymphoma (P, oil)

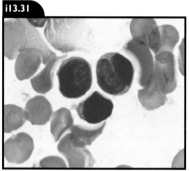

Small cleaved lymphoma (DQ, oil)

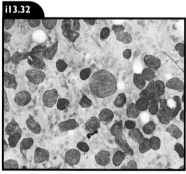

Small cleaved lymphoma—large cell (DQ)

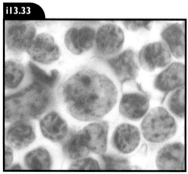

Small cleaved lymphoma—large cell (P, oil)

nuclei (eg, twisted) |i13.30|, |i13.31|. Nuclear membrane irregularity is best appreciated in Papanicolaou stain and is subtle in some cases. The chromatin is usually coarse but not as coarse as that of a small mature lymphocyte—a potential clue to the diagnosis. Nucleoli, if present, are small and inconspicuous. The cytoplasm is scant but may be slightly more abundant than in a small lymphocyte. Mitoses are rare.

Large lymphoid cells, typically noncleaved, also are usually present and may comprise up to 20% of the smear |i13.32|, |i13.33|. Small mature (T) lymphocytes, which are reactive rather than neoplastic, also may be present when the lymphoma is more or less confined to the follicles. TBMs usually are absent or rare. The characteristic immunophenotype is CD19+, CD20+, CD5−, CD23−. CD10 is often positive.

13.4.6 Mixed Lymphoma

Mixed (B-cell) lymphoma refers to the mixture of small cleaved and large cells in roughly equal proportions (see also "T-Cell Lymphoma," p 244). The higher the proportion of large cells, the worse the prognosis. Although in theory there is a two-cell population, in practice there is actually a spectrum of cell sizes ranging from small to large.

The aspirate usually is cellular and consists predominantly of small cleaved and large cells. The small cleaved cells are identical to those described in small cleaved lymphoma. In most cases, the large cells are noncleaved. Plasmacytoid cells and plasma cells are absent or rare. Mitoses are usually few but are increased with diffuse pattern of growth. TBMs usually are sparse but increase with the number of large cells.

Reactive hyperplasia and mixed lymphoma may be particularly difficult to distinguish since both display a range of maturation of cells. Clinical features, eg, age and extent of adenopathy, can be helpful. Reactive hyperplasia is more heterogeneous with a full range of cells, including TBMs, plasmacytoid and plasma cells, and a predominance of small mature lymphocytes. Mixed lymphoma has a more limited range of cells, with fewer small mature lymphocytes and an increased number of cleaved cells, while TBMs are sparse and plasma cells are rare. The immunophenotype is the same as for small cleaved lymphoma.

13.4.7 Large Cell Lymphoma

Large cell lymphomas form a diverse group that includes cleaved and noncleaved, immunoblastic, and true histiocytic lymphomas. Large cell lymphoma occurs in adults and children and is the most common lymphoma occurring in patients with AIDS. Some patients have a history of lymphoreticular malignancy or immune system abnormality, including autoimmune diseases such as Hashimoto thyroiditis or Sjögren syndrome.

Large cell lymphomas present in extranodal locations in many cases, including the gastrointestinal tract, skin, bone, and, especially in AIDS, the brain. Large cell lymphomas are aggressive but potentially curable. Most cases are of B-cell origin. Because there is not a good correlation between immunophenotype and prognosis, for practical purposes it usually is sufficient to classify the tumor simply as large cell lymphoma.

The aspirate is variably cellular but usually plentiful. Large lymphoid cells predominate, although a component of small cleaved cells often is present. The "large" cells vary from slightly larger than a histiocyte nucleus (which is really not very big) to giant (rare). From case to case, the cells range from fairly uniform to markedly pleomorphic.

Small mature lymphocytes usually are rare or absent. However, eosinophils, plasmacytoid or plasma cells, or granulomas can be present. TBMs correlate with the mitotic rate. Necrosis may be apparent but is seldom extensive, in contrast with some epithelial malignancies. Noncleaved large cells usually predominate, although large cleaved cells also can occur in varying proportions and, rarely, predominate.

Large cell noncleaved lymphoma is characterized by large cells with relatively smooth (ie, noncleaved) nuclear membranes |i13.34|, |i13.35|. The nucleus is round to oval. Two to five medium-sized nucleoli are seen in most nuclei, usually in a peripheral location (ie, near the nuclear membrane). The chromatin is relatively fine. The cytoplasm is variable in amount and staining but is usually moderately abundant and moderately basophilic. Vacuoles are occasionally present (Diff-Quik). Plasmacytoid cells, immunoblasts, and plasma cells, as well as small and large cleaved cells, may be present.

Large cell cleaved lymphoma is characterized by large cells primarily distinguished by the presence of irregular deep folds (ie, cleaves) in the nuclear membrane |i13.36|, |i13.37|. The nucleus often is oblong rather than round. One or two small inconspicuous nucleoli may be present, often near the tip of the nucleus. The chromatin is coarser than in noncleaved nuclei. Multilobated nuclei can occur. Cytoplasm is scantier than in large noncleaved cells but also may be vacuolated.

B-immunoblastic lymphoma typically shows a relatively homogeneous population of large plasmacytoid lymphocytes |i13.38|, |i13.39|. The nucleus is large, eccentrically located, and noncleaved, with a characteristic single central macronucleolus. The cytoplasm is deeply basophilic in Diff-Quik stain (more so than in large noncleaved cells), amphophilic in Papanicolaou stain, and often has a perinuclear clear space (hof). Cytoplasmic vacuoles (best appreciated in Diff-Quik stain) are characteristic.

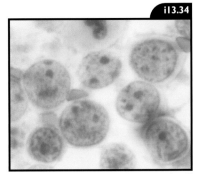

i13.34

Large cell, noncleaved—histiocyte (P, oil)

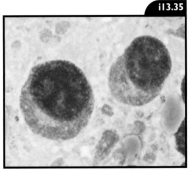

i13.35

Large cell, noncleaved (DQ, oil)

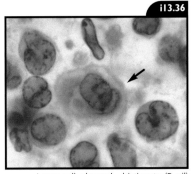

i13.36

Large cell, cleaved—histiocyte (P, oil)

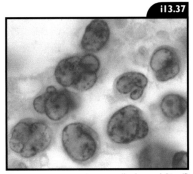

i13.37

Large cell, cleaved (P, oil)

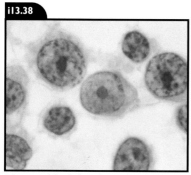

B-immunoblastic lymphoma (P, oil)

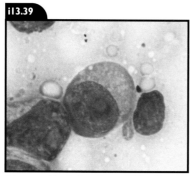

B-immunoblastic lymphoma (DQ, oil)

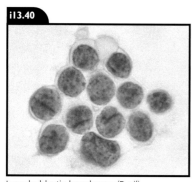

Lymphoblastic lymphoma (P, oil)

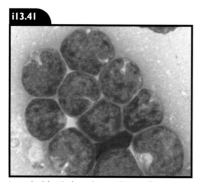

Lymphoblastic lymphoma (DQ, oil)

Follicular center cleaved cells usually are absent (compare with large cell noncleaved lymphoma). Plasmacytoma shows more binucleation, smaller nucleoli, less intense cytoplasmic basophilia, few or no vacuoles, but a more prominent perinuclear hof. IgM expression favors lymphoma; bone lesions and monoclonal gammopathy favor plasmacytoma.

13.4.8 Lymphoblastic Lymphoma

Lymphoblastic lymphoma is a high-grade lymphoma that characteristically affects young adults who frequently present with a mediastinal mass. When lymphoblasts are present in the blood at presentation, the disease is considered leukemia rather than lymphoma (acute lymphoblastic leukemia [ALL]). Most cases show a T-cell phenotype. Nuclear terminal deoxynucleotidyl transferase (TdT) is a highly specific marker for this disease. With modern therapy, cure is possible.

The FNA biopsy consists, in essence, of numerous blasts with frequent mitoses |i13.40|, |i13.41|. The malignant cells are lymphoblasts and prolymphocytes characteristic of ALL and conform to the French-American-British (FAB) classification of acute leukemias as L1 and L2. They are medium-sized and relatively uniform, especially L1, but in contrast to the extreme monomorphism seen in tissue, the cells vary in size in cytology (especially L2). Occasionally, larger cells (macroblasts) may be present. The nuclei are round, and the nuclear membrane varies from smooth to convoluted (a helpful but not essential diagnostic feature). A highly characteristic feature is "blastic" chromatin: fine, delicate, powdery. Nucleoli vary from invisible (L1) to two to three small but conspicuous nucleoli (L2).

The cytoplasm ranges from extremely scant, almost invisible (L1), to slightly more apparent (L2), but is never abundant. It stains dark blue (in Diff-Quik stain) but not as dark as in Burkitt lymphoma. A few cells with periodic acid–Schiff (PAS)–positive cytoplasmic vacuoles are present in most cases. TBMs may be present but usually are not as conspicuous as in Burkitt lymphoma.

13.4.9 Small Cell, Noncleaved Lymphoma: Burkitt and "Non-Burkitt"

Small cell, noncleaved lymphomas are divided into two clinical groups, Burkitt and "non-Burkitt" types. Burkitt lymphoma is further subclassified into endemic ("African," strongly associated with Epstein-Barr virus [EBV]) and sporadic ("American," sometimes associated with EBV) forms. The cells are medium size with high nuclear/cytoplasmic ratios, dark blue, finely vacuolated cytoplasm, many mitoses, and numerous TBMs. These lymphomas are among the fastest growing tumors known |i13.42|, |i13.43|, |i13.44|, |i13.45|.

Burkitt lymphoma is a common lymphoma of children and also is associated with immunosuppression, including in patients with AIDS and transplant recipients. The tumor is aggressive but may respond to aggressive therapy. Sporadic Burkitt lymphoma commonly presents with an abdominal mass and occurs equally in males and females.

Non-Burkitt lymphoma has a wide anatomic distribution. Non-Burkitt lymphoma occurs, on average, in older (middle-aged) patients than does Burkitt lymphoma, although there is considerable overlap of ages. Non-Burkitt lymphoma has no known association with EBV infection.

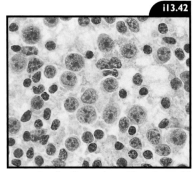

Small cell, noncleaved lymphoma (P)

Cytology of Small Cell, Noncleaved Lymphoma

Burkitt lymphoma is cytologically indistinguishable from ALL, FAB-L3. Non-Burkitt lymphoma is cytologically similar to Burkitt lymphoma, although the cells are larger and more pleomorphic and have coarser chromatin and more prominent nucleoli. The malignant cells are relatively uniform but, particularly in Diff-Quik stain, may not be as monotonous as they appear in tissue. Despite the classification with small cell lymphomas, the cells actually are medium-sized. Occasional Reed-Sternberg–like cells may be seen in some cases.

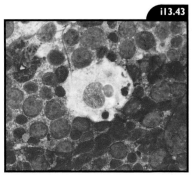

Small cell, noncleaved—"starry sky" (DQ)

The nuclei are round to oval and occasionally multiple. The nuclear membrane is generally smooth (ie, noncleaved) but may be notched or indented. Two to five small but conspicuous nucleoli are present. A characteristic feature is the "blastic" chromatin, which is finely stippled in Papanicolaou stain but not as powdery as in lymphoblastic lymphoma.

The cytoplasm is moderate in amount and deeply basophilic. It characteristically has tiny vacuoles that contain neutral lipid. Rare cells may have PAS-positive granules. TBMs usually are present (resulting in a "starry sky" appearance) but, occasionally, are sparse or absent. Mitotic figures usually are numerous. LGBs are present. Immunophenotypes of Burkitt and non-Burkitt lymphomas are virtually identical. These lymphomas have surface immunoglobulin, usually IgM and occasionally IgD, and are CALLA+. They are CD10+, CD19+, CD20+. Overexpression of c-myc is characteristic.

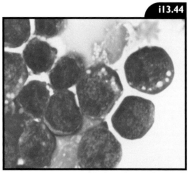

Burkitt lymphoma (DQ, oil)

Except for smaller cell size, the cells are cytologically similar to those of large cell noncleaved lymphoma, which also may have dark blue cytoplasm and cytoplasmic vacuoles. The presence of large bizarre cells suggests large cell lymphoma.

Lymphoblastic lymphoma also is similar but has inconspicuous nucleoli, finer chromatin, and less cytoplasm (which is PAS-positive, lipid-negative), and the clinical features are different (age, leukemia, masses, etc). TdT is positive in most cases of lymphoblastic

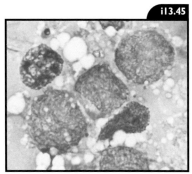

Non-Burkitt lymphoma (DQ, oil)

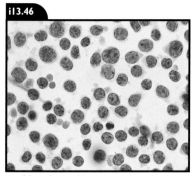

T-cell lymphoma (P)

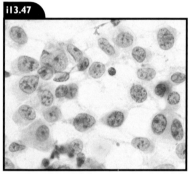

T-cell lymphoma (P)

lymphoma. In addition, lymphoblastic lymphoma is usually a T- or pre–B-cell neoplasm, while Burkitt types are B-cell lymphomas.

13.4.10 T-Cell Lymphoma

T-cell lymphomas form a complex and diverse group of diagnostically difficult neoplasms that account for about 10% to 20% of NHLs. Immunophenotyping or genotyping usually is required to confirm T-cell origin, in contrast with B-cell lymphomas, in which morphology alone is often sufficient.

Unlike B-cell lymphomas, there is no simple method to determine T-cell clonality, and there is no simple model of T-cell differentiation to help classify T-cell lymphomas. Instead, T-cell lymphomas are classified by the anatomic compartment of origin and morphology. The major T-cell compartments are prethymic (ie, bone marrow, associated with ALL), thymic (associated with lymphoblastic lymphoma), and postthymic (associated with peripheral T-cell lymphoma and T-immunoblastic lymphoma). Most (~ 40%-50%) are large cell lymphomas, 30% to 40% are mixed, most of the rest are small cleaved, and a few are small lympho-cytic. Follicular growth is not a feature of T-cell lymphomas.

T-cell lymphomas typically contain a mixture of neoplastic and reactive cells, and the neoplastic cells show a spectrum of sizes and shapes, from small to large, with smooth to convoluted nuclear membranes, resulting in a characteristic polymorphous appearance. B-cell lymphomas, on the other hand, usually are composed almost exclusively of neoplastic cells without a mixed reactive component and usually show limited stages of differentiation, often only one or two cell types.

Peripheral T-cell lymphomas are a heterogeneous group of postthymic lymphoid malignancies with mature T-cell phenotypes that encompasses half a dozen categories in the REAL classifica-tion, as well as several provisional subtypes, including mycosis fungoides, adult T-cell leukemia/lymphoma, lymphoepithelial T-cell (Lennert) lymphoma, angiocentric T-cell lymphoma, hepatosplenic lymphoma, and intestinal T-cell lymphoma.

Peripheral T-cell lymphomas are uncommon. There is a bimodal peak of incidence in the 30s and 70s; males are some-what more commonly affected than females. There is often a history of an autoimmune disorder. Many cases present in the head and neck area, as lymphadenopathy or as nasopharyngeal masses. However, generalized lymphadenopathy, mediastinal masses, and extranodal disease (eg, skin, liver, lung, gastroin-testinal tract, bone, central nervous system), as well as "B" symp-toms (fever, night sweats, weight loss), also are common. Patients are often anemic, and there may be a leukemic phase. The clinical course is variable but can be aggressive.

The aspirate usually is cellular, unless fibrosis is prominent, and is characterized by cellular polymorphism |i13.46|, |i13.47|. There usually is a spectrum of small, medium, and large neoplastic lymphoid cells mixed with benign reactive cells. The lymphomas can be classified as small, mixed, or large cell type, depending on the ratios of the neoplastic cells. Not all cell types are found in all lymphomas.

The small malignant lymphoid cells are slightly larger than mature lymphocytes. The nuclear membranes of neoplastic cells are characteristically highly irregular, grooved, or convoluted but not deeply cleaved. Convoluted nuclei suggest T-cell origin but are not specific. The chromatin is condensed and irregularly dispersed. Nucleoli usually are inconspicuous but occasionally are prominent. The cytoplasm varies from scant to relatively abundant.

Large T cells are more variable in appearance |i13.48|, |i13.49|, They are large atypical lymphocytes, with large round to irregular or convoluted nuclei, vesicular or coarse chromatin, and prominent nucleoli. The cytoplasm ranges from scant to abundant, pale to basophilic. Multilobated nuclei are described in one variant. Some large cells may resemble immunoblasts with eccentric nuclei and prominent nucleoli. Binucleate immunoblasts with prominent nucleoli can mimic Reed-Sternberg (RS) cells |i13.50|. However, classic Reed-Sternberg cells are not present, and the abnormal lymphoid cells in the background are inconsistent with HD.

In addition to the neoplastic cells, an exuberant host response consisting of benign, reactive lymphoid cells, histiocytes (epithelioid and nonepithelioid), eosinophils, neutrophils, and plasma cells usually is present, adding to the characteristic polymorphous appearance of this lymphoma. Benign histiocytes are common; however, TBMs are sparse or absent. Epithelioid histiocytes may be seen (when "high content," designated lymphoepithelioid or Lennert lymphoma), but well-formed sarcoid-like granulomas usually are not present. Perhaps ironically, plasmacytoid cells and even mature plasma cells (terminally differentiated B cells) can be seen in T-cell lymphomas.

Immunocytochemistry and molecular studies help confirm the diagnosis of lymphoma and are essential to identify T-cell lineage. CD45 (leukocyte common antigen) usually is positive. By definition, the tumor cells express one or more T-cell antigens (eg, CD3 or CD43), but no B-cell antigens (CD20 is always negative). T-cell lymphomas usually show an aberrant T-cell phenotype with loss of one or more pan–T-cell markers (CD5, CD7, CD3, or CD2). The malignant cells usually express T-helper phenotype (CD4+, CD8–); suppressor/cytotoxic phenotype (CD4–, CD8+) or aberrant phenotypes also can occur. Rearrangement of the β T-cell receptor gene usually is present.

In theory, peripheral T-cell lymphoma forms a morphologically distinct set of neoplasms, but in practice, the cytologic

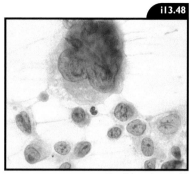
T-cell lymphoma (P)

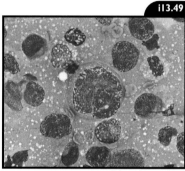
T-cell lymphoma (DQ)

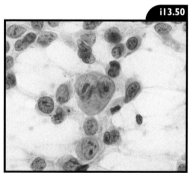
T-cell lymphoma—RS-like cell (P)

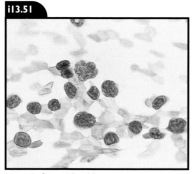

Mycosis fungoides (P)

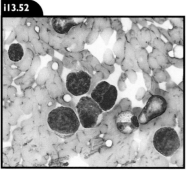

Mycosis fungoides (DQ)

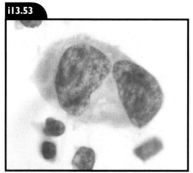

Anaplastic lymphoma (P)

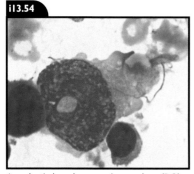

Anaplastic lymphoma—ring nucleus (DQ)

differential diagnosis with B-cell lymphomas can be difficult. In addition, because a mixed population of cells is present, the cytologic differential diagnosis with a benign reactive condition, particularly paracortical hyperplasia, also can be difficult. The presence of highly anaplastic or bizarre cells suggests lymphoma. A spectrum of lymphoid atypia, convoluted nuclei, the presence of eosinophils, and T-cell markers, such as CD3, favor T-cell origin. In summary, in contrast with B-cell lymphomas, T-cell lymphomas generally show more marked anisonucleosis, nuclear membrane irregularity, and hyperchromasia; less conspicuous nucleoli and cytoplasmic basophilia; and fewer LGBs. In addition, many cases have a component of nonneoplastic cells, such as eosinophils, plasma cells, and epithelioid histiocytes.

T-immunoblastic lymphoma is morphologically similar to peripheral T-cell lymphoma (cellular polymorphism with various cell types and a spectrum of atypical lymphocytes with convoluted nuclei) but has a high proportion of large lymphoid cells, ie, T immunoblasts. T immunoblasts are large cells characterized by convoluted nuclei, fine even chromatin, and prominent nucleoli (smaller but more numerous—two to five—than B immunoblasts). The cytoplasm varies from pale to moderately dark and may be vacuolated, but it does not have a plasmacytoid appearance.

13.4.11 Mycosis Fungoides and Sézary Syndrome

Mycosis fungoides, originally thought to be a fungal infection, is a cutaneous T-cell lymphoma. Mycosis fungoides is associated with tumor formation; Sézary syndrome is similar but does not produce tumors.

The FNA biopsy shows a variable mixture of atypical small and large lymphoid cells plus a reactive component of eosinophils, plasma cells, and nonneoplastic lymphocytes |i13.51|, |i13.52|, The small cells have small hyperchromatic nuclei and inconspicuous nucleoli. As the disease progresses, large lymphoid cells with pale, vesicular, convoluted nuclei, prominent nucleoli, and pale scant cytoplasm become more numerous.

13.4.12 Anaplastic Large Cell (CD30/Ki-1) Lymphoma

CD30 (Ki-1)-positive, anaplastic large cell lymphoma is a high-grade malignancy that occurs more commonly in children and young adults and follows an unpredictable course but can have a favorable prognosis. Some tumors previously diagnosed as malignant histiocytosis and true histiocytic lymphoma now are regarded as examples of this lymphoma.

The FNA biopsy obtains large pleomorphic cells, which range in appearance from immunoblast-like to bizarre |i13.53|, |i13.54|. The cells are predominantly single, but occasional clustering may suggest an epithelial malignancy. The cytoplasm is variable in amount, texture, and staining. Cytoplasmic extensions, reminiscent of "hand mirror" cells or rhabdomyoblasts, may be seen. Cytoplasmic inclusion bodies ("hyaline globules"), which correspond to large lysosomes, also can occur.

The nuclei are large, frequently indented or lobulated, and have granular chromatin and conspicuous nucleoli. Binucleated or multinucleated cells can mimic Reed-Sternberg cells. Ring nuclei (wreath-like, donut-shaped, or windows), when present, suggest the diagnosis. There is a heterogeneous population of cells, including a variable number of lymphoid cells, plasma cells, and histiocytes. LGBs may be sparse.

This lymphoma can unexpectedly express epithelial markers and occasionally fails to react with CD45 (LCA), which can be confusing in the diagnosis. Morphologic features and CD30 antigen expression can help establish the proper diagnosis, but not all anaplastic lymphomas are CD30+.

13.4.13 Other Malignant Lymphomas

Marginal Zone B-Cell Lymphoma (Monocytoid B-Cell Lymphoma)

Marginal zone B-cell lymphoma is a low-grade neoplasm of marginal zone lymphoid cells; it includes monocytoid B-cell lymphoma of lymph node and extranodal lymphoma of mucosa-associated lymphoid tissue (MALToma). If the disease is localized, surgical excision can be curative. Patients with marginal zone lymphoma are usually elderly (median age, 60 years) and more commonly women (2:1).

The FNA biopsy usually is cellular |i13.55|, |i13.56|, |i13.57|. Monocytoid B cells are a characteristic feature but are not always present |i13.58|. The monocytoid cells are small to medium lymphoid cells with oval, bean-shaped, or deeply indented "monocytoid" nuclei but clumped "lymphocytoid" chromatin. The nuclear membranes are smooth to slightly irregular. Nucleoli are present but often indistinct. Moderately abundant, pale, gray (in Diff-Quik stain) cytoplasm is a characteristic feature.

Another characteristic feature is the presence of a heterogeneous population of cells, including centrocyte-like cells, plasmacytoid cells and plasma cells, scattered immunoblasts, and, occasionally, neutrophils. CD43 frequently is positive; CD5, CD10, and CD23 usually are negative.

Mantle Cell Lymphoma

Mantle cell lymphoma is a relatively common lymphoma that occurs in elderly adults, more often men (2:1). The disease

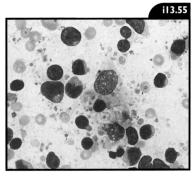
Marginal zone lymphoma (DQ)

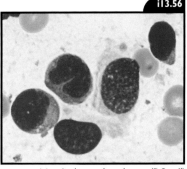
Marginal zone lymphoma (DQ, oil)

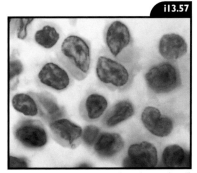
Marginal zone lymphoma (P, oil)

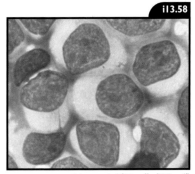
Monocytoid B cells (DQ, oil)

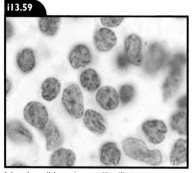

Mantle cell lymphoma (P, oil)

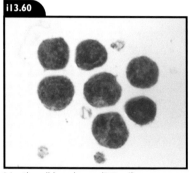

Mantle cell lymphoma (DQ, oil)

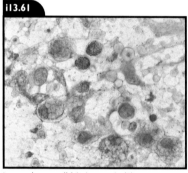

Langerhans cell histiocytosis (P)

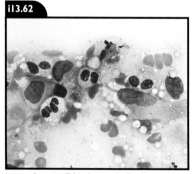

Langerhans cell histiocytosis (DQ)

usually is advanced at the time of diagnosis (ie, high stage). The disease is incurable and is one of the most aggressive malignant lymphomas. Mantle cell lymphoma is thought to arise from a precursor to the normal germinal center, a cell slightly more differentiated than the virgin B-cell small lymphocyte.

The tumor usually is composed of a homogeneous population of small cells with irregular but not deeply clefted nuclear membranes |i13.59|, |i13.60|. The chromatin is condensed but less coarse than in small lymphocytic or small cleaved lymphoma. Nucleoli are inconspicuous. A minor component of small mature lymphocytes and small cleaved cells may be present, but there are usually no large cells unless transformation has occurred (blastic transformation also is possible). Most cases are CD5+; CD10 and CD23 usually are negative. The cytogenetic translocation, t(11; 14) with *bcl-1* gene rearrangement and overexpression of cyclin D1, are characteristic features.

13.5 Histiocytic Neoplasms

13.5.1 Langerhans Cell Histiocytosis

Langerhans cell histiocytosis, formerly known as histiocytosis X, is a group of related nonmalignant immune disorders, characterized by proliferation of differentiated histiocytes, that includes eosinophilic granuloma (localized or multifocal, frequently involves bone), Letterer-Siwe disease (infants), and Hand-Schüller-Christian disease (polyostotic eosinophilic granuloma; a rare disease causing a triad of skull lesions, proptosis, and diabetes insipidus). Langerhans cell histiocytosis may be localized or generalized and commonly involves bone, skin, lungs, and head and neck. Lymphadenopathy can also occur. The behavior is aggressive in some cases. Staging is the most important prognostic factor in these disorders.

In the FNA biopsy, the most characteristic cytologic findings are eosinophils and Langerhans histiocytes, ie, eosinophilic granuloma |i13.61|, |i13.62|. Langerhans histiocytes resemble ordinary macrophages but have characteristic linear folds or grooves in the nuclear membrane and are nonphagocytic. They may be multinucleated; some may have an osteoclast-like appearance. Scattered lymphocytes and plasma cells also may be present. Birbeck ("tennis racket") granules are a characteristic ultrastructural feature of Langerhans cells, and by immunocytochemistry the cells express S-100. Langerhans cells also can be found in a variety of other benign and malignant conditions, including reactive lymph nodes and dermatopathic lymphadenopathy.

13.5.2 Malignant Histiocytosis: True Histiocytic Lymphoma

Malignancies of true histiocytes, malignant histiocytoses, are rare. Malignant histiocytoses occur more often in children and young adults, males more commonly than females. The patients may have fever, weight loss, lymphadenopathy, hepatosplenomegaly, and anemia. Skin and bone also are commonly involved. The clinical behavior is aggressive.

The FNA biopsy usually shows variably sized, dyshesive, single cells, although lymphohistiocytic aggregates may be seen. Most characteristically, the cells are markedly pleomorphic. However, the cells can show a spectrum of differentiation, ranging from relatively well-differentiated and monocyte-like to anaplastic and bizarre.

The nuclei can vary from bean-shaped to irregular to multilobulated. Ring-shaped nuclei or monocytoid chromatin ("salt and pepper" in Papanicolaou stain, "raked sand" in Diff-Quik stain), if present, are characteristic. Many cells are multinucleated and some may resemble Reed-Sternberg cells. Nucleoli usually are medium-sized and often centrally located.

The cytoplasm is abundant and varies from pale (histiocyte-like) to deeply basophilic (B immunoblast–like). Some tumor cells may have cytoplasmic projections, or "handles" (hand mirror appearance). Phagocytosis (RBCs, WBCs, hemosiderin, lipid, debris), when present, is characteristic. Also, cytoplasmic azurophilic granules may be seen in Diff-Quik, which are rare in large lymphocytes. Lymphocytes and plasma cells may be present, but LGBs are not always seen. The cells express typical histiocytic markers, eg, muramidase, α_1-antichymotrypsin, α_1-antitrypsin, and nonspecific esterase.

The differential diagnosis includes large cell lymphoma, particularly anaplastic CD30 (Ki-1) lymphoma, as well as carcinoma, sarcoma, and melanoma. Monocytoid nuclei, with medium-sized nucleoli, abundant and variably stained cytoplasm, and phagocytosis characterize the histiocytic cells. Immunologic markers may be helpful.

13.6 Hodgkin Disease

HD is important because it is one of the most common malignancies in young adults, and it is curable |i13.63|, |i13.64|, |i13.65|, |i13.66|. Males are somewhat more commonly affected than females (4:3) and also have a somewhat worse prognosis. Half of the patients are between the age of 20 and 40 years. Most patients (90%) present with painless supradiaphragmatic lymphadenopathy. Cervical lymph nodes are, by far, the most common primary site, followed by mediastinal and axillary nodes.

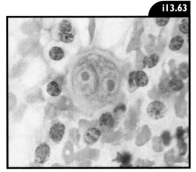

i13.63

Hodgkin disease—RS cell (P)

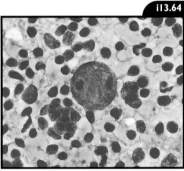

i13.64

Hodgkin disease—RS cell (DQ)

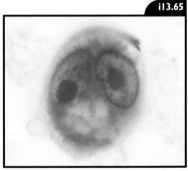

i13.65

HD—Reed-Sternberg cell (P, oil)

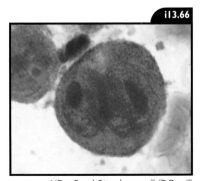

i13.66

HD—Reed-Sternberg cell (DQ, oil)

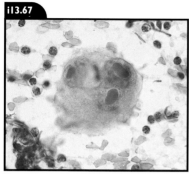

Reed-Sternberg cell (P)

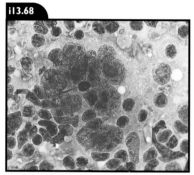

Reed-Sternberg cell—multinucleated (DQ)

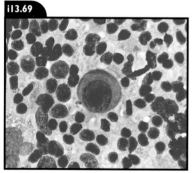

Hodgkin cell (DQ)

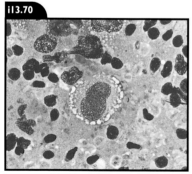

Lacunar cell (DQ)

HD usually arises in a single lymph node or single group of nodes and characteristically tends to spread in contiguity from group to group. This property of HD allows for local therapy and makes staging of HD particularly important. In contrast with NHL, HD virtually never presents in an extranodal site, although it can disseminate later.

Systemic symptoms, so-called "B" symptoms, carry a worse prognosis and may be the presenting complaints. Pruritis also is common. Patients typically have deficient cell-mediated immunity; some cases are associated with EBV. HD tends to occur in upper socioeconomic groups. Because of possible clinical and morphologic similarities, it may be prudent to perform a test for infectious mononucleosis before diagnosing HD in a young patient.

With modern therapy of HD, age and stage at the time of diagnosis are more important clinical factors than the subtype of HD in predicting prognosis. HD is highly curable, especially when low stage. Age may be the single most important prognostic factor (young, favorable; old, unfavorable). Treated patients are now living long enough to develop second malignancies and other medical problems induced by powerful therapeutic agents.

13.6.1 Reed-Sternberg Cells, Variants, and Mimics

Reed-Sternberg cells are large cells that have, at a minimum, bilobed nuclei (but can be multilobed) or are binucleated or multinucleated |i13.65|, |i13.66|, |i13.67|, |i13.68|. The chromatin is coarse and irregular and tends to marginate (especially in Papanicolaou stain), giving the appearance of a thick nuclear membrane. The most characteristic feature, however, is the very large inclusion-like macronucleolus, frequently surrounded by a pale-staining halo. The cytoplasm ranges from scant to abundant and from wispy to dense.

Variants of Reed-Sternberg cells include Hodgkin cells (similar to classic Reed-Sternberg cells, but monolobated and mononucleated) |i13.69|; lacunar cells (large cells with hyperlobated or multiple nuclei and abundant pale to clear cytoplasm) |i13.70|; L&H cells (associated with the lymphocytic and histiocytic lymphocyte-predominant HD, the nuclei are multilobed and resemble a piece of popcorn); pleomorphic Reed-Sternberg cells (bizarre Reed-Sternberg cells associated with lymphocyte-depleted HD); polyploid cells (similar to classic Reed-Sternberg cells, but lack conspicuous nucleoli); and mummified Reed-Sternberg cells (necrobiotic).

Other entities, including poorly differentiated carcinomas, sarcomas, and melanoma, as well as benign conditions such as fat necrosis, can have cells that mimic Reed-Sternberg cells. Binucleate immunoblasts also are common mimickers of Reed-Sternberg cells. Immunoblasts are usually smaller than Reed-Sternberg cells and only rarely binucleated; they have smaller, more rounded nuclei, irregular nucleoli often apposed to the nuclear membrane, and, frequently, plasmacytoid cytoplasm. Immunocyto-chemistry may be helpful: Reed-Sternberg cells tend to be CD45 (leukocyte common antigen) and pan–B cell negative, and CD15 (Leu M1) positive, while the Reed-Sternberg–like immunoblasts may be CD45 and pan–B cell positive and CD15 negative, but these findings are not absolute.

13.6.2 FNA Biopsy of Hodgkin Disease

The aspirate is usually highly cellular, unless there is fibrosis or necrosis, but malignant cells (ie, Reed-Sternberg and variants) may be a minor component. A clue to the diagnosis of HD is finding lymphoid cells that are an order of magnitude larger and "uglier" than ordinary large lymphocytes. These malignant cells seem to "pop out" of the reactive background.

The presence of classic Reed-Sternberg cells is considered a necessary but not sufficient condition to diagnose HD. Because Reed-Sternberg–like cells can be seen in other diseases, the Reed-Sternberg cells also must be found in the proper milieu, ie, a benign reactive background, such as lymphoid cells, plasma cells, histiocytes, granulomas, eosinophils, and neutrophils. Necrosis or fibrosis also can be seen. Granulomas are clues to HD |i13.71|.

Lymphocyte-predominant HD shows mostly small mature lymphocytes. Classic Reed-Sternberg cells are rare by definition, although L&H variants may be numerous. Mixed cellularity HD shows a reactive background in which Reed-Sternberg cells usually are easy to find. Lymphocyte-depleted HD is dominated by anaplastic Reed-Sternberg cells. Nodular sclerosis HD is the most common type and shows collagen bands (as evidenced by metachromatic fibrillar material |i13.72|) and lacunar cells.

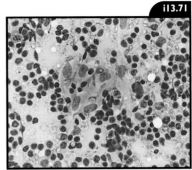
HD—granuloma (DQ)

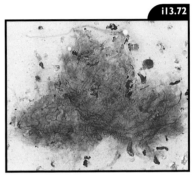
HD—nodular sclerosis (DQ)

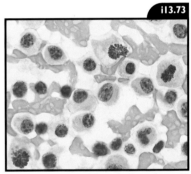
Plasma cell myeloma (P)

13.7 Plasma Cell Myeloma

Plasma cell myeloma is a neoplasm of mature or immature plasma cells that produces a tumorous mass |i13.73|, |i13.74|. The tumors usually present in bone, especially the axial skeleton, skull, or ribs. Extramedullary (soft tissue) myelomas usually occur in the upper airway (nasopharynx, oral cavity) or lung. Multiple myeloma involves lymph nodes only late in the clinical course. The disease is rare in patients younger than 40 years of age; it is the most common lymphoreticular malignancy in blacks.

Patients have a monoclonal gammopathy, resulting in a "spike" on serum protein electrophoresis. About half of the cases secrete IgG, about a quarter IgA, and a fifth Bence Jones light

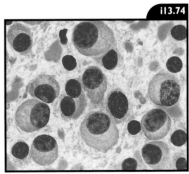
Plasma cell myeloma (DQ)

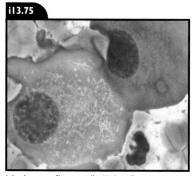

Myeloma—flame cells (DQ, oil)

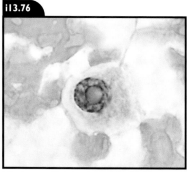

Myeloma—Dutcher body (P)

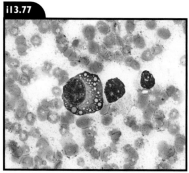

Myeloma—Russell bodies (DQ)

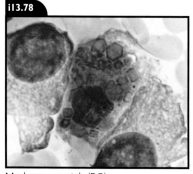

Myeloma—crystals (DQ)

chains (without complete immunoglobulin production). IgM, IgD, or IgE secretion is rare. Clinically, the course is usually one of progressive deterioration, although some cases "smolder." Anemia, bone fractures, renal failure, amyloidosis, repeated infections with encapsulated bacteria (especially *Pneumococcus*), and hypercalcemia often develop.

In essence, the diagnosis is made by finding aggregates of pure plasma cells, often forming loose sheets. Although the aspirate may be cellular, it is frequently diluted with blood. The plasma cells of myeloma are usually fairly mature, but occasionally they are immature or atypical in appearance. |i13.73|, |i13.74|. Mature nuclei have typical coarse clock-face chromatin. Immature nuclei have finer chromatin and prominent nucleoli. Binucleation is particularly common in plasma cell tumors and provides a clue to the diagnosis. Multinucleation and giant and bizarre plasma cells also can be seen.

The cytoplasm typically stains blue (Diff-Quik stain) or amphophilic (Papanicolaou stain) with a perinuclear clearing, or hof. Flame cells, with metachromatic apical cytoplasm, usually are associated with IgA secretion |i13.75|. Cytoplasmic vacuolization is uncommon. Intranuclear (Dutcher) bodies |i13.76| or intracytoplasmic (Russell) |i13.77| bodies, which are collections of immunoglobulin, can be seen. The presence of Dutcher bodies in plasma cells suggests malignancy. Rarely, crystalline intracytoplasmic inclusions occur |i13.78|; these are more common in malignancy.

The differential diagnosis includes lymphoma, particularly lymphoplasmacytic lymphoma or immunoblastic lymphoma, and reactive hyperplasia with prominent plasma cells or lymphoplasmacytoid cells. A mixed inflammatory infiltrate, including mature plasma cells as well as eosinophils, TBMs, and a range of maturation of the lymphoplasmacytic cells, is characteristic of benign reactive lymphoid hyperplasia. Lymphocytes, particularly atypical lymphoid cells, are not seen in plasma cell tumors. Immunologic studies not only can help differentiate benign hyperplasia (polyclonal) from plasma cell neoplasms (monoclonal) but are also useful in determining the plasma cell nature of a poorly differentiated tumor. Myeloma is rarely associated with IgM, in contrast with lymphoplasmacytic lymphoma (Waldenström macroglobulinemia). The differential diagnosis includes other tumors that may have plasmacytoid cells, such as malignant melanoma and adenocarcinomas, eg, some breast cancers.

13.8 Leukemic Lymphadenopathy

Lymphadenopathy is common in patients with leukemia of any category (including lymphoid, myeloid, and monocytic). The tissue phase of some leukemias, including CLL and ALL, has been discussed previously.

The FNA diagnosis usually is fairly straightforward if the history is known and the cells are differentiated. Occasionally, transformation to a higher-grade malignancy occurs, eg, Richter syndrome in CLL |i13.79|. Be cautious diagnosing a leukemic infiltrate in bloody smears: the malignant cells could be contaminants from the blood.

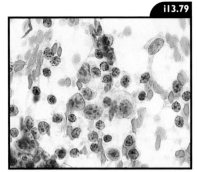

Richter syndrome

13.8.1 Granulocytic Sarcoma

Rarely, granulocytic (myelogenous) leukemia presents as a tumorous mass (granulocytic sarcoma, or chloroma) in virtually any body site, including lymph nodes. Granulocytic sarcoma is more common in children and young adults.

The FNA biopsy is characterized by myeloid cells in various stages of maturation; the cytology depends on the degree of differentiation. If blasts predominate, the aspirate may resemble NHL, particularly in Papanicolaou stain. Myeloblasts are large cells with a moderate amount of pale cytoplasm, large nuclei, fine chromatin, and prominent nucleoli. As the cells mature, a pale area develops in the cytoplasm near the nucleus (ie, in the Golgi apparatus), which in Diff-Quik stain can be seen as the "dawn of neutrophilia" |i13.80|. Look for eosinophilic myelocytes, ie, immature myeloid cells with obvious coarse eosinophilic granulation, which can be seen in both Papanicolaou |i13.81| and Diff-Quik stain. Auer rods support the diagnosis of granulocytic sarcoma, but they also have been identified in circulating lymphoma cells. Cytochemical stains, eg, chloroacetate esterase, Sudan black, or myeloperoxidase, may be helpful in cases dominated by blasts.

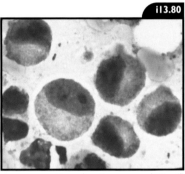

Granulocytic sarcoma (DQ, oil)

The differential diagnosis also includes a benign inflammatory infiltrate or abscess, as well as normal bone marrow, extramedullary hematopoiesis (myeloid metaplasia), and myelolipoma. An abscess usually shows good differentiation to neutrophils and is associated with typical inflammatory signs; organisms may be identified. In hematopoietic tissue, although immature cells are seen, all three cell lines—RBCs, WBCs, and megakaryocytes—are represented.

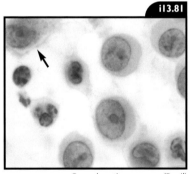

Granulocytic sarcoma (P, oil)

13.8.2 Hairy Cell Leukemia

Hairy cell leukemia is a rare, chronic, lymphoproliferative disorder of characteristic neoplastic lymphocytes with cytoplasmic processes, or "hairs" |i13.82|. The disease may involve lymph nodes, and, rarely, patients may present with a tumorous mass. The cells range up to twice the size of a small lymphocyte, with slightly eccentric round to oval to dumbbell-shaped nuclei. The hairy projections are more evident in Diff-Quik than in

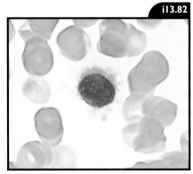

Hairy cell leukemia (DQ, oil)

253

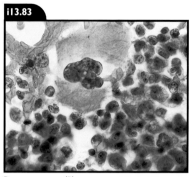

Bone marrow (P)

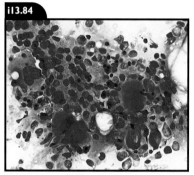

Bone marrow (DQ)

Papanicolaou stain. The cells appear bland and may be misinterpreted as part of a reactive lymphadenitis. Cytochemical staining for acid phosphatase resistant to tartaric acid is characteristic (ie, TRAP positive).

13.9 Extramedullary Hematopoiesis (Myeloid Metaplasia)

Extramedullary hematopoiesis can be seen in a variety of hematologic disorders. It usually involves the liver and spleen, as well as paravertebral and mediastinal sites. Other sites of involvement, such as lymph node and kidney, can occur but are rare. The cytology is similar to normal bone marrow and includes immature blood cells, including all three lineages (erythroid, myeloid, and megakaryocytic) |i13.83|, |i13.84|. Inadvertent puncture of bone marrow, eg, from an osteoporotic vertebral body, can yield an identical picture. The differential diagnosis includes lymphoma, because of the dispersed population of immature cells, and anaplastic carcinoma or sarcoma, because of the presence of "funny looking" giant cells (megakaryocytes).

Masses in the breast should be evaluated by fine needle aspiration (FNA) biopsy. The use of FNA biopsy can reduce not only costs compared with excisional biopsy but also the number of "unnecessary" surgeries for benign disease. In addition, by using FNA biopsy, the patient can be informed, almost immediately, of the most likely diagnosis. This can relieve anxiety if benign, or if malignant, therapeutic options can be discussed at the first visit.

Although FNA biopsy usually can distinguish benign from malignant breast disease, the exact classification of breast masses by cytology can sometimes be a diagnostic problem. Many benign diseases of the breast, particularly the common group of lesions known as fibrocystic disease, are cytologically similar, ie, benign cells all look alike |i14.1|. Specifying the exact type of breast cancer also can be a problem. For example, nearly half of breast cancers are of mixed cell type (ie, not homogeneous), which might not be apparent in a biopsy (due to sampling, etc). Small cell infiltrating ductal carcinoma is cytologically similar to infiltrating lobular carcinoma (ILC), although the prognosis is also similar. The diagnosis of medullary carcinoma requires a "pushing" border, histologically, which cannot be assessed cytologically.

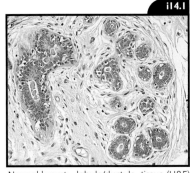

i14.1

Normal breast—lobule/ductule, tissue (H&E)

False-positive diagnoses occur but are rare. Most false positives (or false "suspicious" diagnoses) are due to errors of interpretation and most commonly involve fibroadenomas with atypical features, epithelial proliferations, phyllodes tumors, inflammatory lesions, atypical apocrine cells, and radiation changes.

False-negative diagnoses range from 5% to 20%. Most false-negatives are due to sampling problems, eg, geographic miss of the lesion. Extensive fibrosis, such as seen with a scirrhous ductal carcinoma or ILC, also can cause false negatives owing to sampling problems. Bland, well-differentiated, or small cell tumors, eg, lobular, tubular, papillary, small cell ductal, and in situ carcinomas, can be difficult to diagnose by cytology.

A negative biopsy result does not completely exclude malignancy. A positive diagnosis should correlate with the clinical and mammographic findings. Unfortunately, not all breast lesions can be diagnosed accurately by FNA biopsy. This underscores the importance of the triple test.

14.1 The Triple Test

To summarize, physical examination alone is about 70% to 90% accurate; mammography alone, about 85% to 90% accurate; and FNA biopsy alone, about 90% to 99% accurate in clas-

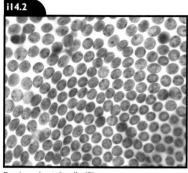

Benign ductal cells (P)

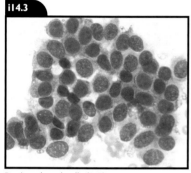

Benign ductal cells (DQ)

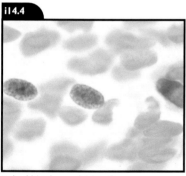

Naked bipolar nuclei (P, oil)

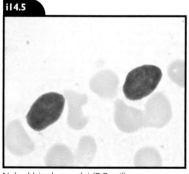

Naked bipolar nuclei (DQ, oil)

sifying breast masses as benign or malignant No single test allows detection of all breast cancers. Consequently, an important clinical approach to the diagnosis and management of patients with breast abnormalities is the combination of all three tests. This diagnostic triad is known as the "triple test."

If all three parameters of the triad (clinical evaluation, mammography, FNA biopsy) are definitively malignant (MMM), there is only about a 1% chance of error, and definitive therapy, including mastectomy, can be considered. On the other hand, if all three are unequivocally benign (BBB), there is about a 98% chance (range, ~ 95%-100%) that the lesion is, indeed, benign, and the patient can be safely followed up. Any other, lesser combination must be carefully evaluated in clinical context and, generally, histologically biopsied.

14.2 The Cells

14.2.1 Ductal Cells

Benign ductal cells are characteristically found in cohesive orderly sheets of uniform cells |i14.2|, |i14.3| but can exhibit mild to moderate crowding. Occasionally, tubular structures ("ductules") or even intact lobules are aspirated. Ordinarily, intact single cells are sparse in benign breast aspirates, although exceptions occur, such as in fibroadenomas, epithelial hyperplasia, or apocrine metaplasia.

Benign ductal cells are usually relatively uniform but can be somewhat variable—within limits—in proliferative diseases. The nuclei are round to oval and range in size up to about twice the diameter of an RBC. Benign ductal nuclei usually have smooth nuclear membranes. The chromatin is fine and even but can be somewhat hyperchromatic. Nucleoli are normally inconspicuous and single.

The cytoplasm is usually scant and delicate but may be more distinct with prominent cells borders ("honeycomb" appearance) and commonly shows variable degrees of apocrine change.

14.2.2 Myoepithelial Cells—Naked Bipolar Nuclei

The presence of myoepithelial cells or the naked bipolar nuclei derived from them is a hallmark of a benign breast aspirate. Naked bipolar nuclei are oval to elongated, about the size of an RBC, and have dark but bland chromatin, smooth outlines, no nucleoli, and no cytoplasm |i14.4|, |i14.5|. They may be found in the background of the smear or attached to sheets or groups of epithelial cells. Be cautious diagnosing malignancy when these sentinel nuclei are present; however, their presence does not guarantee a benign diagnosis.

14.2.3 Foam Cells

Foam cells may be derived from ducts (foam duct cells) or bone marrow monocytes (foamy histiocytes or macrophages) or both (simply, foam cells). Foam cells are found singly or in loose clusters |i14.6|, |i14.7|. They have abundant multivacuolated cytoplasm with relatively distinct cell borders, and they sometimes contain pigments or inclusions. The round to oval nuclei are bland or reactive appearing. Multinucleated giant foam cells also occur. Foam cells usually are associated with benign breast lesions and cysts but can be seen in malignancy.

14.2.4 Apocrine Cells

Apocrine metaplastic cells are frequently found in benign breast aspirates in conditions such as fibrocystic disease, fibroadenomas, and cysts. Apocrine cells often form cohesive, regular, flat sheets or papillae. In contrast with ordinary benign ductal cells, single benign apocrine cells are common.

The principal distinguishing feature of apocrine cells is abundant, finely granular cytoplasm, due mostly to numerous mitochondria—similar to oncocytes. The cytoplasm stains blue to bright orange in Papanicolaou stain |i14.8| and blue-gray to purplish in Diff-Quik stain |i14.9|. Larger lysosome-sized (Lendrum) granules also may be seen.

The nuclei are eccentrically located and may vary in size and shape but usually are fairly uniform. The nuclear membranes are smooth and the chromatin finely granular and evenly dispersed (Papanicolaou stain). Single, round, prominent nucleoli are common.

Because benign apocrine cells can have enlarged nuclei, prominent nucleoli, pleomorphism, and dissociation, "atypical" apocrine cells should be interpreted cautiously. Naked bipolar nuclei may not be conspicuous, particularly in cyst aspirates.

14.3 Nonneoplastic Diseases and Conditions of the Breast

14.3.1 Acute Mastitis and Breast Abscess

Acute mastitis, often associated with lactation, causes pain, swelling, redness, and increased warmth of the breast; fever

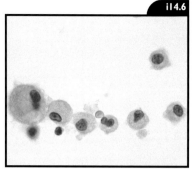
i14.6

Foam cells (P)

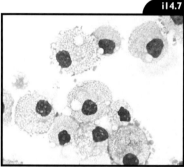
i14.7

Foam cells (DQ)

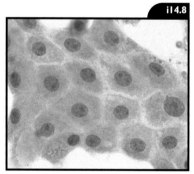
i14.8

Apocrine cells (P)

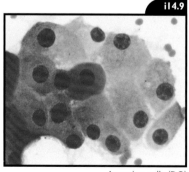
i14.9

Apocrine cells (DQ)

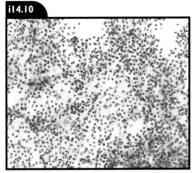

Breast abscess (P)

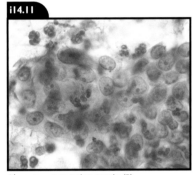

Abscess—reparative atypia (P)

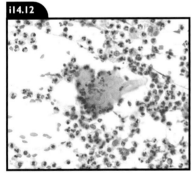

Subareolar abscess (P)

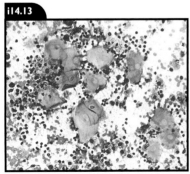

Subareolar abscess (DQ)

and lymphadenopathy also can occur. Acute mastitis can localize, forming a breast abscess. The usual causative organisms are *Staphylococcus aureus* or *Staphylococcus epidermidis*, anaerobic *Streptococcus*, or *Bacteroides* species; mixed anaerobic infections are common.

The clinical differential diagnosis of a breast abscess or its resulting scar includes breast cancer. Acute mastitis could arouse suspicion of inflammatory carcinoma, which also occurs more commonly during pregnancy. Breast cancer and breast infections can coexist, but this is unusual.

The FNA biopsy obtains yellow purulent-appearing material that can be cultured. Thick cellular smears show marked acute inflammation; granulation tissue; macrophages, sometimes including multinucleated giant cells; debris; etc—the usual diagnostic features of an abscess |i14.10|. Epithelial and mesenchymal cells may display inflammatory or reparative atypia, mimicking malignancy |i14.11|. A diagnostic clue, however, is that breast cancer, even so-called inflammatory carcinoma, is seldom associated with acute inflammation.

14.3.2 Subareolar Abscess

Subareolar abscess occurs over a wide age range, is not related to lactation, and can occur even in men. Escape of squamous material from the ducts into the stroma elicits an exuberant foreign body reaction, with abscess and fistulous tract formation, similar to a ruptured epidermal inclusion cyst. Subareolar abscess can mimic breast cancer clinically.

The aspirate is dominated by suppurative granulomatous inflammation. Squamous material, mostly anucleate squames, is the hallmark of this disease |i14.12|, |i14.13|. Giant cells engulfing squames is a particularly characteristic finding |i14.14|. Granulation tissue can be seen and occasionally is prominent. Evidence of cholesterol crystals also may be appreciated. Atypical, reactive ductal or squamous epithelium may suggest malignancy. Note that naked bipolar nuclei may be absent.

14.3.3 Granulomatous Mastitis

The causes of granulomatous mastitis run the gamut from infections (eg, tuberculosis and fungus) to foreign bodies (including sutures and silicon) to sarcoid. Granulomatous mastitis can cause a breast mass that clinically mimics breast cancer.

The FNA biopsy diagnosis rests on finding granulomas or multinucleated giant cells, with or without the specific inciting agent. If an infectious etiology is suspected, culture the aspirate. Acid-fast organisms may or may not be demonstrable in tuberculous mastitis. The differential diagnosis includes fat necrosis and breast abscess with granulation tissue. Rarely, infiltrating carcinoma is associated with a granulomatous response.

14.3.4 Fat Necrosis

Fat necrosis often is found in the subcutaneous tissue of the breast rather than the breast per se. A history of trauma is common but not invariable. Fat necrosis can result in a firm, irregular, fixed mass, sometimes with skin retraction, mimicking malignancy. Fat necrosis and cancer also can coexist.

A gritty sensation, similar to that associated with cancer, is sometimes appreciated during the biopsy procedure. The aspiration obtains greasy material, which tends to bead up on air-dried slides. The cytology shows large foamy macrophages (lipophages), including multinucleated giant cells |i14.15|, |i14.16|. Hemosiderin pigment, evidence of old bleeding, also may be present. Inflammation is variable. Epithelial cells are few but may be reactive or atypical in appearance. Reactive macrophages and fibroblasts also are commonly seen as evidence of mesenchymal repair. These mesenchymal cells can be markedly atypical—even bizarre—in appearance (especially in Diff-Quik stain), with large, pleomorphic nuclei, irregular nuclear membranes, macronucleoli, and mitotic figures, which may suggest a sarcoma |i14.17|. Remember that fat necrosis is relatively common, while breast sarcomas are extraordinarily rare. Also, the smears are not dominated by highly atypical cells in fat necrosis, and, another clue, the atypical cells usually look worse in Diff-Quik than in Papanicolaou stain. Lipid, amorphous material, calcified debris (soaps), or oleic acid crystals (colorless, nonbirefringent, needle-shaped, sunburst pattern) may be present in the background.

14.3.5 Galactocele

Galactocele, or milk cyst, is a retention cyst caused by occlusion of a lactiferous duct. The FNA biopsy obtains milky fluid with few cells—mostly foam cells.

14.3.6 Lactating Adenoma (Lactational Hyperplasia)

Lactational changes normally result in diffuse, symmetric enlargement of the breasts, but occasionally a discrete breast mass is detected clinically—the so-called lactating adenoma. Lactating adenomas are usually the result of focal, exuberant hyperplasia but also can result from lactational change superimposed on a preexisting adenoma, such as a fibroadenoma. Most will spontaneously resolve in the months after delivery or lactation.

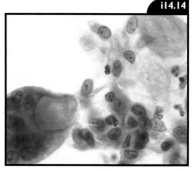

i14.14

Subareolar abscess (P)

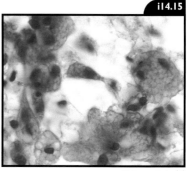

i14.15

Fat necrosis (P)

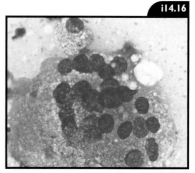

i14.16

Fat necrosis (DQ)

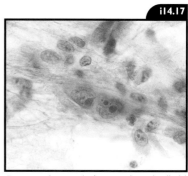

i14.17

Fat necrosis—atypical mesenchymal cells (P)

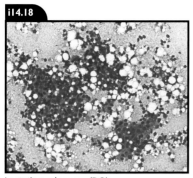

Lactating adenoma (DQ)

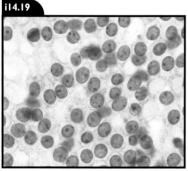

Lactating adenoma (P)

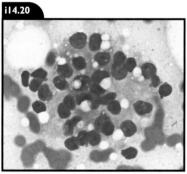

Lactating adenoma (DQ)

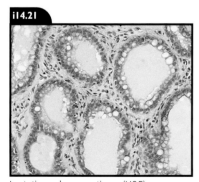

Lactating adenoma, tissue (H&E)

The FNA biopsy is very cellular, and at first blush the cells may appear to be poorly cohesive |i14.18|, |i14.19|, |i14.20|, |i14.21|. Closer inspection reveals that most of the single "cells" are in fact naked epithelial nuclei that have been released from the delicate foamy cytoplasm. In addition, small sheets of cells and, sometimes, intact lobules may be identified. The nuclei are enlarged with smooth nuclear membranes, marginated chromatin, and prominent central nucleoli. Naked bipolar nuclei are present, but they tend to blend into the background of naked epithelial nuclei. Cytoplasmic debris, protein, fat droplets, and occasionally necrosis also can be seen, resulting in a "dirty" background.

High cellularity, apparently dyshesive cells, pleomorphism, hyperchromasia, prominent nucleoli, and possibly even necrosis may strongly suggest malignancy. A history of pregnancy is extremely helpful in pointing to a benign diagnosis. However, breast cancer is the second most common malignancy diagnosed during pregnancy (after cervical carcinoma).

14.3.7 Fibrocystic Disease of the Breast

Fibrocystic disease affects the majority of adult women to some degree and, therefore, is also known as fibrocystic change. Fibrocystic changes usually become clinically evident in early middle age, reaching a peak just before menopause. The etiology is unknown, but hormonal imbalance seems to be involved. Some, but not all, forms of fibrocystic disease are associated with an increased risk of developing breast cancer.

The changes of fibrocystic disease are usually bilateral but not necessarily symmetric and can produce masses suspicious for malignancy. Clinically, bilaterality, multiple nodules, and premenstrual pain favor a benign diagnosis. Fibrocystic disease primarily affects the lobule rather than the large duct system.

It can be difficult by cytology alone to distinguish among the various benign lesions lumped in the category of fibrocystic disease (benign cells all look alike). From a cytologic viewpoint, the benign entities comprising fibrocystic disease (as well as fibroadenomas and papillomas) may be thought of as a triad of cysts, fibrosis, and epithelial proliferation |f14.1|, occurring as pure or mixed lesions. Examples of pure lesions include "blue dome" cysts and areas of fibrosclerosis. Epithelial proliferation can be proliferation of ducts per se (adenosis, eg, microglandular adenosis) or hyperplasia of the intraductal epithelium (epithelial hyperplasia, eg, papillomatosis, epitheliosis).

Mixtures of lesions are the rule rather than the exception. For example, sclerosing adenosis can be thought of as a combination of fibrosis (sclerosis) and epithelial proliferation (adenosis). Papillomas (which are usually of large duct origin and

f14.1 Fibrocystic Disease (FCD)

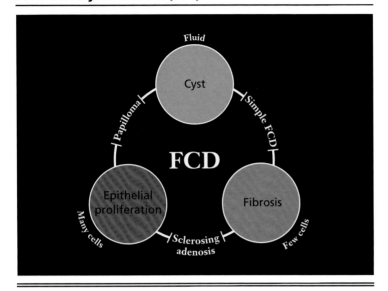

not strictly fibrocystic disease) are the combination of epithelial proliferation growing into an actual or potential cyst. The most common mixture is the combination of cysts and fibrosis or simple fibrocystic disease.

Each point on the triangle has a characteristic cytologic presentation |f14.1|. Areas of epithelial proliferation lead to increased cellularity |i14.22|, while fibrosis is firm and rubbery and yields few cells. Cysts contain fluid.

Cysts

FNA is a simple and safe treatment for cystic disease of the breast. When aspirating a benign cyst, drain the cyst as completely as possible and reaspirate any residual mass. Most breast cysts, by far, are benign, but cystic malignancies can be difficult to diagnose cytologically owing to sampling problems.

The FNA biopsy may obtain yellow, green, brown, bloody, clear, turbid, milky (galactocele), or opaque fluid. Simple cysts have a thin or absent lining and usually yield clear yellow fluid with only a few cells (predominantly foam cells). Cells with hyaline globules, probably giant lysosomes, can be seen |i14.23|. Papillary cysts typically are filled with a turbid fluid containing more cells, which often have apocrine features. Bloody cyst aspirates are more suspicious for neoplasia (papillary neoplasms or cystic cancers). Reactive or degenerative changes may be present.

Fibrosis

When the needle enters an area of dense fibrosis, the mass feels firm, resistant, and rubbery (but usually not gritty). The FNA biopsy is poorly cellular with only a few small groups of

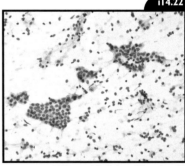

FCD—epithelial proliferation (P)

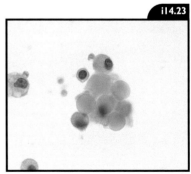

Breast cyst—hyaline globules (P)

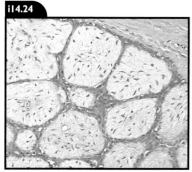

Fibroadenoma, tissue (H&E)

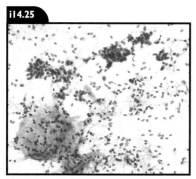

Fibroadenoma (P)

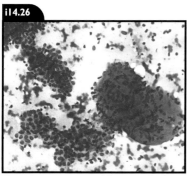

Fibroadenoma—stromal fragment (DQ)

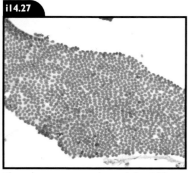

Fibroadenoma—monolayered sheet (P)

cohesive, bland, ductal cells and a few naked bipolar nuclei. It may be difficult to determine that such a poorly cellular biopsy is "satisfactory" based on cytologic findings alone.

Epithelial Proliferation

Epithelial proliferations include epithelial hyperplasias (papillomatosis or epitheliosis) and adenosis; in addition, fibroadenomas and papillomas have a similar cytologic appearance. Although it may be difficult to distinguish among these various entities by cytology alone, the key question—benign or malignant?—usually can be answered by FNA biopsy. The aspirate is typically highly cellular but shows the characteristic features of a benign breast aspirate, including a dual population of cohesive ductal cells and naked bipolar nuclei. Numerous mild to moderately crowded sheets of relatively uniform epithelial cells may be seen. Various other cell types, including foam cells and apocrine cells as well as stromal fragments, adipose tissue, or calcification, may result in a polymorphous appearance. A few, single, intact epithelial cells may be present and occasionally are numerous. Necrosis is absent (or rare and focal).

14.4 Benign Breast Neoplasms

Most benign breast "neoplasms," such as fibroadenomas, papillomas, and lactating adenomas, actually may represent focal exuberant hyperplasias more closely related to fibrocystic disease than to true neoplasms. The cytologic distinction between these neoplasms and ordinary fibrocystic disease can be difficult: the differential diagnosis rests more on quantitative than on qualitative differences in the cells, as well as on the clinical presentation. Traditionally, however, the lesions presented in this section have been regarded as neoplasms, and phyllodes tumors are definitely neoplastic.

14.4.1 Fibroadenoma

Fibroadenoma is a benign fibroepithelial tumor |i14.24|. The classic clinical presentation of fibroadenoma is a rounded, freely mobile mass (like a marble) in the breast of a young woman (in her 20s or 30s). The clinical differential diagnosis includes cysts, lymph nodes, and circumscribed cancers, eg, medullary carcinoma.

The FNA biopsy typically obtains an abundance of glistening mucoid material, although scarified lesions may result in sparse aspirates. The cytology characteristically displays a triad of abundant epithelial cells, numerous naked oval nuclei, and metachromatic stromal fragments |i14.25|, |i14.26|.

Epithelial cells often form large cohesive sheets of honeycombed or moderately crowded but fairly uniform cells |i14.27|. A characteristic feature is the presence of antler-like papillary fronds |i14.28|, which are seen in most fibroadenomas and rarely are seen in fibrocystic disease or cancer. Intact single cells occur in about 20% of aspirates of benign fibroadenomas.

Naked oval nuclei usually are present, often in abundance |i14.29|. Some of these naked nuclei are myoepithelial in origin, but the majority are derived from stromal cells and are larger than myoepithelial nuclei with more open chromatin and conspicuous nucleoli.

Stromal fragments consist of well-demarcated fibro-myxoid material (metachromatic in Diff-Quik stain) containing spindle cells but not adipocytes or inflammatory cells |i14.30|. In young patients, stromal fragments tend to be numerous, but they diminish with age. Myxoid degeneration of the stroma sometimes occurs, which can mimic colloid carcinoma in an aspirate (islands of epithelium in lakes of mucus), except naked oval nuclei are present in fibroadenoma and the age groups are different. Benign multinucleated giant cells can be seen in fibroadenoma, especially in younger patients. Foam or apocrine cells can be found in either fibrocystic disease or fibroadenoma and, therefore, are not particularly helpful in that differential diagnosis.

Fibrocystic disease with epithelial proliferation can be difficult to distinguish cytologically from fibroadenoma. Features favoring fibroadenoma include high cellularity, large flat honeycombed sheets, abundant naked nuclei, antler-like fronds, and numerous stromal fragments, as well as a marble-like breast mass. High cellularity, single cells, and cytologic atypia in fibroadenoma could suggest malignancy. Features favoring a benign diagnosis are stromal fragments, antler horn clusters, honeycomb sheets, fine chromatin, smooth nuclear membranes, apocrine metaplasia, lactational changes, and naked bipolar nuclei. Atypical features in fibroadenoma are usually focal |i14.31|. A definitive diagnosis of carcinoma should be based on the usual malignant criteria, ie, a smear dominated by clearly malignant-appearing cells, including intact single atypical cells, in which naked bipolar nuclei are absent. Rarely, carcinoma arises in a fibroadenoma.

Fibroadenomas with cellular stroma share some cytologic features with phyllodes tumors, but they lack nuclear atypia, have few mitotic figures, and are less cellular than phyllodes tumors. Conservative local therapy seems appropriate.

14.4.2 Phyllodes Tumors

Phyllodes tumors are rare stromal neoplasms with a nonneoplastic epithelial component. The stroma can be benign or malignant. The average age of presentation is the 40s to 50s, older

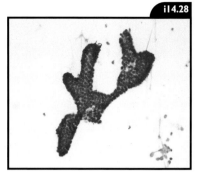

i14.28

Fibroadenoma—"antler" (P)

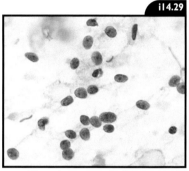

i14.29

Fibroadenoma—naked oval nuclei (P)

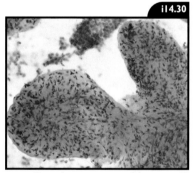

i14.30

Fibroadenoma—stromal fragment (P)

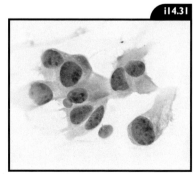

i14.31

Fibroadenoma—focal atypia (P)

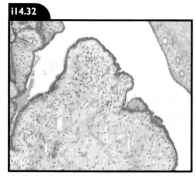

Phyllodes tumor, tissue (H&E)

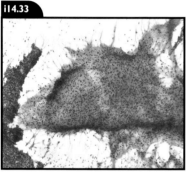

Phyllodes tumor (P)

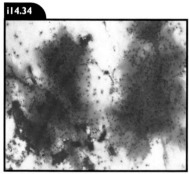

Phyllodes tumor (DQ)

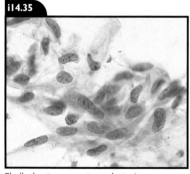

Phyllodes tumor—stromal atypia

than the usual patients with fibroadenoma but similar to those with breast cancer. Phyllodes tumors are usually lobulated and often large. A characteristic histologic finding is leaf-like (phyllode) invaginations of the proliferating stroma into large ducts |i14.32|. Wide local excision or simple mastectomy is usually the therapy of choice.

The FNA biopsy usually obtains a dimorphic population of epithelial and stromal cells |i14.33|, |i14.34|, which may be indistinguishable from fibroadenoma in some cases. The key diagnostic features of phyllodes tumor relate to the stroma. High stromal cellularity, single intact mesenchymal cells, and stromal cell atypia, if present, help differentiate this lesion from fibroadenoma.

The stromal cells range from bland and monomorphic to highly malignant (ie, sarcomatous) appearing |i14.35|. Highly cellular areas may merge with acellular, sclerotic, hyalinized, or cystic zones. Marked stromal overgrowth with little or no epithelium and stromal cell atypia with nuclear enlargement, irregular nuclear membranes, hyperchromasia, irregular chromatin, and multiple nucleoli point to malignancy. Sarcomatous elements can include osteosarcoma, chondrosarcoma, liposarcoma, angiosarcoma, or neurofibrosarcoma.

There also is a benign glandular component similar to that seen in fibroadenomas (including antlers, etc), sometimes forming huge sheets of epithelial cells. Squamous metaplasia, rare in fibroadenomas, can be seen in phyllodes tumors. Conversely, apocrine metaplasia is rare in phyllodes tumors but not in fibroadenomas.

14.4.3 Summary of Features of a Benign Breast Aspirate

A benign breast aspirate is usually characterized by low cellularity, composed of cohesive epithelial cells and naked bipolar nuclei |t14.1|. However, highly cellular smears are not necessarily malignant (eg, epithelial hyperplasia in fibrocystic disease, fibroadenoma), and, conversely, low cellularity does not exclude cancer. The presence of sentinel naked bipolar nuclei is a warning to be cautious in diagnosing malignancy.

Benign epithelial cells are relatively uniform but can show some degree of variability within limits, particularly with epithelial proliferation; intact single cells are usually—but not always—sparse. Benign cells form flat sheets and aggregates that are relatively orderly but may exhibit variable (mild to moderate) crowding or piling up. Benign nuclei can vary in size but usually are no larger than twice the diameter of an RBC. The nuclei are round to oval and have smooth nuclear membranes. Benign nuclei can be somewhat hyperchromatic, but the chromatin is usually fine and the nucleoli small. Macronucleoli are suspicious for malignancy. The cytoplasm ranges from scant and delicate to abundant and apo-

t14.1 General Features of Fine Needle Aspiration Biopsy of the Breast

	Benign Pattern	Malignant Pattern
Cellularity	Usually low, can be high	Usually high, can be low
Cells	Variable within limits; variable cell types	Uniform cells or obvious atypia; single cell population
Groupings	Cohesive clusters; few single cells	Loose clusters vs marked molding; many single cells
Arrangement	Relatively orderly; sheets	Disorderly; single, sheets, or glands
Pleomorphism	Usually little	Usually more
Nuclei	Usually small	Usually enlarged
Nuclear membrane	Smooth	Irregular
Chromatin	Fine, even	Coarse, dark, irregular
Nucleoli	Usually inconspicuous	Often prominent
Naked bipolar nuclei	Present	Usually absent
Background	Usually clean	Often necrotic
Favors diagnosis	Cystic, apocrine	Intracytoplasmic lumens, signet ring cells
Summary	Dual population: epithelial and myoepithelial; cohesive	Homogeneous population: epithelial only; dispersed

crine. In benign lesions, there often is a variability of cell types, including apocrine, ductal, foam, myoepithelial, and histiocytes.

14.5 Malignant Breast Neoplasms

14.5.1 FNA Biopsy of Breast Cancer

The diagnosis of breast cancer often can be suspected, almost immediately, by the characteristic gritty texture—like an unripe pear—encountered by the probing needle |i14.36|. A bloody aspirate also suggests malignancy.

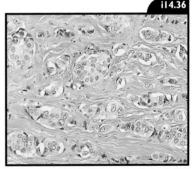
i14.36

Breast cancer, tissue (H&E)

Cytologically, breast cancer usually presents as a homogeneous population of malignant cells. There are two key factors to analyze when contemplating a diagnosis of breast cancer: the cellularity of the smear and the degree of cytologic atypia, which are quantitative and qualitative features, respectively. In essence, there should be "lots of cells to look at" (quantity) and they should all "look malignant" (quality) to make a definitive diagnosis. Unfortunately, not every aspirate of breast cancer follows the rules.

Quantitative Features (Cellularity)
Cancer cellularity means the smear contains an abundance of cells. The cells are present in poorly cohesive groups: importantly, many are single. Be cautious diagnosing malignancy in

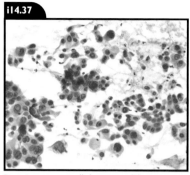

Breast cancer—cellular smear (P)

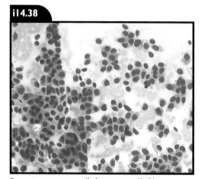

Breast cancer—cellular smear (DQ)

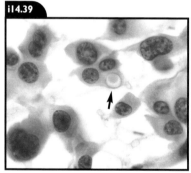

Breast cancer—atypia, ICL (P)

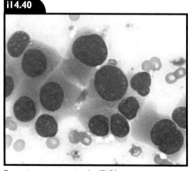

Breast cancer—atypia (DQ)

the absence of intact, single, atypical cells. The presence of "many cells, many single" is a worrisome finding in a breast biopsy |i14.37|, |i14.38|. However, some benign lesions, eg, fibroade-nomas, can yield highly cellular smears, and, conversely, low cellu-larity does not completely exclude the possibility of cancer (due to sampling problems, sclerotic tumors, etc). Groups of cancer cells often are seen in disorderly, piled up heaps or sheets of irregularly arranged, crowded cells. Marked nuclear molding, "cannibalism," "bird's eyes," or marked cellular crowding are clues to malignancy. Naked bipolar nuclei of myoepithelial cells usually are absent in cancer. Thus, in breast cancer there is usually a homogeneous population of epithelial cells, in contrast with the dual population of epithelial cells and naked bipolar nuclei char-acteristic of a benign breast aspirate.

Qualitative Features (Atypia)

Cancer atypia means the cells look malignant, showing the usual features of malignancy, including pleomorphism, enlarged nuclei, coarse and irregular chromatin, prominent nucleoli or macronucleoli, single cell necrosis, and mitotic figures, including atypical forms |i14.39|, |i14.40|, |t14.2|. Nuclear enlarge-ment is an important feature of malignancy. Nuclear enlargement and pleomorphism are usually more obvious in Diff-Quik stain. Nuclei larger than twice the diameter of an RBC are suspicious. Note, however, that some breast cancers have small (ie, normal sized) uniform nuclei that are cytologically bland (eg, some lobular, tubular, papillary, and small cell ductal carcinomas). Irreg-ular nuclear membranes are an important feature of malignancy. Intracytoplasmic lumens (ICLs) also are important in the diag-nosis of breast cancer, but great care must be taken to distinguish them from mere cytoplasmic vacuolization, which is nonspecific. ICLs |i14.39|, |i14.41| are sharply punched-out cytoplasmic vacuoles outlined by a thick rim of cytoplasm, and they contain condensed dots of inspissated mucin ("targetoid appearance"). Their sharp dense outline, as seen with the light microscope, corresponds ultrastructurally to microvilli (see |i8.20|, p 144). ICLs frequently are present in breast cancers but are rarely found in benign breast lesions when using routine stains. In the background of the smear, the presence of necrosis, nuclear and cytoplasmic debris, ghost cells, inspissated secretion, or mucus arouses suspicion of malignancy.

The Problem of Cytologic Atypia

"Atypical" or "suspicious" aspirates, neither clearly benign nor clearly malignant, are being encountered with increasing frequency as FNA biopsy is more widely used. In this gray zone of diagnostic uncertainty, the features of benign and malignant breast aspirates overlap. In some cases, benign- and

t14.2 Typical Features of Breast Cancer

	Features
Clinical	Hard, fixed, irregular mass; dimpled skin, nipple retraction, etc
FNA biopsy	Gritty or bloody
Cells	Abundant, dispersed*; irregular heaps; disorderly groups*; sometimes well-formed acini (vs poorly differentiated glands); pleomorphism; usually enlarged (especially in Diff-Quik stain)
Nuclei	Pleomorphic; hyperchromatic, fine to coarse chromatin; often eccentric; irregular membranes*; crowded, lost polarity; thickened membranes; enlarged nuclei; prominent nucleoli, irregular or multiple; increased mitoses; atypical mitoses*
Cytoplasm	Intracytoplasmic lumens*; mucin positivity; often lipid positive
Background	Cellular smear*; nuclear debris; necrosis; loose cohesion; cytoplasmic debris; mucus; single cells*; ghost cells; no naked bipolar nuclei*; inspissated material

*Particularly useful diagnostic feature.

malignant-appearing cells are seen in the same aspirate, which should probably be regarded as suggestive, rather than diagnostic, of malignancy. Similarly, the presence of only a few abnormal cells in a smear is a "suspicious" rather than a diagnostic finding.

Signs favoring malignancy include disorganized clusters (usually small, crowded), loss of cohesion, nuclear atypia (variable enlargement, greater than two RBC diameters, irregular nuclear membranes, conspicuous nucleoli), ICLs, and necrotic debris. On the other hand, large flat sheets of orderly cells with uniform nuclei that are smaller than two RBC diameters with smooth nuclear membranes and the presence of naked bipolar nuclei favor a benign diagnosis.

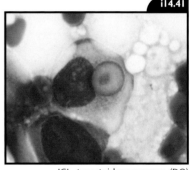
i14.41

ICL, targetoid appearance (DQ)

14.5.2 Infiltrating Ductal Carcinoma

The FNA biopsy of infiltrating ductal carcinoma conforms to the general description of breast cancer already given (ie, cellularity, atypia). Single cells are usually conspicuous. Glands often are poorly formed, but numerous well-formed microacini suggest malignancy. Necrosis is common. There may be foci of squamous, apocrine, or clear cell metaplasia. Stroma varies from scant to abundant (scirrhous carcinomas). Fine to coarse calcifications are common and may allow mammographic detection. ICLs containing mucin are highly suggestive of cancer in routine cytologic preparations. Intracytoplasmic lipid or glycogen is common.

The conventional wisdom is that FNA biopsy cannot distinguish between infiltrating and in situ carcinoma. However, a

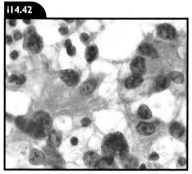

Medullary carcinoma (P)

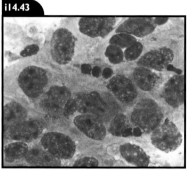

Medullary carcinoma (DQ)

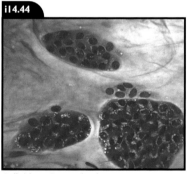

Colloid carcinoma (DQ)

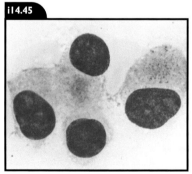

Colloid carcinoma—red granules (DQ, oil)

palpable mass and irregular angulated clusters of atypical cells and irregular stromal fragments suggest invasion.

Various tumor markers, including hormone receptors, B72.3, carcinoembryonic antigen, keratin, α-lactalbumin, Ki-67, proliferating cell nuclear antigen, and tumor suppressor p53 gene, may be positive. Many cases are S-100 positive.

14.5.3 Special Types of Ductal Carcinoma

Medullary Carcinoma

Medullary carcinoma, which accounts for about 5% of breast cancers, is more common in younger patients. It often presents as a soft, rounded, mobile mass that may be mistaken clinically for a fibroadenoma or a cyst. The prognosis is better than ordinary ductal carcinoma when strict criteria are used in diagnosis, in particular, that the tumor is completely circumscribed histologically.

Although the tumor behaves relatively well, it "looks terrible" microscopically, being composed of highly malignant-appearing large cells |i14.42|, |i14.43|. There is little or no gland formation and, by definition, mucin production is absent. The cytoplasm is delicate and syncytial with many naked nuclei. A lymphoplasmacytic infiltrate usually is present.

Medullary carcinoma usually is easy to recognize as malignant, and the specific diagnosis can be suspected by cytology, but histology is necessary for final diagnosis to exclude invasive margins.

Colloid Carcinoma

Colloid carcinoma (aka mucinous or gelatinous carcinoma) usually occurs in older (postmenopausal) patients, and when pure (ie, not mixed with ordinary ductal carcinoma), has a favorable prognosis. Colloid carcinoma may be mistaken clinically for a cyst or fibroadenoma.

The FNA biopsy obtains islands of tumor cells floating in a sea of mucus |i14.44|. The tumor cells usually are found in relatively cohesive sheets, balls, or acini. Single tumor cells usually are present, but naked bipolar nuclei are not. The cells usually are bland and monomorphic. Signet ring cells and large, obviously malignant cells are rare or absent in pure colloid carcinoma. Hemorrhagic foci are common, but necrosis is not seen in pure colloid carcinoma. Fine red (metachromatic) granules may be seen in the cytoplasm with Diff-Quik (possibly neurosecretory granules) |i14.45|. About one quarter of cases show argyrophilia. Intracellular mucin is paradoxically scant.

The differential diagnosis includes mucocele-like lesions (with scant benign-appearing epithelium), papillomas with abundant mucus, and fibroadenoma with myxoid degeneration (see p 265). Be cautious in diagnosing colloid carcinoma in young women.

Tubular Carcinoma

Tubular carcinoma may represent an early stage in the evolution of ordinary breast carcinoma; most of these tumors are less than a centimeter in diameter. When pure, tubular carcinoma has a much better prognosis than ordinary breast cancer. Histologically, the tumor grows as widely patent, angular glands, surrounded by a loose cellular stroma.

The FNA biopsy may be only moderately cellular, and single cells tend to be sparse. A characteristic but not pathognomonic feature is the presence of tubular structures, reminiscent of sections of garden hose |i14.46|. Another characteristic feature is glands with "arrowhead" outlines |i14.47|. The tumor cells usually are well-differentiated and cytologically bland. Irregular nuclear membranes and particularly ICLs, when present, suggest malignancy. Incidentally sampled naked bipolar nuclei may be present in the background, which can confound the diagnosis of this well-differentiated cancer.

Apocrine Carcinoma

Pure apocrine carcinoma is rare, but focal apocrine change is relatively common in breast cancer. Apocrine carcinoma is sometimes regarded as merely descriptive, rather than a separate diagnostic category.

The FNA biopsy usually obtains large, malignant-appearing apocrine cells, which have abundant, finely granular cytoplasm |i14.48|, |i14.49|. The cytoplasm stains variably pink to blue-gray in Papanicolaou stain and gray-purple in Diff-Quik stain. Some cells may have large, PAS-positive, cytoplasmic inclusions (hyaline globules), which are probably lysosomal in origin. Clear cell change also can occur, due to mitochondrial degeneration. Naked tumor nuclei may be conspicuous.

The differential diagnosis with atypical apocrine metaplasia sometimes can be difficult. Malignant features include high cellularity, increased single cells, syncytial tissue aggregates, high nuclear/cytoplasmic ratios (some cells), large nuclei with frankly malignant features, and necrosis, as well as absence of both naked bipolar nuclei and admixed benign elements. As usual, clinical history can be extremely helpful in diagnosis.

"Carcinoid" Tumors

The FNA biopsy of so-called carcinoid tumors (aka argyrophilic carcinoma or carcinoma with endocrine differentiation) usually obtains a monotonous population of small bland cells. The cells occur singly or in loose groups, monolayered sheets, ribbons, or rosette-like structures. Plasmacytoid cells with

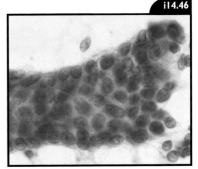

i14.46

Tubular carcinoma (P)

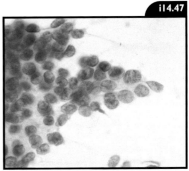

i14.47

Tubular carcinoma (P)

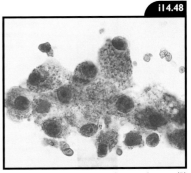

i14.48

Apocrine carcinoma (P)

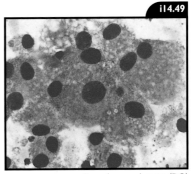

i14.49

Apocrine carcinoma (DQ)

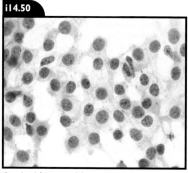

Carcinoid tumor (P)

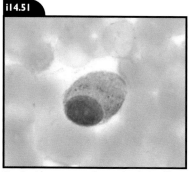

Carcinoid tumor—red granules (DQ, oil)

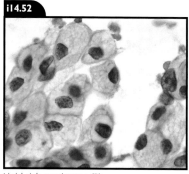

Lipid-rich carcinoma (P)

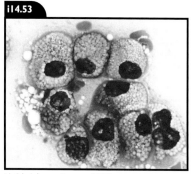

Lipid-rich carcinoma (DQ)

eccentric nuclei or small spindle cells, or both, can be seen. Nuclear pleomorphism and nuclear membrane irregularity are minimal. The chromatin characteristically has a "salt-and-pepper" texture (in Papanicolaou stain) |i14.50|. Nucleoli usually are inconspicuous or absent. The cytoplasm is variable in amount. In Diff-Quik stain, the cytoplasm may show fine red granularity, corresponding to neurosecretory granules |i14.51|. Mitoses are rare. Chromogranin and synaptophysin, among others, may be demonstrable immunocytochemically. This tumor is not associated with the carcinoid syndrome, although serotonin may be produced.

Lipid-Rich Carcinoma

The FNA biopsy of lipid-rich carcinoma obtains cells with relatively small and uniform nuclei, while the cytoplasm contains abundant lipid, resulting in a multivacuolated, clear cell ("hypernephroid") appearance |i14.52|, |i14.53|. The tumor also has been known as "histiocytoid carcinoma" because of the resemblance of the cells to histiocytes. Ordinary breast cancer often shows lipid vacuolization of the cytoplasm; however, in ordinary breast carcinoma, the more lipid in the cytoplasm, the more atypical the nuclei appear. In lipid-rich carcinoma, there is a disparity between the relatively bland nuclei and the marked lipid accumulation.

Metaplastic Carcinoma

In an attempt to simplify a complex subject, the basic types of metaplastic carcinoma are adenocarcinoma with squamous differentiation (adenosquamous carcinoma) and carcinosarcoma (classic metaplastic carcinoma). Spindle cell carcinoma also occurs (sarcomatoid carcinoma).

Adenosquamous Carcinoma: The FNA biopsy obtains malignant glandular and squamous cells |i14.54|. The squamous component is usually minor but occasionally predominates. It also can change to spindle squamous cell carcinoma, thus merging with the sarcomatoid variant of metaplastic carcinoma.

Spindle Cell Carcinoma: The sarcomatoid variant of metaplastic carcinoma can take two forms. The first is spindle cell carcinoma |i14.55|. In this form, the adenocarcinoma cells become spindled (similar to spindle squamous cell carcinoma mentioned previously). The spindle cells can range from relatively bland to obviously malignant appearing. Spindle cell carcinoma mimics spindle cell sarcoma and can even grow in a storiform pattern, histologically. Spindle cell change also occurs in a variety of other adenocarcinomas (eg, carcinomas of the kidney, lung, and pancreas). Immunocytochemistry may be helpful by demonstrating epithelial cell markers.

Carcinosarcoma: The classic form of metaplastic carcinoma is carcinosarcoma. Carcinosarcoma has, in addition to the epithelial malignancy, heterologous sarcomatous elements (eg, malignant fibrous histiocytoma, chondrosarcoma, osteosarcoma, rhabdomyosarcoma, fibrosarcoma) |i14.56|. The sarcomatous elements are apparently metaplastic in origin and derived, at least in some cases, from the epithelium.

Squamous Cell Carcinoma

Pure squamous cell carcinoma (SCC) of the breast is extremely rare. The tumor shows the usual features of SCC, including pleomorphic cells, dark nuclei, and dense squamoid cytoplasm. It often is well-differentiated and keratinizing |i14.57|. The differential diagnosis includes adenosquamous carcinoma (the glandular component may be sparse), metastatic SCC, and SCC arising in the skin of the breast.

14.5.4 Lobular Carcinoma

Lobular carcinoma accounts for about 5% to 10% of breast cancer and occurs at a median age of 45 to 55 years. Pure ILC does not involve the nipple area and, therefore, is not associated with nipple discharge or Paget disease. The prognosis of ILC is similar to infiltrating ductal carcinoma—the major reason for specifically identifying lobular carcinoma is its tendency to be multicentric and bilateral more often than is ductal carcinoma.

Histologically, the tumor tends to grow in rows of single cells and in concentric circles around ducts or lobules ("targetoid" pattern). Note, however, that growth in single file chains of cells is not specific for lobular carcinoma.

The FNA biopsy usually yields a moderately cellular specimen with monomorphic, small, isolated cells and a few loosely cohesive small groups, which may exhibit molding or single file chain arrangements |i14.58|, |i14.59|, |i14.60|. Well-formed glandular acini are absent or rare. Lobular carcinoma is a common source of false negatives, because sometimes only a few bland cells are aspirated, making the diagnosis of malignancy difficult (ICLs and irregular nuclear membranes are diagnostic clues).

The cells are usually 8 to 12 µm in diameter (normal sized, ie, small). They can have angular outlines but occasionally show a striking lymphoplasmacytoid appearance that, particularly when the cells are highly dissociated, may suggest lymphoma or plasmacytoma |i14.61|. (Ductal carcinomas also can have this appearance.) Naked bipolar nuclei usually are not present.

The nuclei are small, round to angular, and eccentrically located and may mold one another slightly. The nuclei are fairly uniform with fine to granular chromatin and little or no hyperchromasia. They may have one or two small nucleoli, which can be prominent. Although the nuclei may appear deceptively bland, on close inspection they frequently have irregular membranes

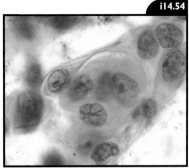
Adenosquamous CA—SCC component (P)

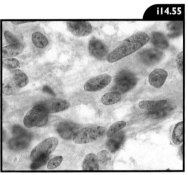
Spindle cell carcinoma (P)

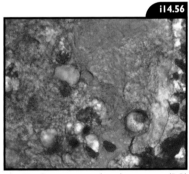
Carcinosarcoma, chondrosarcoma (DQ)

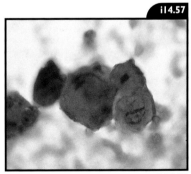
SCC (P)

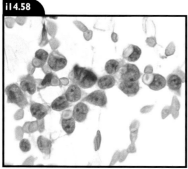

Lobular carcinoma—ICLs (P)

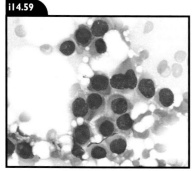

Lobular carcinoma (DQ)

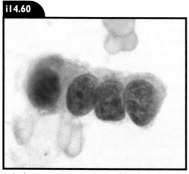

Lobular carcinoma—single file chain (P, oil)

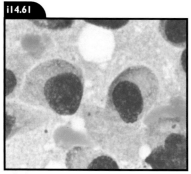

Lobular carcinoma—plasmacytoid cells (DQ)

(best seen in Papanicolaou stain), a useful diagnostic feature of malignancy.

The cytoplasm is small to moderate in amount. It is pale (in Papanicolaou stain) with relatively well-defined cell borders. Cytoplasmic vacuolization is common. From case to case, there is a spectrum from multiple small vacuoles ("bubbly" cytoplasm) to ICLs to well-developed signet ring cells.

Lobular carcinoma can be difficult or impossible to distinguish from ductal carcinoma by cytology alone: small cell ductal carcinomas mimic lobular carcinoma, and, conversely, large cell or pleomorphic lobular carcinomas mimic ductal carcinoma. Small cell size, dispersed cells, minimal pleomorphism and atypia, ICLs, and plasmacytoid appearance all favor lobular carcinoma, but none of these findings are specific.

Signet Ring Carcinoma

Signet ring carcinoma is an aggressive subtype of breast carcinoma, probably a mucinous variant of lobular carcinoma, distinct from colloid carcinoma. The FNA biopsy obtains small, uniform, dissociated cells, similar to ordinary lobular carcinoma. However, cytoplasmic mucin production is prominent and displaces the nucleus, resulting in the characteristic signet ring appearance |i14.62|. Signet ring forms should be numerous to diagnose this variant. Exclude metastatic signet ring cell carcinoma, eg, from the stomach.

14.5.5 Large Duct Tumors

Papillary Neoplasms

Papillary neoplasms, including benign papillomas and papillary carcinomas, are characterized histologically by slender papillae with fibrovascular cores. Papillary neoplasms are fairly rare tumors; most are benign and solitary, and they usually arise in the large duct system beneath the areola.

Benign Papilloma vs Noninvasive Papillary Carcinoma: Benign papillomas are usually smaller than 3 cm and occur in patients who are, on average, 40 years of age. Papillary carcinomas usually are larger than 3 cm and tend to occur in older women who are, on average, in their 50s or 60s. A bloody nipple discharge is a common presenting sign of papillary neoplasms.

The FNA biopsy of a papillary neoplasm is often bloody, and chocolate-colored cyst fluid may be obtained. The presence of a cyst containing nonapocrine papillary clusters or cell balls suggests a papillary neoplasm |i14.63|. Cellularity is variable, depending on the extent of cyst formation. Benign papillomas tend to be less cellular than papillary carcinomas. Strong intercellular cohesion favors a benign diagnosis, and numerous single cells favor malignancy, but single cells also can be seen in benign papillomas. At least a few myoepithelial naked bipolar nuclei are usually present in benign papillomas.

The cytology of benign papilloma may suggest fibroadenoma, except that the stromal component tends to be sparse or absent in papillomas. Collagenous cores, similar to those seen in collagenous spherulosis, are a characteristic but not specific feature of benign papilloma.

A well-known paradox of the histology of papillary neoplasms is that papillary carcinoma can appear more uniform than benign papilloma. The explanation for this is that there are many different kinds of cells in benign papillomas, including ordinary epithelial cells, which can show variability within limits, basal cells, apocrine cells, foam cells, and hemosiderin-laden macrophages, giving the overall impression of pleomorphism. This variation in types of cells is an important clue to a benign diagnosis. On careful scrutiny, the individual benign cells lack malignant features. In contrast, papillary carcinoma is composed primarily of one cell type, and these malignant cells can be fairly bland and uniform in appearance.

Tall columnar cells with distinctive squared-off apical cell borders and oval to elongated nuclei are a characteristic feature of papillary neoplasms |i14.64|, |i14.65|. The nuclei usually show no more than mild to moderate pleomorphism. Nuclear stratification, membrane irregularity, hyperchromasia, and ICLs, if present, suggest carcinoma. Large nucleoli and nuclear pleomorphism can be seen in benign or malignant papillary lesions. Mitotic rate is not particularly useful in the differential diagnosis.

Benign apocrine metaplasia is frequent in papillomas but is not seen in papillary carcinoma. Squamous metaplasia is very rare in papillomas. Mucin production is common in either lesion. An infarcted papilloma can show marked cytologic atypia and necrosis, mimicking malignancy. Invasion in papillary carcinoma can take the form of infiltrating ductal carcinoma or infiltrating papillary carcinoma, which has a better prognosis.

Because it can be difficult to distinguish benign papilloma from papillary carcinoma, when a papillary neoplasm is suspected on needle aspiration, formal tissue biopsy should be recommended for definitive diagnosis (this is, in essence, the same "rule" used for frozen section diagnosis of papillary neoplasms of the breast, ie, "await permanent sections").

14.5.6 Miscellaneous Breast Tumors

Inflammatory Carcinoma

Inflammatory carcinoma presents clinically as acute mastitis, with a red, inflamed, warm, edematous breast. Inflammatory carcinoma is a clinical, not a pathologic, entity. It is usually associated with dermal lymphatic spread of breast cancer of

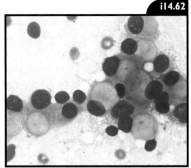

i14.62

Signet ring carcinoma (DQ)

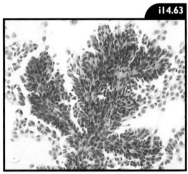

i14.63

Papillary carcinoma—poor cohesion (P)

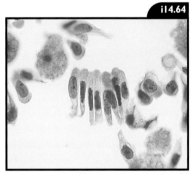

i14.64

Papillary neoplasm, benign (P)

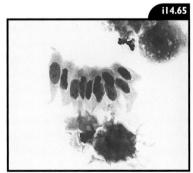

i14.65

Papillary neoplasm, benign (DQ)

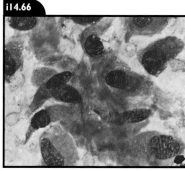

Breast stromal sarcoma (P)

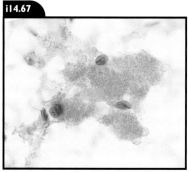

Granular cell tumor (P)

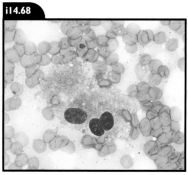

Granular cell tumor (DQ)

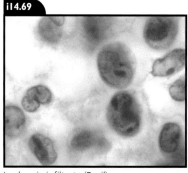

Leukemic infiltrate (P, oil)

various morphologic types. Involvement of the dermal lymphatics is a poor prognostic sign. Inflammatory carcinoma has an unfortunate tendency to occur during pregnancy. Patients with inflammatory carcinoma usually are treated with radiation rather than surgery.

There may not be a distinct mass to aspirate (try using a tangential approach through the skin and subcutaneous tissue). Random samples also may be obtained. The cytology depends on the type of underlying breast cancer but is usually ordinary ductal carcinoma showing typical cytologic features, except that the sample may be sparsely cellular with more cohesive groups than usual and fewer single cells. Despite its name, inflammatory cells usually are sparse.

Salivary and Sweat Gland Analog Tumors

Salivary and sweat gland analog tumors occur, rarely, in the breast. The differential diagnosis includes primary sweat gland tumors of the skin of the breast.

Adenoid Cystic Carcinoma: Primary adenoid cystic carcinoma of the breast is morphologically identical to that occurring in the salivary gland. Metastases are rare, but the tumor may recur with inadequate surgery.

The FNA biopsy obtains a highly cellular smear with a uniform population of small, uniform, basaloid cells and, most characteristically, balls and cylinders of homogeneous mucoid material, which is translucent in Papanicolaou stain and intensely metachromatic (magenta) in Diff-Quik stain. The differential diagnosis includes other lesions that show acellular hyaline bodies, eg, collagenous spherulosis.

Other Salivary-Type Tumors of the Breast: For mucoepidermoid carcinoma, the differential diagnosis is metaplastic and metastatic carcinomas. Apocrine carcinoma is indistinguishable from ordinary apocrine carcinoma. Pleomorphic adenoma is identical to the salivary gland tumor.

Soft Tissue Tumors of the Breast

Although soft tissue tumors of the breast are rare, virtually any kind can occur |i14.66|. Immunocytochemistry may be helpful in differential diagnosis.

Granular Cell Tumor: Granular cell tumor can mimic breast cancer clinically (firm, fixed, irregular mass, may cause skin retraction), grossly (looks and cuts like infiltrating carcinoma), and microscopically (may have irregular margins and atypical cells). Granular cell tumor tends to arise in younger patients and occurs most often in the upper inner quadrant of the breast. The tumor is thought to be of neural origin and related to Schwann cells.

The FNA biopsy obtains a variably cellular specimen with clusters of cells and single cells. The most characteristic feature is the presence of coarse cytoplasmic granules (also found dispersed in the background of the smears owing to cell rupture) |i14.67|, |i14.68|. The granules are PAS-positive and correspond ultrastructurally to tertiary lysosomes.

The nuclei are small, round to oval, and eccentrically located. They have evenly dispersed chromatin and occasional nucleoli. The cells usually lack malignant criteria; malignant granular cell tumor is extremely rare. The presence of marked, coarse, cytoplasmic granularity is a good clue to a benign diagnosis in a breast aspirate.

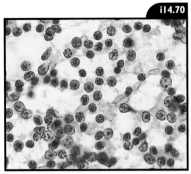
Breast lymphoma

Malignant Lymphoma/ Leukemia

Primary non-Hodgkin lymphoma of the breast is rare; primary Hodgkin disease of the breast is essentially nonexistent. However, secondary involvement by either is more common. Leukemia also can present as a breast mass |i14.69|.

Primary non-Hodgkin lymphomas can be divided into two clinicopathologic groups. One affects young women, is frequently bilateral and diffuse, is often associated with pregnancy, disseminates rapidly to other extranodal tissues, and is a Burkitt-type lymphoma. The second, more common group, which accounts for about 80% of primary breast lymphomas, presents clinically like breast cancer, ie, unilateral breast mass in an older woman. Most of these lymphomas are high-grade, B-cell type |i14.70|. Some may be lymphomas of the mucosa-associated lymphoid tissue (MALT).

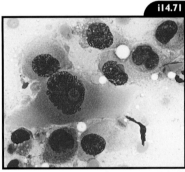
Metastatic melanoma—INCI (DQ)

The primary diagnostic features of lymphoma in FNA biopsy are a dispersed cell pattern, without formation of true tissue aggregates, and lymphoglandular bodies in the background. The cells have typical lymphoid morphology, best appreciated in Diff-Quik stain. Occasionally, ordinary breast carcinoma presents a highly dispersed cell pattern reminiscent of malignant lymphoma or plasmacytoma. Mucin production excludes lymphoma and plasmacytoma, and conspicuous lipid production is rare in lymphoma.

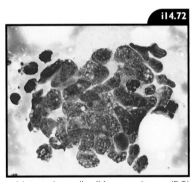
Metastatic small cell lung carcinoma (DQ)

Metastases

In FNA biopsy, metastatic malignancy accounts for up to 5% of all malignant breast tumors. Among the most common tumors to metastasize to the breast are melanoma |i14.71|; lymphoma; carcinomas of the lung |i14.72|, ovary, gastrointestinal tract, and genitourinary system |i14.73|; and soft tissue sarcomas. Metastasis of breast carcinoma to the other breast is probably the most common source, but a new primary tumor must be excluded. In men, prostatic carcinoma is a relatively common source of breast metastases.

Metastases are usually freely mobile, well-circumscribed masses that ordinarily do not cause changes in the overlying skin.

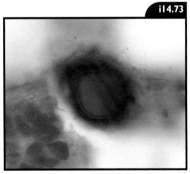
Metastatic endometrial carcinoma (P)

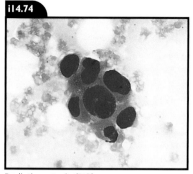

Radiation atypia (DQ)

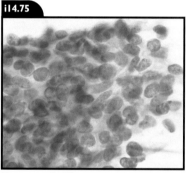

Gynecomastia (P)

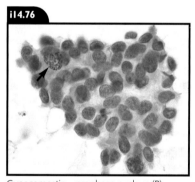

Gynecomastia—prophase nucleus (P)

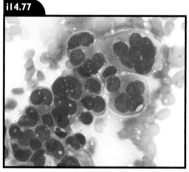

Gynecomastia—multinucleation (DQ)

A metastasis may be mistaken clinically and mammographically for a benign lesion, such as a cyst or fibroadenoma.

When encountering a breast cancer with benign mammography or unusual cytologic features (eg, psammoma bodies |i14.73|, melanin, small [oat] cell, squamous cell, or clear cell pattern), consider the possibility of metastasis. Ancillary studies may be helpful in some cases, but clinical history often is critical. Note that breast cancer can be S-100–positive and, rarely, even contains melanin, complicating the differential diagnosis with melanoma.

14.5.7 Irradiated Breast and Posttherapy Breast Masses

Breast-conserving surgery with radiation is increasingly common treatment for breast cancer. After therapy, even in nonirradiated patients, a variety of lesions may occur that must be differentiated from recurrent carcinoma, eg, suture granuloma, fat necrosis, and scars.

Radiation-induced epithelial atypia may be difficult to distinguish from recurrent malignancy. However, highly atypical irradiated cells usually are sparse, and nuclear detail is typically lacking (smudgy chromatin) |i14.74|. Naked bipolar nuclei favor a benign diagnosis. The clinician must provide the history of radiation therapy, and diagnostic conservatism is appropriate in this setting.

14.6 Male Breast

14.6.1 Gynecomastia

Gynecomastia is common, particularly at puberty and in old age. Gynecomastia usually is bilateral, particularly when puberty- or hormone-related, but may be more prominent on one side. However, unilateral disease may be more common in patients selected for needle biopsy.

Clinically, there are two forms of gynecomastia. One, mammoplasia, presents as a firm rubbery mass beneath the areola. The mass is resistant to the needle, and the biopsy is painful. In the other form, true gynecomastia, the contour and consistency of the male breast are similar to that of the female breast, and the biopsy is relatively painless. The cellularity varies from scant (usual) to abundant. The smears show sparse to numerous sheets of cohesive, moderately crowded or tightly packed ductal cells with relatively few single, intact epithelial cells |i14.75|. However, nuclear atypia, including nuclear enlargement and pleomorphism as well as mitotic activity, is common in gynecomastia, especially mammoplasia |i14.76|. Apocrine and cystic changes can occur. Naked bipolar nuclei are present. Multinucleated epithelial cells |i14.77| and giant stromal cells may be seen, and squamous metaplasia can be extensive.

14.6.2 Cancer of the Male Breast

Cancer of the male breast is an uncommon but important disease that usually can be easily identified by FNA biopsy. Risk factors include Klinefelter (XXY) syndrome, family history, radiation, head trauma, gonadal injury (including mumps), estrogens, cirrhosis, and obesity. There is no proven link between gynecomastia and breast cancer. Other than its rarity, cancer of the male breast is otherwise similar to cancer of the female breast regarding epidemiology, natural history, diagnosis, staging, and response to therapy. Furthermore, breast cancers often are hormonally dependent in men. The overall prognosis is somewhat worse in the male, in part because of its tendency to involve the skin or chest wall muscle early in the course of the disease (ie, high stage).

The cytology of male breast cancer is essentially identical to that of cancer of the female breast. As in women, the quantity |i14.78| and quality |i14.79| of the cells are diagnostically important. Virtually all types of breast cancer have been reported in the male. Ductal carcinoma is, by far, most common; lobular carcinoma is particularly rare. Among metastatic cancers, it can be difficult to distinguish metastatic prostatic carcinoma from primary breast cancer, particularly if the prostate primary is clinically unknown. Note that prostate-specific antigen can be expressed in breast cancer.

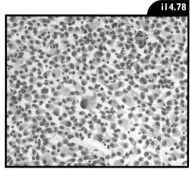

Male breast cancer—cancer cellularity (P)

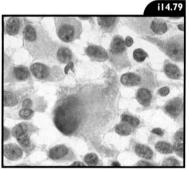

Male breast cancer—cancer atypia (P)

CHAPTER FIFTEEN

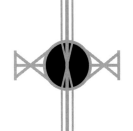

This chapter is divided into three sections: lung, pleura, and mediastinum. Exfoliative cytology of lung (see Chapter 2) and pleura (see Chapter 3) are discussed elsewhere. Although there are numerous similarities between the aspiration and exfoliative cytology of these sites, there are also significant differences.

LUNG

Presumptive clinical diagnosis of primary or metastatic malignancy is the usual indication for fine needle aspiration (FNA) biopsy of the lung, but the cytologic method also can be used to diagnose benign tumors such as hamartomas and inflammations such as granulomas. FNA biopsy is particularly indicated when sputum cytologic and bronchoscopic findings are negative but tumor remains a strong clinical possibility. For most patients, the diagnostic benefit of the procedure far outweighs the risk of complications (see Chapter 7), particularly when thoracotomy can be avoided.

FNA biopsy is highly accurate in distinguishing between small cell carcinoma and non–small cell carcinoma. False-negative results are related primarily to inadequate sampling, usually due to geographic miss of the lesion, but also can occur with well-differentiated tumors, such as bronchioloalveolar carcinoma or carcinoids. False-positives can result from marked reactive atypia, which can be associated with a wide variety of pulmonary insults ranging from inflammation to radiation. The unsatisfactory rate ranges from about 5% to 20%.

15.1 Transbronchial (Wang) Needle Biopsy

Transbronchial ("Wang") needle biopsy is a modification of FNA biopsy performed through the bronchoscope. The procedure originally was used to detect mediastinal metastases (ie, for staging), but its use has been extended to facilitate diagnosis of other lesions that can be reached with a bronchoscope. Complications, such as pneumothorax, are less likely than with transthoracic FNA biopsy. To reduce contamination with blood or mechanically exfoliated cells, Wang needle biopsy should be performed before taking brushings or biopsies. Cytodiagnostic criteria are essentially identical to those used for transthoracic FNA biopsy.

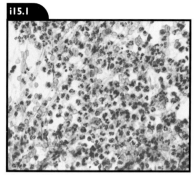

Abscess (P)

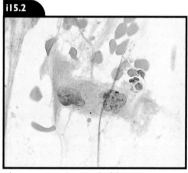

Abscess—reactive atypia (P)

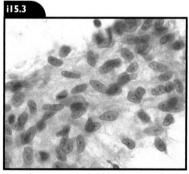

Granuloma—epithelioid histiocytes (P)

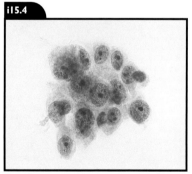

Granuloma—reactive pneumocytes (P)

Failure of the needle to penetrate tracheal cartilage or deflection of the needle from the target are common problems. False negatives primarily result from failure to sample the lesion. If the target is a lymph node, lymphocytes are an important criterion of adequacy; ciliated cells or macrophages are insufficient. A false-positive diagnosis (of metastasis) can occur if, eg, endobronchial tumor is inadvertently sampled.

15.2 The Cells

The various types of cells were described in Chapter 2.

15.3 Benign Diseases of the Lung

15.3.1 Inflammatory Disease

Abscess

Most abscesses result from aspiration of foreign or infective material, commonly by alcoholic or debilitated patients. Because the right main-stem bronchus is more vertical, most abscesses occur in the right lobe. Abscesses also can occur due to embolic seeding (usually multiple nodules) or pneumonia. Note that patients with a lung abscess can have underlying lung cancer.

The FNA biopsy usually obtains purulent material (which often can be recognized grossly and cultured). Foul-smelling specimens suggest anaerobic infections. The cytologic studies show the expected features of an abscess, including acute inflammation, macrophages, and necrosis |i15.1|. Bacteria, other organisms, or aspirated vegetable matter may be identified microscopically. Later, chronic inflammation and granulation tissue, as well as atypical metaplastic cells, evidence of repair and regeneration, or foreign body reactions, may be seen. Reactive atypia and necrosis may suggest malignancy |i15.2|.

Granuloma

Granulomatous disease can be caused by a wide variety of agents; one of the most common is tuberculosis. The radiologic appearance of granulomas can mimic lung cancer.

The diagnostic features of granulomas consist of nodular collections of epithelioid histiocytes, characteristically forming loose syncytial aggregates of cells with elongated, often cleaved, bland nuclei, eccentrically located in the cytoplasm, which often appears fibrillar in the Papanicolaou stain |i15.3|. Giant cells may or may not be present. Langhans giant cells with peripheral nuclei are characteristic of tuberculosis but not specific. Acute or chronic inflammation or necrosis also may be present. When amorphous, granular, necrotic-appearing material is aspirated, suspect granulomatous inflammation but exclude cancer. Necrosis may obscure the diagnostic cells. To arrive at a specific diagnosis, the causative organism, agent, or cells must be demonstrated. Special stains, cultures, and polarized light can be helpful.

Reactive atypia associated with granulomas, particularly due to tuberculosis or *Aspergillus*, together with a radiologic appearance suggesting a neoplasm, may lead to a false-positive diagnosis of cancer |i15.4|. On the other hand, granulomas can coexist with cancer, particularly cancers with squamous differentiation. When an infectious disease is suspected, some of the aspirate can be submitted for cultures and special stains.

Lipid Pneumonia

Lipid, or lipoid, pneumonia can result from endogenous or exogenous lipids. Exogenous lipid pneumonia, eg, due to oily nose drops, is now rare. Endogenous lipid pneumonia is due to lipids released with cell death. It often is associated with bronchial obstruction (postobstructive pneumonia), including obstruction caused by malignancy. The chest x-ray may resemble pneumonia or cancer.

The FNA biopsy obtains many lipid-laden histiocytes, or lipophages, with abundant, vacuolated cytoplasm |i15.5|, |i15.6|. Special stains, such as oil red O, can be used to demonstrate lipid in the vacuoles in fresh specimens. Multinucleated giant cell histiocytes usually are present. Variable degrees of inflammation and evidence of fibrosis (fibroblasts, collagen) can be seen.

Pulmonary Infarct

Pulmonary infarcts usually are the result of thromboemboli, typically from the leg veins of bedridden patients. Although relatively common, the diagnosis may not be made during life because many are asymptomatic or mimic other pulmonary diseases. The classic chest radiographic appearance of a pulmonary infarct is a wedge-shaped abnormality, with the base on the pleural surface, but the most common radiologic finding is nonspecific elevation of a hemidiaphragm with basal atelectasis. A pulmonary infarct also can present as a coin lesion or localized mass that must be differentiated from cancer, infection, or granuloma.

The sequence of events in pulmonary infarcts is hemorrhage, necrosis, inflammation, organization, scar. The FNA biopsy findings depend on when the biopsy is taken and where it is taken from. The periphery of the lesion can show marked reactive atypia of glandular cells, closely mimicking adenocarcinoma |i15.7|, |i15.8|. The center of the lesion may show reactive squamous metaplasia and repair/regeneration, mimicking squamous

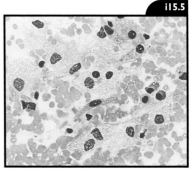

Lipid pneumonia (DQ)

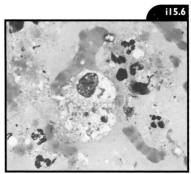

Lipid pneumonia (DQ)

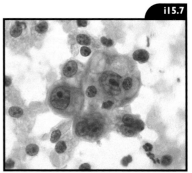

Pulmonary infarct—reactive atypia (P)

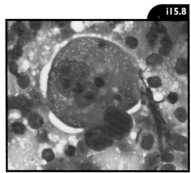

Pulmonary infarct—reactive atypia (DQ)

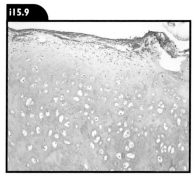

Hamartoma, tissue (H&E)

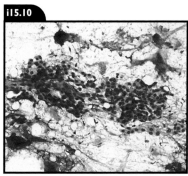

Hamartoma (DQ)

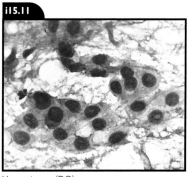

Hamartoma (DQ)

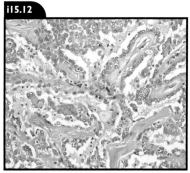

Sclerosing hemangioma, tissue (H&E)

cell carcinoma (SCC). In reactive atypia, there is usually a spectrum from clearly benign to the most atypical cells; highly atypical cells are usually sparse. Numerous histiocytes, which may contain hemosiderin, lipid, or RBCs, may be present. Acute or chronic inflammation, reactive fibroblasts, granulation tissue, or necrosis can also be seen. When the lesion scars, few or no cells are obtained.

15.3.2 Benign Neoplasms of the Lung

Hamartoma

Pulmonary hamartoma, also known as fibrochondrolipoma, is a benign mesenchymal tumor that, although rare, accounts for 75% of all benign lung neoplasms. Hamartomas occur most commonly in middle-aged men. They usually present as asymptomatic, solitary, well-circumscribed, peripheral lung masses, less than 4 cm in diameter, but also can present as a coin lesion mimicking cancer.

The FNA biopsy diagnosis of hamartoma may be immediately suspected by the impact of the needle as it impales a rubbery to hard, cartilaginous tumor |i15.9|. The amount of aspirated material ranges from sparse (potentially nondiagnostic) to abundant and often is mucoid or gelatinous. The cytologic findings are reminiscent of pleomorphic adenoma of the salivary gland: intensely metachromatic chondroid matrix with embedded cells |i15.10|, |i15.11|. The cartilage can range from immature (fibromyxoid) to mature (with lacunar chondrocytes); mixtures are common. Reactive bronchial cells; adipose, muscle, or fibrous connective tissue; and inflammation also may be seen in a clean background. Reactive atypia of bronchial cells could be misinterpreted as evidence of malignancy.

Inflammatory (Myofibroblastic) Pseudotumors

Inflammatory pseudotumors are a rare group of benign lesions that include fibroxanthoma (xanthogranuloma) and plasma cell granuloma. Inflammatory pseudotumors occur predominantly in younger patients (average, 30 years of age). Inflammatory pseudotumors usually are asymptomatic, slow-growing, well-circumscribed, small peripheral lung masses that can produce coin lesions mimicking malignancy. Recently, clonality has been demonstrated in these tumors, suggesting they may be true neoplasms (myofibroblastoma).

The FNA biopsy findings in inflammatory pseudotumor are nonspecific, but suggest a benign reactive process. The aspirate may include plasma cells, lymphocytes, eosinophils, neutrophils, mast cells, histiocytes, and myofibroblasts in varying proportions. The stroma can range from edematous to myxoid to fibrous to hyalinized. Myofibroblasts, which are spindle- to stellate-shaped cells with plump oval nuclei, fine chromatin, and conspicuous nucleoli, are characteristic findings. Reactive alveolar macrophages and giant cell histiocytes also may be present. The cytoplasm may contain lipid (xanthoma or foam cells) or hemosiderin. When histiocytes are prominent, the diagnosis of fibroxanthoma or xanthogranuloma has been used. Plasma cells also are characteristic of inflammatory pseudotumors; when abundant, the lesion has been designated plasma cell granuloma. Occasionally, mast cells are prominent (mast cell granuloma or mast cell tumor).

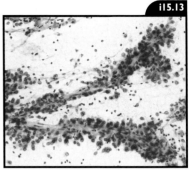
Sclerosing hemangioma (P)

Sclerosing Hemangioma (Pneumocytoma)

Sclerosing hemangioma, or type II pneumocytoma, is a rare benign tumor of the lung |i15.12|. The tumor cells are epithelial and do not express factor VIII, but they do demonstrate surfactant apoprotein antigen. Thus, they are probably type II, or granular, pneumocytes rather than endothelial cells. The lesion is closely related to (identical with?) papillary adenoma. The average patient is a middle-aged woman. The tumor produces an asymptomatic peripheral lung mass that can mimic cancer.

The FNA biopsy obtains abundant material; a characteristic finding is aggregates of cells surrounding small blood vessels or sclerotic cores |i15.13|. The aspirate shows a biphasic cell population (stromal cells and reactive bronchial or alveolar cells) without obvious malignant features |i15.14|, |i15.15|, |i15.16|. Intranuclear cytoplasmic invaginations, giant cells, and hemosiderin-laden macrophages may be seen. Mitotic figures are rare. The differential diagnosis encompasses well-differentiated adenocarcinomas, including bronchioloalveolar and papillary carcinomas (primary, metastatic), and carcinoid tumor. Clear-cut malignant features exclude a diagnosis of sclerosing hemangioma.

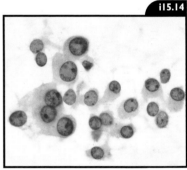
Sclerosing hemangioma, biphasic (P)

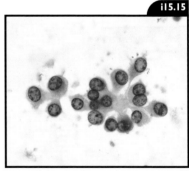
Sclerosing hemangioma—rosette (P)

15.4 Lung Cancer

Lung cancer is the number one cancer killer of men and women. The overall 5-year survival rate is only about 5% to 10% and has remained relatively unchanged for decades. Tobacco smoking is the main cause of lung cancer. Other associated factors include genetic predisposition, virus, radiation, radon gas, air pollution, occupational exposure to various metals, chemicals, and, at least in smokers, asbestos.

The peak incidence is around 60 years; men are more commonly affected than women. Patients are also at increased risk for the development of head and neck cancers. Signs and symptoms of lung cancer appear relatively late in the course of the disease. Weight loss and cough are the most common

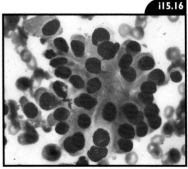
Sclerosing hemangioma (DQ)

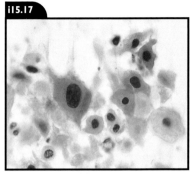

Keratinizing SCC (P)

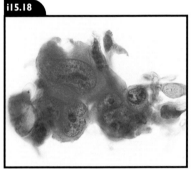

Keratinizing SCC (P)

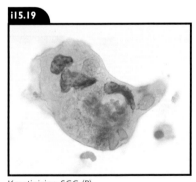

Keratinizing SCC (P)

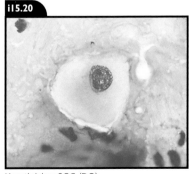

Keratinizing SCC (DQ)

presenting symptoms. Dyspnea, weakness, chest pain, and hemoptysis also are relatively common.

About 20% of patients have paraneoplastic syndromes, particularly patients with small cell carcinoma. Patients may present with symptoms related to a paraneoplastic syndrome rather than directly related to the cancer itself. These syndromes include endocrine, hematologic, cutaneous, neuromuscular, and connective tissue disorders.

As many as three quarters of the cases of lung cancer have spread beyond the lung by the time of diagnosis. Metastases occur first to the hilar lymph nodes, followed by mediastinal, lower cervical, and axillary lymph nodes. Distant metastases to the liver, lung, adrenal, bone, kidney, and brain are all too common. Lung cancer, along with breast cancer and melanoma, is notorious for its ability to metastasize to virtually any site in the body.

Although stage of the tumor is probably the most important factor in prognosis, there may be some correlation with cell type. In general, SCC has the best prognosis, while small cell and giant cell carcinomas have the worst prognosis.

Lung cancer, ie, bronchogenic carcinoma, is thought to arise from a multipotential primitive cell; mixed tumors are very common. In fact, the majority of lung cancers are heterogeneous in cell type when studied extensively. The mixed nature of tumors often is more apparent in cytologic than in histologic studies (see p 294).

15.4.1 Squamous Cell Carcinoma

SCC occurs predominantly in men, is strongly associated with cigarette smoking, and is decreasing in incidence. Most cases arise in the large bronchi and are centrally located.

Keratinizing (Well-Differentiated) SCC

Although primary SCC of the lung is common, it is relatively unusual for it to be highly keratinized. Therefore, consider a metastasis, particularly from the head and neck area, when well-differentiated, keratinizing SCC is seen in a lung aspirate.

The two most characteristic features of keratinizing SCC are marked pleomorphism, including bizarre cells (eg, snakes, tadpoles), and marked keratinization (eg, dense, refractile cytoplasm, cytoplasmic rings, and spirals) |i15.17|, |i15.18|, |i15.19|. Pearls are pathognomonic of keratinization. In Papanicolaou stain, keratinized cells stain bright yellow or orange; in Diff-Quik stain, keratinized cells stain glassy "robin's egg" blue |i15.20|. Keratinized cells often are large, and some cells have low nuclear/cytoplasmic ratios.

The nuclei are irregular and angular, with coarse to pyknotic (ink dot) chromatin. Nucleoli often are obscured by the dense chromatin. Cells without nuclei (ghosts) are common. Look for fragments of less-differentiated, nonkeratinized, malignant cells to help diagnose a tumor composed predominantly of highly differentiated squamous cells or anucleate squames.

The background of keratinized SCC often is necrotic and granular. In some cases, the tumor is cystic; the needle obtains pearly yellowish fluid that looks like pus but contains keratin debris. In other cases, abundant inflammation is present, which can obscure tumor cells and mimic a benign abscess.

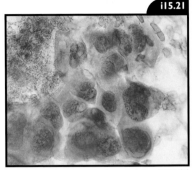

Nonkeratinizing SCC (P)

Nonkeratinizing (Moderately to Poorly Differentiated) SCC

Nonkeratinizing SCC lacks squamous pearls and bizarre cells, although an occasional dyskeratotic cell may be seen. Cells deriving from nonkeratinizing SCC are more uniform and have higher nuclear/cytoplasmic ratios than those of keratinizing SCC. The cytoplasm is relatively dense and well-defined; it often is cyanophilic (ie, blue-green) in the Papanicolaou stain, but the staining reaction is variable |i15.21|, |i15.22|. The cytoplasm stains blue or purple in Diff-Quik stain |i15.23|, |i15.24|. In poorly differentiated nonkeratinizing SCC, the only clues to squamous differentiation may be a tendency to sheet-like arrangement of cells with dense cytoplasm and distinct cell borders.

The nuclei of nonkeratinizing SCC are located centrally and have irregular nuclear membranes. The chromatin is coarse and dark but somewhat more open than that of keratinizing SCC. The chromatin is irregularly distributed with areas of chromatin clearing. Nucleoli are usually more prominent than in keratinizing SCC but less so than in adenocarcinoma.

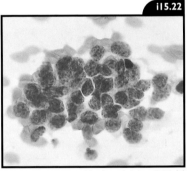

Nonkeratinizing SCC (P)

Mixtures of keratinized and nonkeratinized cancer cells are common. Keratin, even from a so-called nonkeratinizing SCC, often elicits a granulomatous reaction, a clue to squamous differentiation in a poorly differentiated tumor.

Pseudokeratosis, ie, dense, orangeophilic cytoplasm, caused by degeneration, can occur in adenocarcinoma, mimicking SCC. Cytoplasmic vacuolization is nonspecific and can be seen in either adenocarcinoma or SCC.

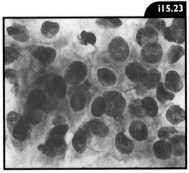

Nonkeratinizing SCC (DQ)

Poorly differentiated SCC may be difficult to distinguish from small cell carcinoma. SCC has denser cytoplasm than small cell carcinoma, and the cells resist being crushed. Molding is usually more prominent in small cell carcinoma. The nuclear chromatin is usually coarser and nucleoli more prominent in SCC than in small cell carcinoma. The presence of granulomas favors SCC. Either tumor may be associated with necrosis, but inflammation or cavitation favors SCC.

Benign reactive changes, such as those due to infectious agents, particularly tuberculosis or fungi, or infarction, can mimic SCC. Features favoring a reactive process include evidence of degeneration, such as smudgy chromatin and cytoplasmic vacuo-

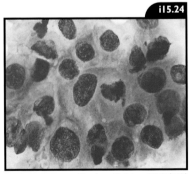

Nonkeratinizing SCC (DQ)

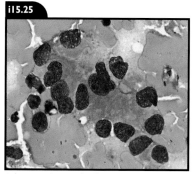

Adenocarcinoma (DQ)

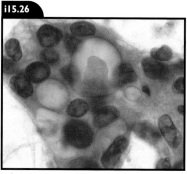

Adenocarcinoma (P)

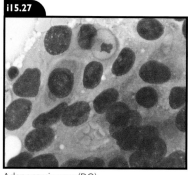

Adenocarcinoma (DQ)

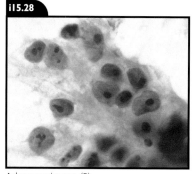

Adenocarcinoma (P)

lization, the presence of foamy or hemosiderin-laden macrophages, and a spectrum of benign to atypical cytologic changes.

15.4.2 Adenocarcinoma

Adenocarcinoma has become the most common type of lung cancer in both sexes. Although associated with cigarette smoking, adenocarcinoma is also the most common type of lung cancer in nonsmokers. Adenocarcinoma typically arises in a peripheral location; it is sometimes associated with a scar. Occasionally, adenocarcinoma diffusely coats the lungs, mimicking mesothelioma (see p 297).

There are two basic morphologic types of adenocarcinoma of the lung: (1) bronchogenic, the more common, or usual type, associated with bronchial glands or mucous goblet cells, and (2) bronchioloalveolar carcinoma (BAC). There is overlap in the morphology of the two types, which are sometimes regarded as basically the same entity, and stage-for-stage the prognosis is also similar. It also can be difficult to determine whether adenocarcinoma is primary or metastatic.

Bronchogenic Adenocarcinoma

The key diagnostic feature of adenocarcinoma is, of course, definite glandular differentiation, ie, formation of glands |i15.25| or mucin production by malignant cells |i15.26|. Sheets of disorderly, crowded, atypical cells usually are present. Palisading of cells around the edges of tissue fragments provides another diagnostic clue to glandular differentiation.

The cells characteristically exhibit nucleocytoplasmic polarity (basal nuclei, apical cytoplasm). The cytoplasm is delicate and finely vacuolated and tends to stain basophilic (in Papanicolaou stain). It often contains mucin. Mucin is metachromatic in Diff-Quik stain |i15.27|, but special stains (mucicarmine, PAS with diastase) can help demonstrate it. Intracytoplasmic lumens also indicate glandular differentiation. Hyalin cytoplasmic globules are present in some cases.

The nuclei typically have more open delicate chromatin and more prominent nucleoli than in SCC. The classic finding in adenocarcinoma is a large "owl's eye" nucleus, with pale chromatin and a single, cherry-red macronucleolus (in Papanicolaou stain) |i15.28|. However, the quality of the chromatin and the size and number of nucleoli can vary significantly from this classic picture. Binucleation or multinucleation can occur. Irregular nuclear membranes are usually present and provide a clue to a malignant diagnosis.

The differential diagnosis includes BAC, large cell undifferentiated carcinoma, metastatic adenocarcinoma, and poorly differentiated SCC. Benign reactions, eg, due to pneumonia, infarcts, physical or chemical agents, also can closely mimic adeno-carcinoma in some cases. Malignant cells form a discrete population of atypical cells, while in benign conditions there usually is a spectrum from benign to the most atypical. Clinical history, as always, is crucial in proper diagnosis.

Bronchioloalveolar Carcinoma

BAC is defined as primary adenocarcinoma of the lung in which most of the tumor grows as a single layer of cells along alveolar and bronchiolar walls without invading the stroma or causing tissue destruction. On chest x-ray, BAC can be seen as a single solitary mass (coin lesion), multiple masses (simulates metastases), or diffuse (pneumonia-like infiltrate).

BAC has been increasing in incidence. Although more common in later life, BAC can occur in young adults. Men and women are affected equally. Although BAC is associated with cigarette smoking, many cases occur in patients who have never smoked. BAC has the longest median survival of primary pulmonary adenocarcinoma and may be curable if localized.

BAC can arise from or mimic bronchiolar epithelial cells, including Clara cells (most cases) and mucous cells, or alveolar cells, primarily granular type II pneumocytes. However, the exact cell type cannot be reliably determined by light microscopy. Therefore, the combined term bronchioloalveolar carcinoma is usually used.

Two basic morphologic subtypes of BAC can be recognized by light microscopy: mucinous (secretory |i15.29|) and non-mucinous (nonsecretory or serous |i15.30|); mixtures are common. BAC also can occur as a scar cancer (sclerosing BAC). BAC is usually, but not always, well-differentiated.

The general cytologic features of classic well-differentiated BAC include abundant clusters, large sheets, or papillae of deceptively bland glandular cells without cilia, with relatively few single cells, in a clean background. The nuclei are uniform, round, or oval with some crowding. Irregular nuclear membranes are a clue to malignancy. Numerous intranuclear cytoplasmic invaginations (INCIs) favor BAC over ordinary bronchogenic carcinoma |i15.31|. The chromatin is finely granular. Macronucleoli, if present, suggest malignancy. Mitoses are rare; necrosis is absent. Abundant histiocytes may be present, which can be atypical in appearance and confused with tumor cells.

Mucinous BAC is composed of crowded or honey-combed sheets of goblet cells, usually found floating in pools of mucus. Terminal bar–like apical borders or false cilia, due to microvilli, and prominent nucleoli may be appreciated, but multi-nucleation, intracytoplasmic lumens, or signet ring cells are absent or rare. Intranuclear cytoplasmic invaginations are infrequent (compared with nonmucinous BAC). Little or no inflammation is present in the background.

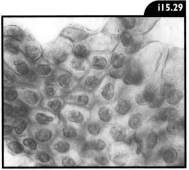
BAC—mucinous (P)

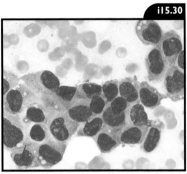
BAC—serous (DQ)

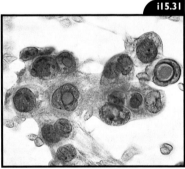
BAC—INCI (P)

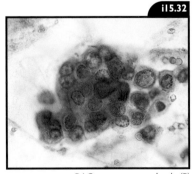
BAC—psammoma body (P)

289

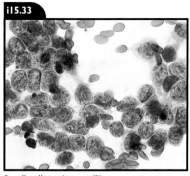

Small cell carcinoma (P)

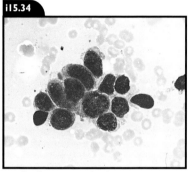

Small cell carcinoma (DQ)

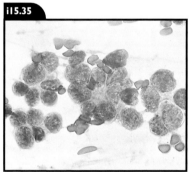

Small cell carcinoma—rosette (P)

Nonmucinous BAC is composed of sheets or papillae of smaller cells that can resemble either alveolar pneumocytes or mesothelial cells. Occasional cases contain abundant cytoplasmic glycogen, but mucin is scanty or absent. Intranuclear cytoplasmic invaginations are characteristic but not specific. Psammoma bodies are present in some cases |i15.32|. Nonmucinous BAC accounts for a significant number of scar cancers.

Poorly differentiated BAC has the usual features of malignancy and is difficult to distinguish from ordinary bronchogenic or metastatic adenocarcinoma. The presence of intranuclear cytoplasmic invaginations, psammoma bodies, and a component of very well-differentiated tumor cells favors BAC. Be cautious diagnosing BAC when there is a history of another primary adenocarcinoma, including lung cancer, or in patients with multiple lung nodules. Reactive bronchial or alveolar cells can be mistaken for BAC. Reactive cells usually are present in small flat sheets, and highly atypical cells are usually few. The presence of true cilia is a benign feature. A conspicuous background of inflammation also favors a reactive process. Be careful in diagnosing BAC in a patient who is febrile or has a reasonable explanation for reactive changes in respiratory cells.

15.4.3 Small Cell (Neuroendocrine) Carcinoma

Small cell carcinoma is thought to arise from primitive cells that have the capacity for Kulchitsky (neuroendocrine) cell differentiation. It no longer is considered an undifferentiated form of cancer. Small cell carcinoma is more common in men than women, but its incidence may be rising in women. Small cell carcinoma rarely occurs in nonsmokers. The tumor usually is widely disseminated at the time of diagnosis. Surgery is so ineffective in therapy that tumors of this cell type usually are considered unresectable. However, some patients respond to intensive medical therapy (radiation, combination chemotherapy), although the overall 5-year survival rate remains less than 5%.

Small cell carcinoma usually is centrally located. The tumor characteristically metastasizes extensively to hilar and mediastinal lymph nodes. A hilar or perihilar mass is seen radiologically in up to 75% of patients. Metastatic deposits often are more prominent than the primary lesion.

Small cell carcinoma is divided into three morphologic types. The first is pure small cell carcinoma, which includes classic oat cell (or lymphocyte-like) and intermediate cell subtypes (as previously defined by the World Health Organization). The other two types are considered variants of pure small cell carcinoma: combined (with squamous or adenocarcinoma) and mixed (small and large cell) types.

Immunocytochemically, small cell carcinoma usually expresses neuroendocrine markers such as neuron-specific enolase, synaptophysin, and sometimes chromogranin, as well as epithelial markers such as keratin. Ultrastructurally, the tumor cells often have small desmosomes and characteristic features of neuroendocrine differentiation such as microtubules and neurosecretory granules (NSGs).

The FNA biopsy shows numerous isolated cells, syncytial aggregates, sheets of cells |i15.33|, |i15.34|, and, occasionally, rosettes |i15.35|. At low power, the cells appear relatively uniform; however, at high power, within their small size range, the cells of small cell carcinoma are quite pleomorphic. Spindle cells also may be seen |i15.36|.

Although classically composed of small neuroendocrine cells, cell size and NSGs are not the key diagnostic features of small cell carcinoma. On the one hand, many other tumors, including poorly differentiated squamous carcinomas or adenocarcinomas, are composed of "small blue cells." On the other hand, the "small" cells of small cell carcinoma may be unexpectedly large, particularly in air-dried biopsy material. There is also a large cell neuroendocrine carcinoma (see below). Similarly, NSGs are neither necessary nor sufficient for the light microscopic diagnosis of small cell carcinoma. NSGs can be found in other lung neoplasms, particularly carcinoid tumors.

The key diagnostic features of small cell carcinoma pertain to chromatin, nucleoli, and cytoplasm. The nuclei are hyperchromatic, but in well-preserved cells the chromatin is relatively fine without prominent clumping or chromocenter formation. Nucleoli are invisible or small and inconspicuous. The cytoplasm is delicate and scant, resulting in an extremely high nuclear/cytoplasmic ratio: the cell is composed almost entirely of its nucleus. Paranuclear cytoplasmic inclusions, blue bodies or BBs (collections of intermediate filaments), are found in many cases but are not specific |i15.37|.

The tumor cells are delicate and easily crushed; thus, nuclear streaming or crush artifact is another characteristic feature |i15.38|. Nuclear degeneration is common in small cell carcinoma and frequently results in the chromatin having a coarse rather than fine texture, as seen in well-preserved cells.

15.4.4 Large Cell Neuroendocrine Carcinoma

Large cell neuroendocrine carcinoma refers to non–small cell carcinomas that demonstrate neuroendocrine features by electron microscopy or immunocytochemistry. Although neuroendocrine differentiation in non–small cell carcinoma cannot be reliably determined by light microscopy alone, some cases have paraganglioma-like features (eg, rosettes, long

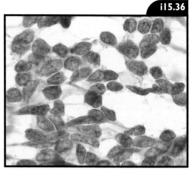

Small cell carcinoma—spindle cells (P)

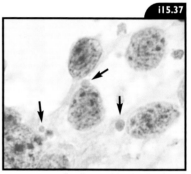

Small cell CA—blue bodies (P, oil)

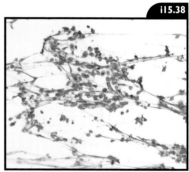

Small cell CA—crush artifact (P)

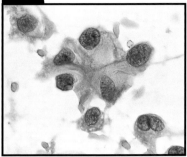

Large cell neuroendocrine CA (P)

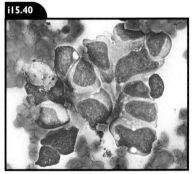

Large cell neuroendocrine CA (DQ)

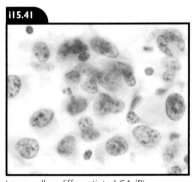

Large cell undifferentiated CA (P)

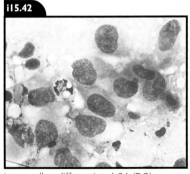

Large cell undifferentiated CA (DQ)

neurite-like cytoplasmic processes) |i15.39| and others resemble small cell carcinoma, except that the cells appear larger, as if magnified |i15.40|.

15.4.5 Large Cell Undifferentiated Carcinoma

Large cell undifferentiated carcinoma amounts to something of a "wastebasket" category for poorly differentiated, non–small cell tumors that are difficult to classify. Although some of these carcinomas may, in fact, be undifferentiated, most tumors in this category will show evidence of squamous or glandular, and even neuroendocrine, differentiation on close scrutiny, eg, using electron microscopy or immunocytochemistry.

Most large cell undifferentiated carcinomas occur in men and are associated with smoking. Like adenocarcinoma, they usually occur in a peripheral location. The tumor grows rapidly and has a poor prognosis. However, when confronted with a poorly differentiated or undifferentiated neoplasm, particularly in a young person, consider the possibility of a germ cell tumor or the syndrome of undifferentiated carcinoma/poorly differentiated adenocarcinoma, which are potentially treatable tumors. Sometimes large cell carcinoma, as well as giant cell carcinoma, is associated with secretion of human chorionic gonadotropin or with other paraneoplastic syndromes.

The FNA biopsy of large cell undifferentiated carcinoma obtains obviously malignant cells that, by definition, lack light microscopic evidence of specific differentiation (eg, squamous, glandular) |i15.41|, |i15.42|. The cells are large but not necessarily enormous. A few giant tumor cells may occur but are not numerous (see "Giant Cell Carcinoma," below). The nuclei may be very abnormal with irregular nuclear membranes, coarse irregularly distributed chromatin with parachromatin clearing, and prominent macronucleoli, often with perinucleolar clearing. Binucleation and multinucleation are common. Mitoses, including abnormal forms, may be frequent. The cytoplasm varies from fine and delicate to granular and dense. By definition, the cells are mucin-negative and do not show glandular or squamous differentiation by light microscopy. Hyalin cytoplasmic globules are seen occasionally.

In cytologic studies, it is rare to find a tumor that shows no evidence whatsoever of specific cellular differentiation. Tumors considered histologically to be undifferentiated frequently show evidence of specific differentiation cytologically.

15.4.6 Giant Cell Carcinoma

Giant cell carcinoma, like large cell carcinoma, comprises a heterogeneous group of tumors. Most occur peripherally. Giant cell carcinoma can be a "dedifferentiated" squamous or adenocarcinoma, a subset of large cell undifferentiated carcinoma, or a specific entity not directly related to other types of lung cancer. The prognosis is usually dismal.

The FNA biopsy specimen of giant cell carcinoma is characterized by the presence of a "significant number" of multinucleated malignant tumor giant cells, often with spectacular malignant atypia. Large but not giant malignant tumor cells also are present. Glandular or squamous differentiation or both may be apparent in some cases. Mitoses, including markedly abnormal ones, may be frequent. A neutrophilic infiltrate is common in the background, and neutrophils are frequently present in the cytoplasm of the giant tumor cells |i15.43|.

The differential diagnosis of giant cell carcinoma includes metastases from other giant cell carcinomas, eg, from the pancreas, or pleomorphic sarcomas. Some cases of giant cell carcinoma have a significant spindle cell component (giant and spindle cell carcinoma), suggesting the possibility of a pleomorphic or spindle cell sarcoma |i15.44|.

15.4.7 Carcinoid Tumors

Carcinoid tumors account for about 5% of cases of lung cancer. The average age at diagnosis is the 40s (younger than ordinary lung cancer), with an equal sex distribution. Typical carcinoids are not associated with smoking but may be part of the inherited syndromes of multiple endocrine neoplasia. Carcinoids are low-grade malignancies; some cases metastasize locally and a few distantly, especially to the liver. If the tumor can be completely resected, the patient is usually cured.

Carcinoids are morphologically divided into typical and atypical forms. There are also mixed patterns. Other variants include papillary, cystic, oncocytic, clear cell, spindle cell, signet ring, and adenocarcinoid. Bronchial carcinoids rarely produce the carcinoid syndrome unless there are extrathoracic metastases. Immunocytochemically, these tumors demonstrate neuroendocrine and epithelial markers.

Typical carcinoid tumor, usually centrally located, is by far the most common type of lung carcinoid. It frequently presents as an endobronchial polyp covered by an intact mucosa. Histologically, the tumor grows in nests, ribbons, cords, rosettes, or, rarely, papillae.

The FNA biopsy usually obtains numerous loosely cohesive, small, monotonously uniform cells with a lymphoplasmacytoid appearance |i15.45|. Rosettes, palisades, or small clusters may be seen. A few larger atypical cells may be present ("endocrine atypia"). The nuclei have smooth nuclear membranes, "salt-and-pepper" chromatin, and inconspicuous nucleoli. The cytoplasm is

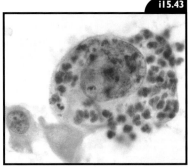

Giant cell CA—neutrophils (P)

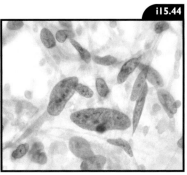

Giant and spindle cell CA—spindle cells (P)

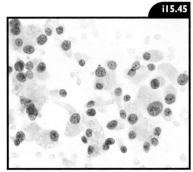

Typical carcinoid (P)

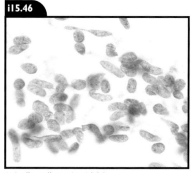

Spindle cell carcinoid (P)

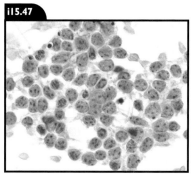

Atypical carcinoid (P)

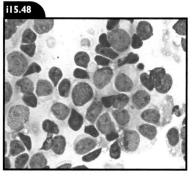

Atypical carcinoid (DQ)

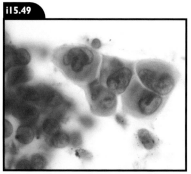

Mixed carcinoma—sharp contrast (P)

finely granular. Argyrophilic NSGs are characteristically present (metachromatic in Diff-Quik stain). There is no necrosis, few or no mitoses, and crush artifact is not common.

Spindle cell carcinoids usually occur subpleurally, with a predilection for the right middle lobe in adults. Peripheral carcinoids tend to be small (< 2 cm) and well circumscribed but not encapsulated. They may be accompanied by carcinoid tumorlets (cytologically identical to spindle cell carcinoid, but the tumors are tiny). Peripheral carcinoids tend to be more aggressive than central carcinoids, although metastases are unusual.

The FNA biopsy obtains spindle-shaped tumor cells, usually in disorderly aggregates |i15.46|. Compared with typical carcinoid, the cells may be somewhat more pleomorphic with some degree of nuclear molding, nuclear membrane irregularity, and mitotic activity, but they have finer chromatin. Nucleoli are usually small and inconspicuous. Necrosis is not seen, and the background usually is clean. Argyrophil stains may be focally positive, but argentaffin is negative. Amyloid stroma may be prominent.

Atypical carcinoid is intermediate in appearance and behavior between typical carcinoid and small cell carcinoma |i15.47|, |i15.48|. Atypical carcinoids are distinguished from typical carcinoids by any of the following: increased mitotic rate; larger, more atypical nuclei, with more hyperchromasia, coarser chromatin, more pleomorphism, and prominent nucleoli; and the presence of necrosis. Spindle cells are prominent in some cases. Rosettes and palisades are characteristic of atypical carcinoids. In essence, the more the tumor resembles small cell carcinoma, the worse the prognosis.

15.4.8 Tumor Heterogeneity and Cell of Origin

It is currently thought that all of the cells lining the bronchial tree, including neuroendocrine Kulchitsky cells, and by extension, all of the common types of lung cancer, including small cell carcinoma, arise from a common, primitive endodermal cell. Therefore, it would not be surprising if lung cancer were heterogeneous in cell type. And in fact, on thorough examination, the majority of lung cancers are of mixed cell type. Mixture of cell types is often more apparent in cytology than in histology. A characteristic feature of mixed glandular and squamous carcinoma is a sharp contrast between the delicate glandular cytoplasm and the dense squamoid cytoplasm |i15.49|, |i15.50|, |i15.51|. Endocrine differentiation usually requires special studies such as immunocytochemistry to demonstrate.

Stage for stage, all four common types of lung carcinoma, including small cell carcinoma, behave clinically more or less similarly (although low-stage "small cell carcinomas" actually may be atypical carcinoids). Thus, stage, not cell type, is the most important predictor of survival, and patients with stage I resected lung cancers may do relatively well, with 5-year survival rates reported to be as high as 70% to 80%.

In summary, the clinical value of subclassification of lung cancer, particularly non–small cell types, is questionable. Non–small cell lung carcinomas are frequently heterogeneous and exhibit mixed features of squamous, glandular, and/or neuroendocrine differentiation. Indeed, even single cells may show all three lines of differentiation (tripartite). In practice, a cytodiagnosis of small cell carcinoma or non–small cell carcinoma of the lung usually is sufficient for current clinical purposes.

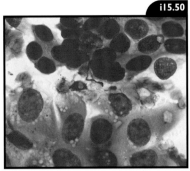

Mixed carcinoma—sharp contrast (P)

15.4.9 Clear Cell Tumors

Clear cell tumors can be benign or malignant, primary or metastatic. Primary clear cell carcinoma is not a specific tumor type but rather represents clear cell change that can occur in most of the usual primary lung cancers, including carcinoids, but not small cell carcinoma. Focal clear cell change is common; however, tumors composed predominantly or exclusively of clear cells are rare. Cytoplasmic clarity is usually due to glycogen accumulation |i15.52|. Also consider metastatic renal clear cell carcinoma.

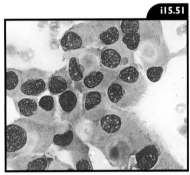

Mixed CA—dense cytoplasm, secretion (DQ)

15.4.10 Salivary Gland Analog Tumors

Salivary gland analog tumors probably arise from submucosal bronchial glands, the pulmonary counterpart of minor salivary glands. They can occur at any age. These tumors are rare, and metastases from a salivary gland primary tumor must be excluded. Adenoid cystic carcinoma is the most common member of this group. It is morphologically identical to the salivary gland tumor of the same type. Mucoepidermoid carcinoma also occurs and may be difficult to distinguish from primary adenosquamous carcinoma of the lung, especially when high-grade. The presence of intermediate cells favors mucoepidermoid carcinoma. Rarely, other salivary gland–like tumors, including pleomorphic adenoma, acinic cell tumor, and oncocytoma, arise in the lung.

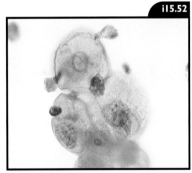

Clear cell CA—yellowish glycogen (P)

15.4.11 Biphasic Epithelial and Mesenchymal Tumors

Mixed epithelial and mesenchymal tumors are rare, but when a biphasic pattern is seen, the differential diagnosis is limited. There are two basic types of biphasic lung cancers: pulmonary blastoma and carcinosarcoma.

Pulmonary blastoma occurs predominantly in middle-aged women. It is usually peripherally located, well-circumscribed, and variable in size. The overall 5-year survival rate is less than 20%.

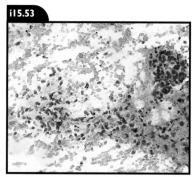

Pulmonary blastoma—biphasic pattern (P)

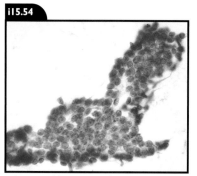

Pulmonary blastoma—adenocarcinoma (P)

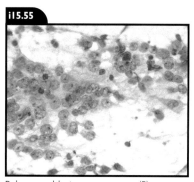

Pulmonary blastoma—sarcoma (P)

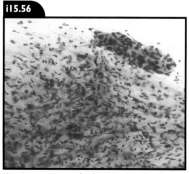

Carcinosarcoma—biphasic

Microscopically, the tumor resembles fetal lung and is the pulmonary counterpart of nephroblastoma (Wilms tumor). The aspirate shows a biphasic pattern of epithelial and spindle cells, often with sharply defined transitions |i15.53|. The adenocarcinomatous component can range from well to poorly differentiated |i15.54|. Squamous differentiation also can occur. The sarcomatous component, which may be predominant, is represented by a myxoid to highly cellular stroma composed of monotonous, small, spindle, mesenchymal cells (blastema) |i15.55|. Benign- or malignant-appearing skeletal muscle, cartilage, or bone may be seen in some cases.

Carcinosarcoma usually occurs in older adults, more often men, on average about 25 years later than pulmonary blastomas. In contrast with pulmonary blastoma, most cases of carcinosarcoma are located centrally, often as an endobronchial polyp. Carcinosarcoma usually has a worse prognosis than pulmonary blastoma, more like ordinary lung cancer, but sometimes pursues an indolent course, particularly when endobronchial.

The aspirate shows a biphasic pattern of epithelial and spindle elements |i15.56|. In most cases, the epithelial component is nonkeratinizing SCC. The sarcomatous component usually is reminiscent of fibrosarcoma or malignant fibrous histiocytoma. Areas of gradual transition are more common in carcinosarcoma than in pulmonary blastoma. The spindle cells are larger than those of pulmonary blastoma and may be bizarre in appearance. A myxoid stroma may be seen. Occasionally, foci of chondrosarcoma, osteosarcoma, rhabdomyosarcoma, or angiosarcoma may be present; osteoclastic giant cells alwo may be seen.

15.4.12 Sarcomas

Virtually any sarcoma can arise in the lung, but metastatic sarcomas are far more common. Solitary lesions favor primary; multiple, metastasis. However, it is unusual for a sarcoma to present as a metastasis from an occult primary tumor. Metastatic sarcomatoid carcinomas, especially of renal origin, can present a diagnostic challenge, particularly since the primary renal tumor may be occult.

15.4.13 Malignant Lymphoma

The bronchus contains mucosa-associated lymphoid tissue (MALT). Low grade B-cell lymphomas of small lymphoid cells, including MALTomas or marginal zone, mantle cell, lymphoplasmacytic, and small cleaved types, are the most common primary pulmonary lymphomas. High-grade lymphomas, which are less common, include large cell and immunoblastic, small noncleaved, and anaplastic lymphomas. Secondary involvement of the lung by lymphoma is more common than primary disease.

15.4.14 Metastases

The most common sources of lung metastases are breast, colon, pancreas, stomach, melanoma, kidney, and sarcomas, but almost any malignant tumor can metastasize to the lung. Multiple, sharply circumscribed, rapidly growing metastases are most common. Endobronchial metastasis can closely mimic a primary lung tumor. Growth along preexisting alveoli may be indistinguishable from BAC, particularly when the tumor is well-differentiated adenocarcinoma.

There are no reliable cytologic features that can distinguish primary from metastatic adenocarcinoma. Features that favor a primary lung tumor include a solitary lesion, mixed adenosquamous differentiation, and no other primary tumor.

In patients with lung cancer and a second primary tumor, about 20% of the cancers occur in the head and neck area. The head and neck cancer usually precedes the lung tumor. Thus, the question frequently arises, is SCC in the lung primary or metastatic? The answer is usually multiple primary tumors.

Melanin pigment in malignant cells is essentially diagnostic of malignant melanoma. Monoclonal antibodies to tumor-associated antigens may help to distinguish primary from metastatic adenocarcinomas, as well as help to determine site of origin. Metastases are discussed in detail in Chapter 8.

PLEURA

Neoplasms of the pleura can be benign (usually solitary) or malignant (usually diffuse). Malignant mesothelioma is considered in this section.

15.5 **Malignant Mesothelioma**

Malignant mesothelioma usually occurs in older adults, more often men (4:1). There is a strong association with asbestos exposure; there also may be a relationship to the simian virus (SV40). Patients often present with chest pain, shortness of breath, pulmonary osteoarthropathy, and weight loss. Pleural effusions are common, and pleural fluid is frequently submitted for diagnosis (see Chapter 3). However, a number of patients do not have an effusion at presentation or have metastases, and these

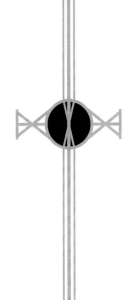

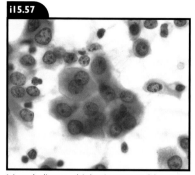

Mesothelioma—biphasic pattern (P)

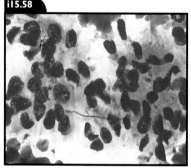

Mesothelioma—biphasic pattern (DQ)

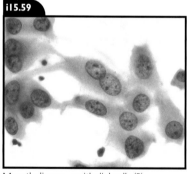

Mesothelioma—epithelial cells (P)

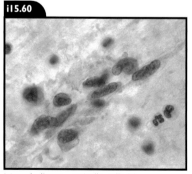

Mesothelioma—spindle cells (P)

cases may be amenable to diagnosis by FNA biopsy. Besides pleura, mesotheliomas also can arise in the peritoneum, pericardium, or tunica vaginalis testis.

Pleural malignant mesothelioma usually produces a diffusely thickened, nodular rind of tissue encasing the lung. A nodular mass in the parenchyma of the lung favors carcinoma over mesothelioma. However, carcinomas can sometimes coat the lung in a manner similar to mesothelioma. Malignant mesothelioma frequently metastasizes to regional lymph nodes, and, occasionally, a patient with mesothelioma presents with cervical or axillary lymph node metastases. Distant metastases also occur but usually late. The prognosis of malignant mesothelioma is poor; most patients die within a year of diagnosis.

The FNA biopsy smears are usually cellular; highly desmoplastic tumors are uncommon. A biphasic pattern of epithelial and spindle cells is most characteristic but not always present |i15.57|, |i15.58|, |i15.59|, |i15.60|, |i15.61|, |i15.62|. Spindle cells may have long cytoplasmic processes. High cellularity, numerous papillae, biphasic combination of epithelioid and spindle cells, and clinical findings help make the diagnosis. The key diagnostic feature of mesothelioma is the strong family resemblance—morphologic kinship—of the malignant cells to ordinary mesothelial cells. Giant tumor cells |i15.63|, granulomas, psammoma bodies, and asbestos bodies sometimes occur. Mesenchymal mucus, principally hyaluronic acid, can also be seen as a coarse metachromatic precipitate in Diff-Quik stain |i15.64|. The cells characteristically express both low and high molecular weight keratins, and are negative for at least two epithelial markers such as CD15 (Leu M1), Ber-Ep4, and carcinoembryonic antigen (CEA). Most adenocarcinomas are positive for CD15 and Ber-Ep4, and those of foregut origin are CEA positive.

MEDIASTINUM

The mediastinum is customarily divided into four compartments: superior, anterior, middle, and posterior. Thyroid and parathyroids and their diseases can also be found in the mediastinum (see Chapters 10 and 12). A variety of cysts also occur; many are developmental, most are benign |i15.65|, |i15.66|.

15.6 Thymoma

Thymoma is a primary neoplasm of thymic epithelial cells. Lymphocytes, predominantly mature T cells, are a secondary element, but at least a few are usually present. Specifically excluded from this definition are other neoplasms occurring in the thymus, such as carcinoids, lymphomas, and germ cell tumors. Although rare, thymoma is the most common primary tumor of the anterior mediastinum. Most thymomas occur in adults, at an average age of about 50 years, with no sex predilection. They usually are asymptomatic but can be associated with a wide variety of paraneoplastic syndromes, such as myasthenia gravis. Thymomas often are relatively large (5-10 cm) by the time of diagnosis, unless they are accidentally discovered during investigation of another disease.

Most thymomas are well-encapsulated. A characteristic, though uncommon, radiologic sign is peripheral calcification (of the tumor's capsule). Cystic change is relatively frequent but usually focal. Extrathoracic metastases are rare but can occur; sites include cervical lymph nodes and liver.

Thymomas are composed of mixtures of neoplastic epithelial cells and reactive lymphocytes. Thymomas traditionally are classified according to the proportion of epithelial cells and lymphocytes. In epithelial thymomas, epithelial cells predominate (defined as more than two thirds of the cells); in lymphocytic thymomas, lymphocytes predominate; in mixed thymomas, the proportions of epithelial cells and lymphocytes are more or less equal; and in spindle cell thymomas, spindle cells predominate.

Another classification system also is used, based on cortical and medullary differentiation of epithelial cells, recapitulating the normal thymus. Cortical thymomas contain epithelioid epithelial cells, and medullary thymomas show spindle epithelial cells. In this classification system, mixed thymomas are diagnosed if both epithelioid and spindle epithelial cell types are present. Aggressive behavior is associated more often with cortical (or mixed) differentiation.

Invasion through the capsule or into the surrounding tissue is the most important factor in prognosis. Unfortunately, invasion cannot be assessed by cytology. Cases that appear cytologically benign can invade and metastasize. Thymic carcinoma is defined as a thymoma showing malignant cytologic characteristics; these tumors show a marked tendency to invade and metastasize.

The FNA biopsy specimen shows a dual population of epithelial cells and lymphocytes in variable proportions. This dimorphic cellular pattern is the key diagnostic feature. The epithelial cells form cohesive aggregates of cells that may be epithelioid |i15.67|, |i15.68|, spindle |i15.69|, |i15.70|, or clear. The epithelial (cortical) cells have bland nuclei with prominent nucleoli and scant to moderate amounts of cytoplasm that ranges from delicate to dense. Spindle (medullary) cells have elongated nuclei with granular chromatin and inconspicuous nucleoli. The lymphocytes are predominantly small mature T cells with a minor component of "immature" lymphocytes but not plasma cells.

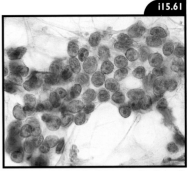
Mesothelioma—epithelial cells

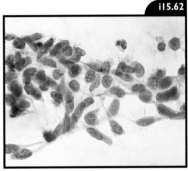
Mesothelioma—spindle cells (P)

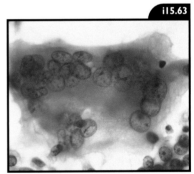
Mesothelioma—giant tumor cell (P)

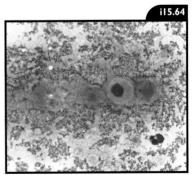
Mesothelioma—myxoid stroma (DQ)

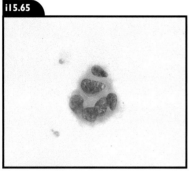

Thymic cyst (P)

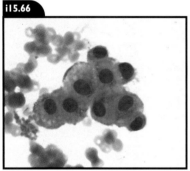

Thymic cyst (DQ)

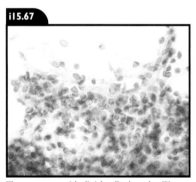

Thymoma—epithelioid cells, lymphs (P)

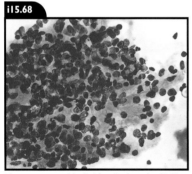

Thymoma—epithelioid cells, lymphs (DQ)

Hassall corpuscles (squamous pearls) are characteristic but infrequently seen and not necessary for diagnosis. Metastatic thymoma is cytologically similar to the primary neoplasm, including the dimorphic cell population |i15.71|, |i15.72|.

Thymic carcinoma is a general term for a "mixed bag" of obviously malignant tumors arising in the thymus. The vast majority are SCCs, either keratinizing or lymphoepithelioma-like; other rare morphologies include small cell carcinoma, clear cell carcinoma, and carcinosarcoma. The presence of pronounced cytologic atypia, necrosis, or mitoses suggests a diagnosis of thymic carcinoma. Except for the lymphoepithelioma-like pattern, thymic carcinomas usually lack the dual cell population characteristic of thymomas.

15.7 Thymic Carcinoid

Thymic carcinoid is a mediastinal endocrine neoplasm of the thymus, which like its pulmonary counterpart is of foregut origin and probably arises from primitive cells with the capacity for neuroendocrine Kulchitsky cell differentiation. It is primarily a disease of adults. Many patients have endocrine manifestations; corticotropin (ACTH) production, sometimes producing Cushing syndrome, is most common. The carcinoid syndrome is rare. A small minority of cases are associated with multiple endocrine neoplasia, usually type I.

Thymic carcinoids are solid unencapsulated tumors that may show delicate central calcification (compare with thymoma). Thymic carcinoids average about 5 to 6 cm in diameter at diagnosis. If the tumor is well circumscribed, it has a good prognosis, but thymic carcinoids are generally more aggressive than their typical pulmonary counterparts and more frequently show local invasion or distant metastasis. However, complete resection usually results in complete cure, which is not always the case with thymoma (eg, myasthenia gravis may persist).

Microscopically, the tumor usually is composed of a dispersed population of small, uniform, round to oval cells with classic salt-and-pepper chromatin, inconspicuous nucleoli, and a modest amount of cytoplasm, as is typical of carcinoids in general. A few larger tumor cells with abundant granular cytoplasm or prominent nucleoli often are present (endocrine atypia). Spindle cells are relatively common in otherwise typical carcinoids (see "Spindle cell carcinoids," p 294). True rosettes (with lumens) may be seen. Lymphocytes usually are not present; thus, carcinoid has a single rather than a dual cell population, in contrast with thymoma. Spindle cell and atypical carcinoids, as well as small cell carcinoma, also can occur in the thymus.

15.8 Germ Cell Tumors

The mediastinum is the second most common site of origin of germ cell tumors, albeit a distant second to gonadal germ cell tumors. Metastasis from a primary gonadal tumor must be excluded. Mediastinal germ cell tumors usually arise in or near the thymus in the anterior mediastinum. Any type of germ cell tumor (GCT) can occur in the mediastinum. Except for mature teratomas (benign germ cell tumor), men, usually in their 20s or 30s, are far more commonly affected than women. Rapid growth and invasion by the tumor results in clinical symptoms. Elevated β-human chorionic gonadotropin or α-fetoprotein may be found in the serum, depending on the tumor type (see Chapter 20).

Germinoma (dysgerminoma or seminoma) is the most common malignant germ cell tumor in the mediastinum; it occurs almost exclusively in men, usually young adults. Like testicular seminoma, it is sensitive to radiation therapy. Microscopically, there is a dual cell population of malignant germinoma cells and reactive lymphoid cells, including plasma cells. The germinoma cells are poorly cohesive, obviously malignant-appearing, and have clear cytoplasm due to glycogen accumulation. A tigroid (striped) background, consisting of interwoven, lacy, PAS-positive material, is characteristic. Granulomas also may be present. Isolated syncytiotrophoblast-like multinucleated giant cells also may be seen but are not associated with cytotrophoblasts as in choriocarcinoma.

Mature cystic teratoma is the most common mediastinal germ cell tumor. It usually occurs in adults and, unlike other germ cell tumors, occurs equally between the sexes. Mature teratoma is predominantly cystic and may grow very large. Calcification is common. The tumor is essentially identical to the ovarian counterpart, filled with cheesy keratinous material, hair, and sometimes even teeth. The FNA biopsy obtains skin and its appendages (eg, squamous cells, anucleate squames, sebaceous cells) |i15.73|, |i15.74|, and possibly neural, gastrointestinal (including pancreas), cartilage, and ciliated respiratory cells. Granulomas with foreign body giant cells, formed in response to keratin, may be seen.

Other germ cell tumors, including immature teratoma, embryonal carcinoma, endodermal sinus tumor, and choriocarcinoma |i15.75|, also arise, very rarely, in the mediastinum. They are identical to their gonadal counterparts (see Chapter 20).

15.9 Malignant Lymphoma

Most primary lymphomas of the mediastinum are Hodgkin disease (usually nodular sclerosis), large cell lymphoma (often associated with sclerosis), and lymphoblastic lymphoma

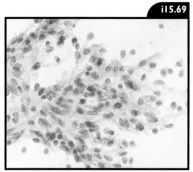
Thymoma—spindle cells, lymphs (P)

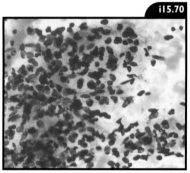
Thymoma—spindle cells, lymphs (DQ)

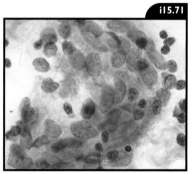
Thymoma metastatic to liver (P)

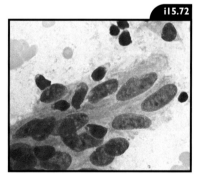
Thymoma metastatic to liver (DQ)

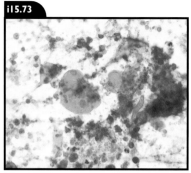

Mixed GCT—mature teratoma (P)

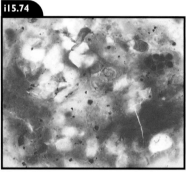

Mixed GCT—mature teratoma (DQ)

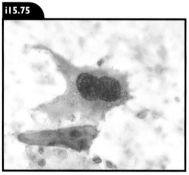

Mixed GCT—choriocarcinoma (P)

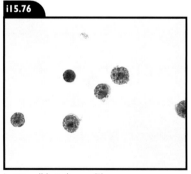

Large cell lymphoma (P)

(often associated with acute leukemia). Secondary mediastinal involvement by lymphoma is common.

15.9.1 Hodgkin Disease

Hodgkin disease can arise in the thymus or lymph nodes. The disease usually affects young adults, women more commonly than men. Reed-Sternberg cells and Reed-Sternberg variants may be rare. The background cellularity is a reactive inflammatory cell infiltrate consisting of lymphocytes, plasma cells, eosinophils, and histiocytes. Cystic change can occur, mimicking cystic thymoma or developmental cysts.

15.9.2 Non-Hodgkin Lymphoma

Large cell lymphoma in the mediastinum occurs most commonly in young adult women, but older men may also be affected. The lymphoma commonly produces superior vena cava syndrome. Most are extranodal B-cell lymphomas, but many cases are primary (B-cell) lymphomas of the thymus.

Microscopically, the nuclei are large and vesicular with irregular or smooth (cleaved or noncleaved) membranes |i15.76|, |i15.77|. The large cells may be mixed with small cleaved lymphocytes. Sclerotic large cell lymphomas are relatively common in the mediastinum, which may mimic Hodgkin disease and also limit the cellularity of the aspirate.

Lymphoblastic lymphoma is the most common malignant lymphoma of children and is particularly common in teenage boys. Most cases of lymphoblastic lymphoma arise in the thymus and are usually of pre–T-cell origin. The classic clinical presentation is acute respiratory distress in an adolescent. Acute lymphoblastic leukemia eventually develops in most patients. There is a high mortality rate.

Microscopically, lymphoblastic lymphoma is composed of blastic lymphoid cells; the most characteristic features are very fine, powdery chromatin and high nuclear/cytoplasmic ratios |i15.78|. The nuclear membranes can be smooth or, more characteristically, convoluted. Nucleoli are invisible or inconspicuous. Numerous tingible body macrophages and mitoses are present. Necrosis may be extensive; eosinophils or granulomas also can be seen.

15.10 **Neurogenic Tumors**

Neurogenic tumors are the most common cause of a posterior mediastinal mass. In children, most arise from the sympathetic nervous system, and many are malignant. Females are somewhat more commonly affected than males. Adults are more likely to develop nerve sheath tumors and paragangliomas. Benign neurogenic tumors may yield few diagnostic cells, making cytologic interpretation difficult or impossible. Paragangliomas are discussed in this section. Other neuroendocrine tumors, including carcinoids and small cell carcinoma, are discussed elsewhere.

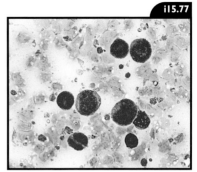

Large cell lymphoma (DQ)

15.10.1 Sympathetic Nervous System Tumors

Although most common in the adrenal gland, a quarter of all sympathetic nervous system tumors arise in the mediastinum. Malignant sympathetic nervous system tumors are found predominantly in children (who tend to be somewhat older than those with adrenal tumors). Diagnostically elevated concentrations of catecholamine metabolites may be detected in the urine.

Neuroblastoma is a classic small blue cell tumor composed of monotonously uniform, somewhat cohesive cells, usually with necrosis and frequently with calcification. Homer Wright rosettes may be seen (see p 356). Neuroblastoma usually occurs in children. Primitive neuroectodermal tumors (PNETs) also can occur in the mediastinum.

Ganglioneuroblastoma is essentially neuroblastoma with ganglion cell differentiation. Ganglioneuroblastoma is more common than neuroblastoma in the mediastinum (see p 356).

Ganglioneuroma, a benign tumor of adults, is composed of mature ganglion cells plus benign spindle (Schwann) cells; neuroblasts are absent. Ganglion cells are large, have prominent nucleoli, and may be multinucleated |i15.79|. Foci of lymphocytes could be mistaken for neuroblasts.

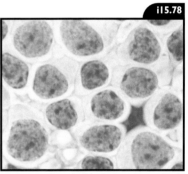

Lymphoblastic lymphoma (P, oil)

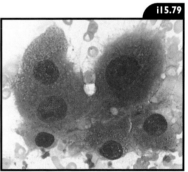

Ganglioneuroma (DQ)

15.10.2 Peripheral Nervous System

Aspiration of neural tumors may cause pain, a clue to the diagnosis.

Neurofibroma accounts for about 10% of all neural tumors of the mediastinum. Most cases are associated with von Recklinghausen disease (neurofibromatosis). In contrast with other body sites, neurofibromas of the mediastinum usually are encapsulated.

Schwannoma is the most common neurogenous tumor of the mediastinum. Schwannomas, or neurilemomas, may show cystic change or calcification. They are generally solitary but may grow large. Microscopically, the tumor has cellular (Antoni A) and degenerated or myxoid (Antoni B) areas. The cells are elongated to spindle-shaped and may form palisades. Regressive or degenerative changes (ancient schwannoma, with bizarre cells), as well as increased cellularity, may be seen in mediastinal schwannomas,

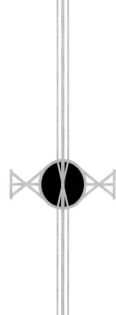

which could be mistaken for sarcoma. Diffuse, prominent, cytologic atypia or mitoses suggest actual malignant change.

Malignant schwannoma can occur sporadically or can be associated with von Recklinghausen disease or radiation exposure. The tumor tends to occur in young adults but is rare in children. Spindle, pleomorphic, epithelioid, and pigmented variants occur. The main features of malignancy are the presence of prominent cytologic atypia, numerous mitoses, and necrosis. Malignant change can be focal; thus, sampling may be a problem in diagnosis.

15.10.3 Paraganglioma

Paragangliomas can occur in the anterior or posterior mediastinum, arising from aorticosympathetic chemoreceptors or the branchiomeric apparatus, respectively. About half of posterior mediastinal paragangliomas produce catecholamines with intermittent hypertension (ie, extra-adrenal pheochromocytoma). Few anterior or superior paragangliomas secrete catecho-lamines. Mediastinal paragangliomas sometimes occur in association with multiple endocrine neoplasia, type II. Anterior mediastinal paragangliomas often are aggressive clinically.

The tumors are highly vascular. The cells usually are large and polygonal and grow in organoid nests (Zellballen). The cytoplasm is abundant, acidophilic, and slightly granular. The nuclei can be markedly atypical and pleomorphic yet benign. Focal necrosis is common, even in benign tumors. Mitoses usually are sparse or absent, but their presence does not necessarily indicate malignancy. Glycogen is negligible, but occasionally pigmented cells are seen. Mast cells may be present. Sustentacular cells, unique to paragangliomas, may be demonstrated with electron microscopy and are S-100 positive.

The differential diagnosis includes carcinoids, eg, of the thymus, which are neuroendocrine tumors of epithelial origin. Carcinoids, including atypical carcinoids, usually have more uniform cells. Rosette formation favors carcinoid tumor. Either tumor may have NSGs and express neuroendocrine markers, but keratin expression favors carcinoid tumor.

15.11 Mesenchymal Tumors

Virtually any mesenchymal neoplasm can arise in the soft tissue of the mediastinum. Neural and neuroendocrine tumors were previously described. Benign lipomas (rule out thymolipoma), lymphangiomas (usually in children), and hemangiomas (usually cavernous) are also relatively common. Other sarcomas, such as liposarcoma, are rare (see Chapter 9).

15.12 Metastases

Metastases are the most common cause of a mediastinal abnormality diagnosed with FNA biopsy. The usual sources of metastases include carcinomas of lung, particularly small cell carcinoma, breast, thyroid, head and neck, kidney, prostate, and testis, as well as malignant melanoma (see Chapter 8).

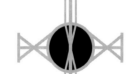

Liver

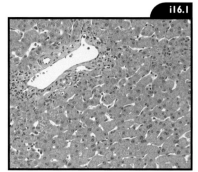

Liver, tissue (H&E)

Λ Visualized as the classic liver lobule, the architectural unit of the liver has at its center a central vein; at the periphery are approximately six portal triads, each containing an artery, vein, and bile duct, as well as nerves and lymphatics |i16.1|. Plates of hepatocytes, one or two cells thick, radiate from the central vein. These liver cell plates are lined on either side by endothelial cells and Kupffer cells (histiocytes). Between the trabeculae are vascular spaces, the liver sinusoids, in which blood flows (portal to central), bathing the hepatocytes. Between adjacent hepatocytes, a minute gland-like opening, the bile canaliculus, is formed, into which the bile is secreted by the hepatocytes. Bile flows in the canaliculi toward the portal space, in the opposite direction of the blood.

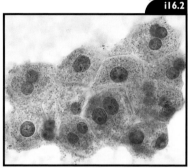

Hepatocytes (P)

16.1 The Cells

16.1.1 Hepatocytes

Hepatocytes are relatively large cells that are found in aspirates as single cells, flat sheets of cells, or occasionally endothelial-lined trabeculae. Individual hepatocytes have abundant distinctly granular cytoplasm, polygonal outlines, and centrally located nuclei, with low nuclear/cytoplasmic ratios. Various cytoplasmic pigments, particularly lipofuscin, also are frequently present. In Papanicolaou stain, hepatocytes typically stain red-orange, orange-brown, or blue-green |i16.2|, and in Diff-Quik stain, blue to purple |i16.3|, |i16.4|. Vacuolization or clearing of the cytoplasm, due to glycogen or fat accumulation |i16.5|, also is common. The nuclei are round, with smooth membranes and moderately granular, evenly distributed chromatin. Nuclear clearing (due to glycogen |i16.6|, eg, in diabetes mellitus or intravenous glucose administration) or well-formed intranuclear cytoplasmic invaginations (INCIs) |i16.7| may be seen. Nuclear variation in size (but not shape), binucleation, multinucleation, hyperchromasia, and prominent nucleoli are commonly observed due to polyploidy or reactive changes.

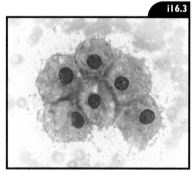

Hepatocytes (DQ)

16.1.2 Bile Duct Cells

Bile duct cells range in size from low cuboidal to tall columnar. Flat, cohesive sheets of orderly cells, reminiscent of endocervical cells, are most common, but tubules and acini also can be seen |i16.8|, |i16.9|. The nuclei are round with smooth membranes, fine chromatin, and inconspicuous nucleoli. Bile duct

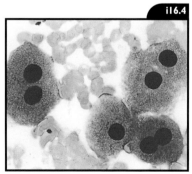

Hepatocytes (DQ)

307

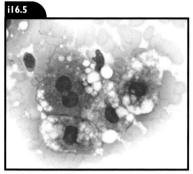

Lipid accumulation, steatosis (DQ)

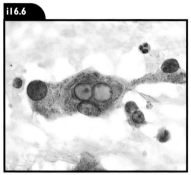

Glycogen nuclei (P)

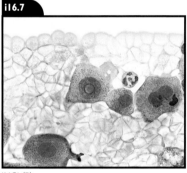

INCI (P)

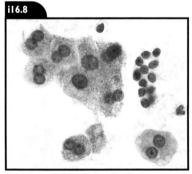

Hepatocytes, bile duct cells (P)

cells usually are present in aspirates of nonneoplastic liver but are characteristically absent in aspirates of liver cell adenoma and hepatocellular carcinoma (HCC).

16.2 Inclusions and Pigments

16.2.1 Hyaline Globules

Hyaline globules may contain α_1-antitrypsin or α-feto-protein (AFP) and are commonly observed in HCC. However, identical bodies can be seen in a number of other tumors, as well as in nonneoplastic conditions of the liver, such as α_1-antitrypsin deficiency, cirrhosis, and regeneration. Giant mitochondria and giant lysosomes also resemble hyaline globules.

16.2.2 Mallory Bodies

Mallory bodies are elongated, ropy to hyaline, cyto-plasmic inclusions that tend to surround the nucleus. They are particularly associated with alcoholic liver disease but also can be seen in a variety of other liver diseases, including HCC.

16.2.3 Lipofuscin

Lipofuscin is the "wear-and-tear" pigment of hepato-cytes and increases with age. It is composed of tertiary lyso-somes, or residual bodies, that are the leftovers of intracellular digestion. Lipofuscin granules are relatively fine and nonrefractile, and they stain golden to dark brown in Papanicolaou stain |i16.10| and dark green in Diff-Quik stain. Lipofuscin pigmentation is extremely common, except in children, although the amount of pigment is variable. Decreased or absent lipofuscin should arouse suspicion of an abnormal process, especially in older patients, including active liver disease, such as hepatitis or cirrhosis, or HCC.

16.2.4 Bile

Bile is an irregular, amorphous, nonrefractile pigment produced only by hepatocytes. It stains various shades of green in Papanicolaou |i16.11| and Diff-Quik |i16.12| stains. Bile can be seen intracellularly or extracellularly and may be associated with hepatitis, obstructive jaundice, and primary or metastatic tumors.

16.2.5 Iron

Iron occurs in the liver as the pigment hemosiderin. Hemosiderin can be seen in hepatocytes, Kupffer cells, or bile duct cells. It is coarse, golden brown, and refractile in Papanicolaou stain. In Diff-Quik stain, it is nonrefractile and stains dark blue-green. Simple iron overload is designated *hemosiderosis*. However, when associated with cirrhosis, the disease is known as *hemochromatosis*. Hemochromatosis can be primary (iron overload causes cirrhosis) or secondary (cirrhosis causes iron overload).

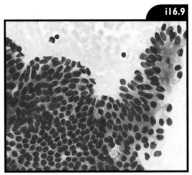
i16.9

Bile duct cells (DQ)

16.3 Diffuse Liver Diseases

Diseases of the liver can be divided into two broad categories: diffuse and nodular. Fine needle aspiration (FNA) biopsy is not used routinely to evaluate diffuse liver diseases, such as hepatitis or cirrhosis. However, diffuse liver disease, particularly cirrhosis, may enter into the differential diagnosis of nodular liver disease. FNA biopsy is frequently used to evaluate nodular (ie, space-occupying) lesions of the liver, such as cysts, abscesses, granulomas, and particularly tumors.

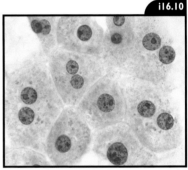
i16.10

Lipofuscin, golden brown pigment (P)

16.3.1 Cirrhosis

In essence, cirrhosis is due to degeneration and regeneration of hepatocytes, resulting in diffuse nodular fibrosis of the liver. The nodules can be small and uniform, about the size of a lobule (micronodular cirrhosis), or relatively large and pleomorphic (macronodular cirrhosis). Large nodules may arouse clinical suspicion of malignancy, particularly HCC.

The FNA biopsy of cirrhotic liver shows reactive hepatocytes and bile duct proliferation. Some hepatocytes may show marked reactive atypia, including nuclear pleomorphism with coarse chromatin, occasional slightly irregular nuclear membranes, frequent binucleation, large round macronucleoli, and INCIs. The hepatocytes frequently display lipid or glycogen vacuolization. Lipofuscin pigmentation ranges from absent to abundant. Bile duct proliferation, a characteristic feature of cirrhosis, results in an increased number of bile duct cells, which can be somewhat pleomorphic and show reactive atypia. HCC and liver cell adenoma typically lack bile duct cells. Chronic inflammation, connective tissue fragments, and bile pigment commonly are observed in FNA biopsies of cirrhosis. Note that necrosis and mitosis can occur in benign cirrhosis; necrosis and fibrosis are unusual in HCC.

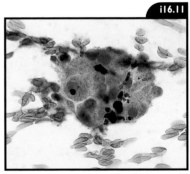
i16.11

Bile, cholestasis (P)

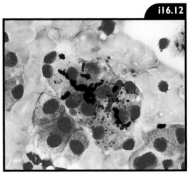
i16.12

Bile, cholestasis (DQ)

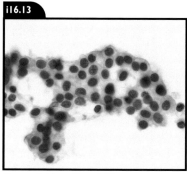

Congenital hepatic cyst (P)

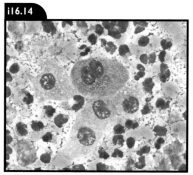

Liver abscess (DQ)

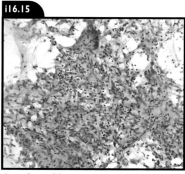

Granuloma (P)

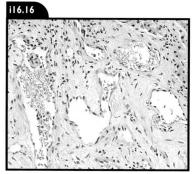

Hemangioma, tissue (H&E)

16.4 Nodular Liver Diseases

16.4.1 Cysts

Cysts of the liver can be congenital or acquired, solitary or multiple. Congenital cysts are by far the more common type; the FNA biopsy is nonspecific and usually shows only a few bile duct–like cells and histiocytes |i16.13|. Acquired hepatic cysts encompass abscesses, hydatid cysts, hematomas, and neoplastic cysts, including primary cystic neoplasms, cystic metastases, and necrotic tumors.

16.4.2 Abscess

Liver abscess can be a serious disease with a high mortality rate. It often is caused by enteric or pathogenic bacteria, especially *Escherichia coli, Klebsiella, Streptococcus, Staphylococcus,* or pneumococci; mixed flora are common. *Candida* is also a relatively common cause. In addition, *Actinomyces,* parasites (such as *Schistosoma*), or *Entamoeba histolytica* can cause liver abscesses. The cytologic findings are as expected for an abscess, including neutrophils, inflammatory cells, and reactive epithelial changes |i16.14|. A careful search for tumor cells is warranted, because the inflammatory cells may dilute and obscure malignant cells of infected metastases.

16.4.3 Granuloma

The causes of liver granulomas are legion and include infections, sarcoid, and neoplasms (eg, lymphomas, metastatic carcinomas). Nodular collections of epithelioid histiocytes (elongated nuclei, fine chromatin, tiny nucleoli with eccentric, often fibrillar cytoplasm) are diagnostic of granulomatous inflammation. Multinuclear giant cells may be present but are neither necessary nor sufficient for diagnosis |i16.15|. The granulomas can be minute and focal; hence, sampling may be a problem in diagnosis.

16.4.4 Benign Tumors

Hemangioma

Hemangioma is the most common benign tumor of the liver |i16.16|. Patients are often multiparous women, suggesting a hormonal influence in the etiology. Cavernous hemangiomas are more common than capillary types. Hemangiomas are usually asymptomatic but may be detected incidentally in the workup of another disease and can be difficult to distinguish from primary or metastatic carcinoma, although angiography may be diagnostic. A biopsy is usually performed more to rule out malignancy than to diagnose the hemangioma, per se. There is a small but real risk of serious hemorrhage, which increases with the caliber of the needle used to obtain the biopsy.

The most characteristic cytologic features of cavernous hemangioma are aspiration of fresh blood, presence of benign endothelial cells, and absence of malignant cells. Unfortunately, in many cases, only blood is obtained (nondiagnostic aspirate). A few variously spindle- or polygonal-shaped endothelial cells, usually single or in small clusters, may be seen in the aspirate. The cells have single nuclei with longitudinal folds or grooves, fine chromatin, and delicate cytoplasm. Fragments of fibrovascular connective tissue or smooth muscle may be obtained |i16.17|. In some cases, diagnostic aggregates of interconnecting capillaries are found. Cell blocks may increase the diagnostic yield.

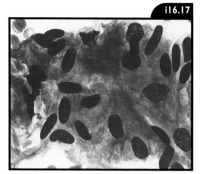

Hemangioma (DQ)

Focal Nodular Hyperplasia

Focal nodular hyperplasia (FNH) is a benign liver tumor, probably nonneoplastic, that is at least twice as common in women as men. The patients are usually in their 20s to 40s, but FNH can occur at any age. Most cases (~ 90%) are asymptomatic, and significant bleeding is rare. Liver function test results usually are normal.

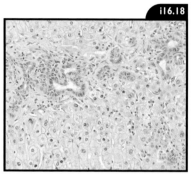

FNH, tissue (H&E)

Grossly, FNH is well-circumscribed, but not encapsulated, and usually solitary. The nodule can vary in size but averages about 5 cm. The most characteristic gross feature is a central stellate scar, which can sometimes be imaged radiologically. Characteristic angiographic findings, together with radionuclide scan demonstrating Kupffer cells, can be virtually diagnostic, but equivocal cases occur. Malignant change is very rare, but FNH may be related to the fibrolamellar variant of HCC (see p 315).

Microscopically, the lesion resembles cirrhosis, ie, nodules of hepatocytes surrounded by fibrous connective tissue, with bile duct proliferation |i16.18|. In contrast with cirrhosis, however, FNH affects the liver focally rather than diffusely ("focal cirrhosis").

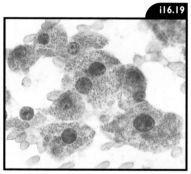

Consistent with FNH—hepatocytes (P)

The most important feature of the FNA biopsy is that all of the normal cell types of the liver lobule are present, including hepatocytes and bile duct cells. The liver cells are small to normal sized without significant atypia |i16.19|, although glycogen, fat, or sometimes hyaline bodies may be seen in the cytoplasm. Bile duct cells also are characteristically present and may appear reactive or proliferative |i16.20|. Bile stasis may occur, but it is not prominent. Spindle-shaped Kupffer cells also can be seen. A variable degree of chronic inflammation may be present; fibrous tissue usually is sparse in aspirate specimens.

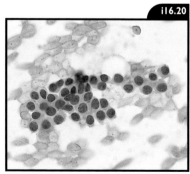

Consistent with FNH—bile duct cells (P)

Liver Cell Adenoma

Liver cell adenoma is a benign neoplasm of hepatocytes. Liver cell adenomas have a strong association with long-term use

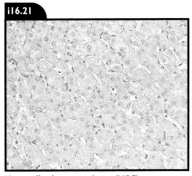

Liver cell adenoma, tissue (H&E)

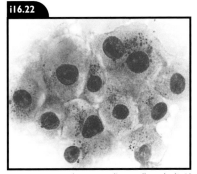

Consistent w/adenoma—liver cells only (DQ)

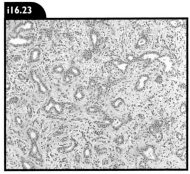

Bile duct hamartoma, tissue (H&E)

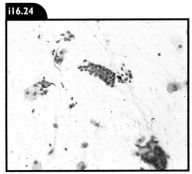

Bile duct hamartoma (P)

of contraceptive steroids (birth control pills). Adenomas are far more common in women than men but also may be associated with androgenic-anabolic steroids, possibly including illicit use by athletes. Clinically, adenomas can occur at any age but usually are diagnosed in the patient's 20s or 30s. Symptoms (pain, mass, bleeding) are common. Most adenomas are highly vascular and have a tendency to rupture, resulting in hemorrhage, which can be fatal. Malignant transformation is rare but occurs more commonly than in FNH.

Grossly, in contrast with FNH, adenomas often have a partial capsule, but there is no central scar. Adenomas are usually solitary but can be multiple. They vary in size, but on average are larger than FNH (about 10 cm). Microscopically, the tumor is composed primarily of liver cells; there are neither portal fields nor central veins in the lesion |i16.21|.

The FNA biopsy specimen consists, in essence, of hepatocytes only, without bile duct cells |i16.22|. The smears are cellular, often forming large, three-dimensional, cohesive groups of hepatocytes. The hepatocytes are usually normal or mildly reactive appearing but may be somewhat enlarged, as if magnified, with more cytoplasm, more vacuolization, and more cytoplasmic granularity than normal. Occasionally, granulomas may be seen. Bile production or stasis is uncommon but can occur. Hemorrhage and necrosis may be prominent.

Liver cell adenoma and particularly FNH are difficult to diagnose conclusively with cytologic studies alone. The cytologic findings usually consist simply of benign or reactive hepatocytes with or without bile duct cells. The diagnosis requires the presence of a mass, proper clinical setting, and—this is crucial—that the needle was in the mass and sampled only the mass. The differential diagnosis of liver cell adenoma with very well-differentiated (minimal deviation) HCC can be difficult or impossible, even in resected specimens (see "Hepatocellular Carcinoma," p 313).

Bile Duct Adenomas and Hamartomas

Bile duct adenomas usually are small (< 1 cm), solitary, and located beneath the liver capsule. Bile duct hamartomas (aka von Meyenburg complexes) are similar but can be found anywhere in the liver |i16.23|. Both of these lesions are composed of well-formed bile ducts in mature fibrous connective tissue stroma and could be confused with primary cholangiocarcinoma or metastatic adenocarcinoma.

The FNA biopsy specimen may be sparse due to fibrosis. The aspirate shows cohesive clusters of orderly bile duct cells, often columnar in shape |i16.24|. The cells usually are bland, but occasionally reactive changes are noted; however, malignant features are absent. There is no cholestasis, and hepatocytes are not present (unless contaminated by surrounding liver tissue).

16.4.5 Malignant Tumors

Hepatocellular Carcinoma

HCC is one of the most common cancers in the world, particularly in parts of Asia and Africa. While HCC is not common in America, it also is not rare and is increasing in frequency. At least 80% of all primary liver cancers are HCC |i16.25|. Most of the rest are cholangiocarcinoma.

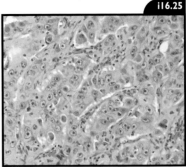

HCC, tissue (H&E)

The development of HCC is associated with, among other things, cirrhosis, alcoholism (particularly in the United States), chronic hepatitis B or C infection, anabolic and contraceptive steroids, metabolic disorders such as α_1-antitrypsin deficiency and tyrosinemia, Thorotrast, and aflatoxin (particularly in Asia and Africa).

In the United States, the vast majority of cases of HCC arise in cirrhosis, usually macronodular type; about one patient in 10 with cirrhosis will eventually develop HCC. However, in many cases, the cirrhosis is undocumented before diagnosis of HCC. The largest single group of cases of HCC occurs in patients with alcoholic liver disease. There is also a strong association between developing HCC and chronic hepatitis B or C infection. Hemochromatosis is intermediate risk and biliary cirrhosis is low risk for development of HCC. Only about 10% of patients with HCC have a normal liver and no serologic evidence of chronic hepatitis; some of these cases may be associated with the use of contraceptives or anabolic steroids. In summary, 90% of patients with HCC have underlying cirrhosis, often due to alcoholism or viral hepatitis (B or C).

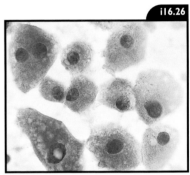

HCC, bone metastasis (P)

Serum AFP is an important clinical marker of HCC that is elevated in most patients. However, elevated serum AFP is nonspecific, unless the levels are very high (at least 500 ng/mL; > 2000 ng/mL is more specific), and some patients with HCC have normal serum AFP levels, particularly those with small (< 5 cm) or well-differentiated tumors.

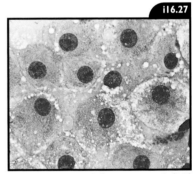

HCC, bone metastasis (DQ)

Most patients with HCC are men (at least 4:1), particularly when associated with cirrhosis, and usually are older than 60 years of age, but younger persons, even children, may be affected. Younger patients (younger than 45 years of age) are less likely to have concomitant cirrhosis, and they have a better prognosis. Patients with HCC usually present with abdominal pain, hepatomegaly, and weight loss. Although ascites is common (due to underlying cirrhosis), peritoneal metastases are rare, accounting for low diagnostic yield of ascitic fluid cytology in HCC. Jaundice is a poor prognostic sign. Metastases occur in about two thirds of cases, primarily to regional lymph nodes, but also to distant sites, particularly lung, adrenal, and bone |i16.26|, |i16.27|. HCC has a propensity to grow in vessels and may reach the heart. Unfortunately, by the time the patient has symptoms, the tumor is usually large and metastatic. At this late stage, patients generally experi-

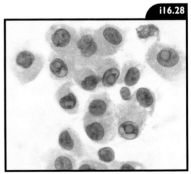

HCC—INCIs (P)

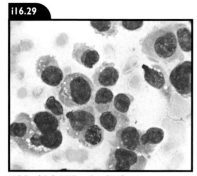

HCC—high N/C ratios (DQ)

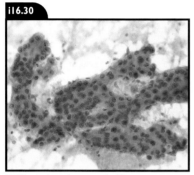

HCC—trabecular growth (P)

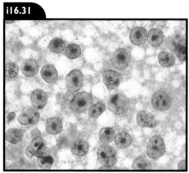

HCC—naked nuclei (P)

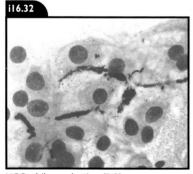

HCC—bile production (DQ)

ence a rapid downhill course (months). This has resulted in the false impression that HCC is a rapidly growing multicentric cancer that is invariably fatal. In fact, HCC is relatively slow-growing and may be cured with surgery if detected early.

Grossly, HCC has three different growth patterns: single/massive (single large tumor mass, most common), multiple/nodular (several nodules), and diffuse. Thus, the gross appearance can mimic other types of liver disease, notably metastatic malignancy.

Microscopically, HCC can range from very well-differentiated (minimal deviation) to an anaplastic giant and spindle cell malignancy. Most HCCs, however, particularly small tumors, are well to moderately differentiated |i16.28|, |i16.29|. Very well-differentiated HCC can be very difficult to diagnose: a rare atypical mitosis or (in cell blocks) thickened liver cell plates (more than two cells thick) or vascular invasion may be the only clues to malignancy.

The FNA biopsy specimen of HCC usually is very cellular; the aspirate characteristically is composed of liver cells only and lacks bile duct cells (unless inadvertently sampled from surrounding liver). The key diagnostic feature of classic HCC is the obvious morphologic kinship of the malignant cells to ordinary liver cells, ie, the malignant cells look like hepatocytes. There are no "foreign" cells as seen in metastatic carcinoma.

The tumor cells usually have polygonal outlines, dense granular cytoplasm, and central nuclei, similar to ordinary hepatocytes. However, many of the cells have high nuclear/cytoplasmic ratios, a clue to malignancy. A characteristic feature of HCC that helps distinguish it from metastatic carcinoma is a trabecular pattern of growth, represented by thick plates or balls of hepatocytes lined by endothelial cells |i16.30|. Reticulin stain can highlight the thick cell plates in cell blocks.

Nuclear pleomorphism is common, but unequal size of hepatocytic nuclei is not diagnostic of HCC. Binucleation or multinucleation also is common but can be seen in benign conditions. Naked nuclei are sometimes so numerous as to suggest malignant lymphoma or anaplastic small cell carcinoma |i16.31|, but again they are not diagnostic of malignancy. Nuclear membrane irregularity is an important clue to malignancy; however, INCIs are common in both benign and malignant hepatocytes. The chromatin usually is coarse and irregularly distributed but may be fine. Paradoxically, very fine chromatin is not a usual feature of benign hepatocytes and suggests malignancy in this setting. Multiple nucleoli or extremely prominent macronucleoli are characteristic of HCC; however, nucleoli are variable and may be inconspicuous in some cases of HCC, while prominent nucleoli can be seen in benign reactive hepatocytes. Mitotic figures, particularly when atypical, suggest malignancy, but mitoses are unusual in well-differentiated tumors, and mitotic figures can occur in benign hepato-cytes. Bile production by malignant cells is considered pathogno-monic of HCC but is seen only in a minority of cases, and bile stasis, which can mimic bile production, is common in other benign and malignant conditions of the liver |i16.32|.

Cytoplasmic hyaline inclusions of various kinds (α_1-antitrypsin, AFP, Mallory bodies) are found in some cases but are not specific |i16.33|, |i16.34|. Councilman bodies, which are degenerated or mummified hepatocytes, also can be seen, but again they are not specific. Fatty change may occur, which can result in a signet ring appearance, mimicking signet ring cell carci-noma. Mucin production, when specifically looked for, may be an unexpectedly common feature of HCC. Glycogen can be demon-strated in most cases of HCC, occasionally resulting in a clear appearance of the cytoplasm (see "Clear Cell HCC," p 316). Lipo-fuscin and iron pigments are notably absent from malignant hepa-tocytes. The background of the smear is usually clean. Necrosis, fibrosis, and inflammation are unusual in HCC.

Pericanalicular carcinoembryonic antigen (CEA) immunostaining is unique to liver cells but does not distinguish between benign and malignant hepatocytes; diffuse CEA staining is seen in many metastatic adenocarcinomas. Expression of AFP is somewhat specific (rule out germ cell tumors and some anaplastic carcinomas) but not very sensitive for the diagnosis of HCC. Albumin gene expression also can be helpful in diagnosis.

Fibrolamellar Variant of HCC: Fibrolamellar HCC is a rare variant of HCC that occurs predominantly, though not exclu-sively, in younger patients (younger than age 35) and has a better prognosis than ordinary HCC. Women are somewhat more commonly affected than men, in sharp contrast with the usual type of HCC. Fibrolamellar HCC is not associated with under-lying liver disease, such as cirrhosis or hepatitis, nor is it thought to be significantly associated with birth control pills. However, a central scar may be present, similar to FNH. Serum AFP usually is not elevated significantly in fibrolamellar HCC. Because the tumor is often localized and typically arises in a noncirrhotic liver, surgical resection may be possible, resulting in cure in some cases. Microscopically, fibrous bands composed of layers of connective tissue (lamellar fibrosis) surround groups of malignant hepatocytes, forming islands of tumor.

The two key cytodiagnostic features of this variant of HCC are oncocytic cytoplasm |i16.35| and lamellar fibrosis |i16.36|. The malignant cells are polygonal with dense, finely granular cyto-plasm, owing to abundant mitochondria, that is deeply eosinophilic (in Papanicolaou stain). If this oncocytic feature is absent, the tumor behaves as ordinary HCC. The tumor cells are otherwise similar to differentiated HCC. Lamellar fibrosis consists of abundant, dense, fibrous connective tissue with parallel (ie, lamellar) rows of benign-

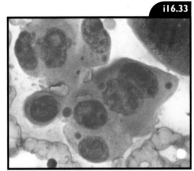

i16.33

HCC—metachromatic hyaline globules (DQ)

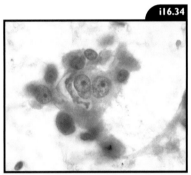

i16.34

HCC—Mallory body (P)

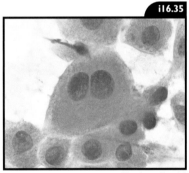

i16.35

HCC, fibrolamellar (P)

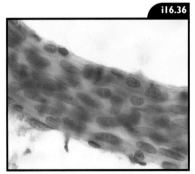

i16.36

HCC, fibrolamellar

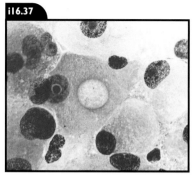

HCC, fibrolamellar—pale body (DQ)

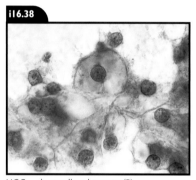

HCC—clear cells, glycogen (P)

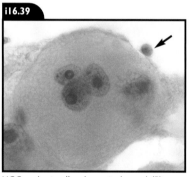

HCC—giant cell, microcyte (arrow) (P)

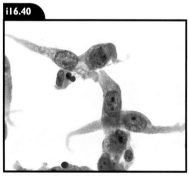

HCC—spindle cells (P)

appearing spindle cell fibroblasts. Ordinary HCC usually has little or no fibrosis. Pale bodies (well-defined intracytoplasmic vacuoles, possibly dilated bile canaliculi) are characteristic of this variant of HCC |i16.37| and are seen in about half of the cases.

Other Variants of HCC: In addition to the classic and fibrolamellar types of HCC, there are several other variants. Except for fibrolamellar HCC, no consistent correlation has been found between cell type and prognosis. Most of the special categories of HCC will have an admixture of the ordinary type, which facilitates recognition of the tumor as a variant of HCC.

Acinar or Adenoid HCC: It is not too unusual for HCC to grow, at least focally, in a pseudoglandular pattern, mimicking adenocarcinoma. Moreover, the malignant hepatocytes sometimes assume a columnar shape with basal nuclei and apical cytoplasm, like adenocarcinoma cells. Features favoring HCC include acini outlined by endothelium, dense granular cytoplasm, hyaline inclusions, bile production, and INCIs.

Clear Cell HCC: About 5% to 10% of cases of HCC are composed of a significant proportion of clear cells, but they are usually mixed with cells of classic HCC. The cytoplasmic clarity is due predominantly to glycogen |i16.38|, but lipid also may be present. Some cells may have a signet ring appearance. This tumor resembles other clear cell carcinomas, such as renal cell carcinoma.

Giant Cell HCC: Many HCCs contain a few tumor giant cells; therefore, a significant proportion of giant tumor cells must be present to diagnose this variant |i16.39|. (Giant hepatocytes also can be seen in certain benign liver conditions.) Osteoclastic giant cells may be present (osteoclastic HCC). Malignant spindle hepatocytes (spindle cell HCC) also can occur |i16.40|. The differential diagnosis includes primary or metastatic sarcomas. A clue to diagnosis of sarcomatoid HCC is the presence of cells transitional to the usual type of HCC.

Small Cell HCC: Small cell HCC is reminiscent of small cell carcinoma but with slightly more abundant, granular cytoplasm and conspicuous nucleoli.

Sclerotic HCC: This is a rare variant of HCC that usually arises in noncirrhotic liver. It may be associated with pseudohyperparathyroidism and hypercalcemia. The cytologic findings are similar to those of ordinary HCC, but giant cells usually are present and there is increased connective tissue stroma, which may result in a poorly cellular aspirate. The main differential diagnosis is with cholangiocarcinoma, which is commonly sclerotic.

Hepatoblastoma

Hepatoblastoma, although rare, is the most common primary malignant neoplasm of the liver in children, who tend to be younger than 4 years old. However, hepatoblastoma can occur in older patients, while classic HCC can affect very young children. Because there is overlap in age of the patient and morphologic appearance between these two tumors, occasionally it can be difficult to distinguish hepatoblastoma from HCC. The distinction is important, however, because hepatoblastoma, particularly the fetal cell type, has a better prognosis.

Hepatoblastoma has no relationship to cirrhosis but often is associated with congenital anomalies. Hepatoblastoma affects twice as many boys as girls. Marked elevations of AFP, much higher than those in ordinary HCC, can be seen in hepatoblastoma. Hepatoblastoma is usually solitary and well circumscribed but is capable of metastasis.

Hepatoblastoma is an embryonal tumor arising from multipotential blastema with the ability to differentiate along epithelial or mesenchymal lines. There are three basic types of hepatoblastoma: epithelial, mixed (epithelial and mesenchymal), and anaplastic types.

Epithelial cells can show a range of differentiation from anaplastic to embryonal to fetal. Anaplastic tumor cells are "small blue cells" similar to those of other pediatric tumors, such as neuroblastoma and Ewing sarcoma |i16.41|. Embryonal cells are small oval to spindle-shaped cells that have large nuclei with coarse dark chromatin, prominent nucleoli, and a small amount of cytoplasm |i16.42|. They can be arranged in cords, rosettes, or papillae; mitotic figures are frequent. Fetal cells are larger than embryonal cells but smaller than mature hepatocytes |i16.43|, |i16.44|. Usually, there is little or no pleomorphism. Fetal cells can have granular or clear cytoplasm, which is more abundant than that of embryonal cells. The fetal cells are typically arranged in loosely cohesive small sheets and acini or large disorderly clusters, cords, or trabeculae. The nuclei are round to oval, moderately hyperchromatic, and have occasional nucleoli. Fetal cells, but not embryonal cells, may contain bile, fat, or glycogen and may be associated with foci of extramedullary hematopoiesis, characterized by megakaryocytes, nucleated RBCs, and other immature blood cells.

The mesenchymal component, when present (ie, mixed hepatoblastoma), characteristically has a primitive, undifferentiated, cellular appearance. Osteoid may be present. Less frequently, other differentiation, including squamous, skeletal muscle, and cartilage, may occur. These metaplastic elements strongly favor a diagnosis of hepatoblastoma over HCC.

In contrast with HCC, marked pleomorphism and giant tumor cells are never seen in hepatoblastoma. Hepatoblastoma or HCC can have hyaline inclusions in the tumor cell cytoplasm.

Cholangiocarcinoma

Cholangiocarcinoma is the second most common primary liver cancer of adults, albeit a distant second to HCC. Patients usually are older than 60 years, and unlike HCC, cholan-

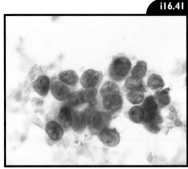

i16.41

Hepatoblastoma—anaplastic cells (P)

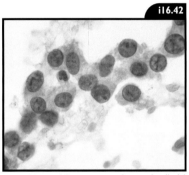

i16.42

Hepatoblastoma—embryonal cells (P)

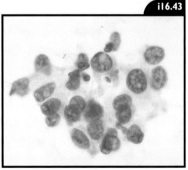

i16.43

Hepatoblastoma—fetal cells (P)

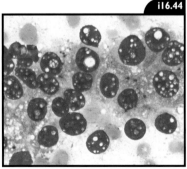

i16.44

Hepatoblastoma—fetal cells (DQ)

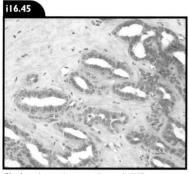

Cholangiocarcinoma, tissue (H&E)

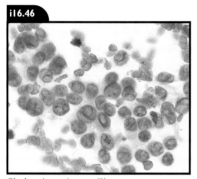

Cholangiocarcinoma (P)

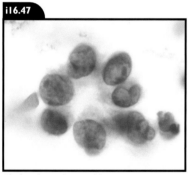

Cholangiocarcinoma (P)

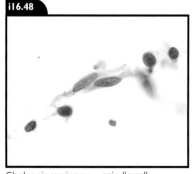

Cholangiocarcinoma—spindle cells

giocarcinoma affects men and women equally. Cholangiocarcinoma is associated with parasites (*Clonorchis sinensis* in the Far East), Thorotrast, intrahepatic lithiasis, pyogenic cholangitis, sclerosing cholangitis (may occur in a young patient), chronic inflammatory bowel disease, and Caroli disease (rare autosomal recessive trait characterized by cystic dilatation of the intrahepatic biliary tree). Cholangiocarcinoma is radiologically indistinguishable from HCC. The clinical symptoms and prognosis also are similar. However, cholangiocarcinoma is not associated with either pre-existing cirrhosis (although secondary biliary cirrhosis may result) or elevated serum AFP levels.

Microscopically, the cells grow in glandular or sometimes papillary configurations, typically in an abundant sclerotic stroma |i16.45|, which may result in a poorly cellular aspirate. Characteristically, in liver cell neoplasms, there are no bile duct cells; in bile duct neoplasms, there are no hepatocytes.

Cholangiocarcinoma is morphologically indistinguishable from adenocarcinoma arising from pancreaticobiliary ductal epithelium; it often is well-differentiated |i16.46|, |i16.47|. Well-differentiated cholangiocarcinoma is reminiscent of normal bile duct epithelium but shows disorderly growth (ie, piling up, crowding, loss of nuclear polarity, irregular or "drunken" honeycombs), microacinar formation, large cells with irregular nuclear membranes, and prominent nucleoli. Less-differentiated tumor cells typically display some squamous features (density, distinct borders) in their cytoplasm. There frequently is a wide range of differentiation of the cells from bland to distinctly malignant appearing, even among cells in the same cluster. Spindle or giant tumor cells occur occasionally |i16.48|. The cells usually are mucin-positive and may form signet rings. Bile stasis is common.

The differential diagnosis with HCC is usually straightforward, but mucin staining and immunocytochemistry (CEA, AFP) can help in a difficult case. However, the differential diagnosis with metastatic carcinoma, particularly from the pancreas or biliary tract, may be impossible on morphologic grounds alone. Clinical history may be helpful. The differential diagnosis also includes benign reactive atypia of biliary cells, mimicking malignancy, such as may be seen in cholangitis. Orderly cohesive sheets of cells with little or no nuclear crowding, regular ranks and files of cells, smooth nuclear membranes, and fine chromatin are the characteristics of reactive cells.

Mixed hepatocellular/cholangiocarcinoma, despite a common cellular ancestor, is rare. The cytologic studies show features of cholangiocarcinoma and HCC.

Sarcomas

Primary sarcomas of the liver are rare; metastatic sarcomas are far more common. Also consider spindle cell HCC in the differential diagnosis (look for cells more typical of ordinary HCC).

Angiosarcoma of the liver is associated with exposure to polyvinyl chloride, Thorotrast, radium, or arsenic compounds, as well as steroids, copper sulfate, and phenelzine. Angiosarcoma is frequently associated with cirrhosis, including hemochromatosis. The tumor is similar to HCC in the affected age group, male predominance, and clinical findings. Results of liver function tests often are abnormal but are nonspecific. Serum AFP is not elevated. Thrombocytopenia and disseminated intravascular coagulation are characteristic of this tumor. Angiography helps in diagnosis. The lesions are usually multiple; thrombosis and infarction are common. Exsanguinating hemorrhage has been reported at biopsy, but the risk is reduced with use of fine needles. The prognosis is poor.

The aspirate is bloody and necrosis is common. The cytologic findings consist of loose groups and single, variably pleomorphic, malignant endothelial cells, which are spindle to polygonal shaped and have ill-defined cell borders, oval to elongated hyperchromatic nuclei, and small nucleoli. Tubular structures (reminiscent of glands) or whorls of cells |i16.49| recapitulate vessels. Occasional bizarre tumor cells also may occur. Intracytoplasmic hemosiderin is common and erythrophagocytosis by tumor cells is suggestive of the diagnosis. Factor VIII positivity supports the diagnosis.

Malignant Lymphoma

Primary lymphoma of the liver is rare; most are non-Hodgkin lymphomas, large B-cell type. However, the liver is commonly involved, secondarily, by malignant lymphoma of various types, including Hodgkin disease.

The FNA biopsy specimen is characterized by a dispersed cell pattern of small to large lymphoid cells with round or cleaved nuclei, variable nucleoli, etc, depending on the particular type of lymphoma. Lymphoglandular bodies are characteristically seen in the background (see Chapter 13).

Metastases

The liver is one of the most common recipients of metastatic malignancy; in fact, metastases are far more common than primary liver cancer. The serum alkaline phosphatase level is characteristically elevated in metastatic disease. The most common source of liver metastases is carcinoma of the gastrointestinal tract, including colon/rectum (in particular) |i16.50|, stomach |i16.51|, and pancreas. Carcinomas of lung, breast, and kidney are also common sources. Adenocarcinoma is the most common metastatic tumor diagnosis.

Many metastatic malignancies, eg, small cell carcinoma |i16.52|, lymphoma, and squamous cell carcinoma, present little problem in diagnosis. However, in some cases, the differential

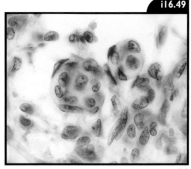
i16.49

Angiosarcoma (P)

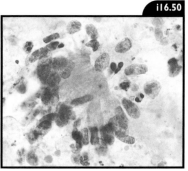
i16.50

Colorectal carcinoma (P)

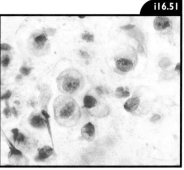
i16.51

Signet ring cell carcinoma, stomach (P)

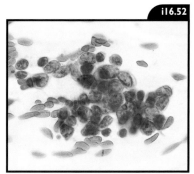
i16.52

Small cell carcinoma, lung (P)

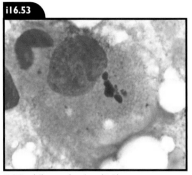

HCC—bile production (DQ)

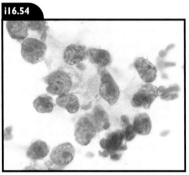

HCC—acini, hyaline globules

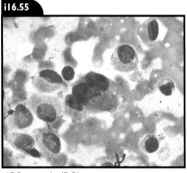

HCC—mucin (DQ)

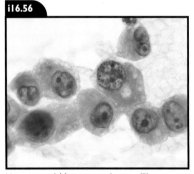

Hepatocytoid breast carcinoma (P)

diagnosis of metastatic adenocarcinoma with HCC may be difficult, and with cholangiocarcinoma, impossible.

The key features favoring metastatic adenocarcinoma over HCC are columnar cells with polar nuclei, acinar formation, and evidence of mucin production. The key features favoring primary HCC are polygonal cells with granular cytoplasm, central nuclei, trabecular arrangement with endothelial lining, and evidence of bile production |i16.53|. Intranuclear cytoplasmic invaginations are more common in HCC than in metastatic carcinomas but also are common in benign hepatocytes. Hyaline bodies are much more common in HCC than in metastatic tumors |i16.54|. Mucin production favors metastatic adenocarcinoma but does not completely exclude HCC (or cholangiocarcinoma) |i16.55|. Necrosis is the rule in metastatic adenocarcinoma but the exception in HCC. Elevated serum levels or cellular expression of AFP favors HCC. A diffuse pattern of cytoplasmic CEA staining is typical of adenocarcinomas, while HCC characteristically shows a predominantly pericanalicular pattern (unique to benign or malignant liver cells).

Hepatocytoid (hepatoid) adenocarcinomas with abundant granular cytoplasm, sometimes containing hyaline globules, arise rarely in various organs, such as stomach, ovary, and breast, and may metastasize to the liver, mimicking HCC |i16.56|.

Renal cell carcinoma can closely resemble HCC, including the presence of granular or clear cytoplasm, INCIs, and lipid or glycogen in the cytoplasm. Polar nuclei and an overall lower nuclear/cytoplasmic ratio in clear cells favor renal origin. Look for a renal mass. Mucin positivity excludes ordinary renal cell carcinoma. Immunocytochemically, AFP expression and canalicular CEA staining support a diagnosis of HCC.

Metastatic melanoma also can closely mimic HCC; similarities include granular cytoplasm, INCIs, and scattered giant cells. Melanin pigment, when present, may resemble various liver cell pigments. Predominance of single cells favors melanoma; endothelial-lined groups of cells (trabeculae) favor HCC. Bile or melanin production, if present, is diagnostic of HCC or melanoma, respectively. S-100 and HMB-45 usually are positive in melanoma, CEA and AFP in HCC. Keratin is positive in HCC but not in melanoma.

Pancreas

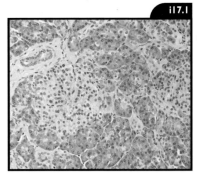

il7.1

Pancreas, tissue (H&E)

Exocrine and endocrine functions are performed by the pancreas, by acinar and islet cells, respectively |i17.1|. The pancreas, particularly the ductal system, is closely related, embryologically, to the extrahepatic biliary tract and the gallbladder. Most pancreaticobiliary neoplasms are adenocarcinomas that arise from the ductal epithelium and are morphologically similar regardless of exact site of origin. Acinar and islet cell neoplasms are rare.

17.1 FNA Biopsy of the Pancreas

Without fine needle aspiration (FNA) biopsy, the differential diagnosis of chronic pancreatitis and pancreatic carcinoma can be difficult—clinically, surgically, and even histologically (particularly frozen sections). Tissue biopsy has a relatively high false-negative rate, and false positives occur in up to 3% of frozen sections. Furthermore, taking tissue for biopsy is associated with serious complications in a number of cases, including hemorrhage, fistula formation, pancreatitis, and, rarely, even death. The accuracy of FNA biopsy is at least as good as tissue biopsy, and probably better, with considerably less morbidity and mortality. Because of its safety and reliability, preoperative or intraoperative FNA biopsy has become widely accepted as the standard pancreatic biopsy technique.

17.2 The Cells

17.2.1 Acinar Cells

The normal pancreas is predominantly made up of acinar cells, which are the parenchymal cells of the exocrine pancreas. Acinar cells are similar in appearance to serous acinic cells of the salivary gland; they are pyramidal or polygonal in shape and are present mostly in cohesive aggregates. The aggregates form microacinar structures that recapitulate the normal pancreatic acini.

The cytoplasm is abundant and characteristically coarsely granular owing to the presence of zymogen granules, ie, proenzymes of trypsin, elastase, lipase, and chymotrypsin, etc |i17.2|, |i17.3|. However, degranulation of the cytoplasm is common, which results in a clear or vacuolated appearance |i17.4|. The nuclei are usually smooth, round, and uniform, about the size of an RBC, and eccentrically located. The chromatin is moderately gran-

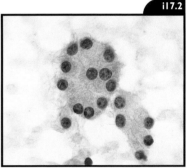

il7.2

Acinar cells (P)

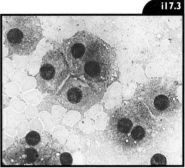

il7.3

Acinar cells, granules (DQ)

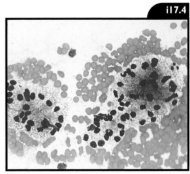

il7.4

Acinar cells, degranulated (DQ)

323

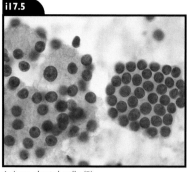

Acinar, ductal cells (P)

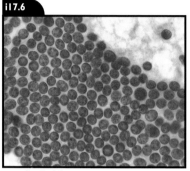

Ductal cells (P)

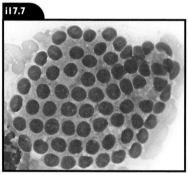

Ductal cells (DQ)

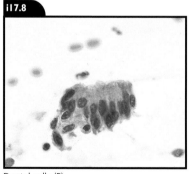

Ductal cells (P)

ular and evenly distributed, and there is a distinct or prominent nucleolus. Naked acinar nuclei are common in aspirate specimens.

17.2.2 Ductal Cells

Ductal cells usually are present, albeit as a minor component |i17.5|. Ductal cells form cohesive sheets of uniform cells in "honeycomb" arrangements with little or no nuclear overlap or crowding |i17.6|, |i17.7|. Ductal cells range from low cuboidal to tall columnar as the ducts get larger |i17.8|. The nuclei are basal, round, and uniform. An important aspect of benign ductal cells is their smooth nuclear membranes. The chromatin of benign ductal cells is fine and evenly distributed. Nucleoli are inconspicuous. The cytoplasm is delicate, pale, and finely vacuolated and may contain mucin. A few goblet cells may be present.

Reactive ductal cells show nuclear enlargement, occasional binucleation, some variation in size and shape, and prominent nucleoli, but usually they maintain smooth nuclear outlines. The chromatin can range from pale ("repairish") to somewhat coarse and dark, due to degeneration. Atypical changes usually are focal in benign reactive conditions.

17.2.3 Islet Cells

Islets of Langerhans, the endocrine cells of the pancreas, account for only 1% to 2% of the pancreatic mass and are concentrated in the tail of the pancreas. Although functionally diverse, islet cells are morphologically identical and cannot be distinguished with routine stains. In fact, islet cells are seldom specifically recognized at all in FNA biopsies without special stains (see "Pancreatic endocrine neoplasms," p 333).

17.2.4 Miscellaneous

Because of its anatomic relationships, miscellaneous cells, eg, hepatocytes, gastric or intestinal cells (as well as partially digested food), occasionally are found in FNA biopsies of the pancreas. Mesothelial cells, which may show reactive changes, also are seen commonly.

17.3 Diseases of the Pancreas

17.3.1 Pancreatitis

Pancreatitis is associated with, among other things, alcoholism; biliary tract disease, including obstruction and stones; trauma; and malignancy.

Acute Pancreatitis

The classic presentation of acute pancreatitis is sudden onset of severe abdominal pain, which may radiate to the back, accompanied by a characteristic increase in the serum amylase level. It is often preceded by heavy eating or drinking (alcohol). Trypsin activation seems to be the key inciting factor, leading to activation of other pancreatic digestive enzymes. This results in autodigestion of the pancreas, with acute suppurative inflammation, granulation tissue, and hemorrhage accompanied by parenchymal and fat necrosis. Fat necrosis occurs not only in the pancreas but also in the mesentery and omentum. Calcium salts react with the released triglycerides, forming soaps (saponification). Acute pancreatitis heals by chronic inflammation and fibrosis, which may result in the formation of pseudocysts.

Acute pancreatitis usually is clinically obvious and, therefore, biopsy seldom is performed. However, FNA biopsy provides a safe and reliable method of diagnosing various sequelae of acute pancreatitis, including pancreatic abscess.

The FNA biopsy of acute pancreatitis is dominated by amorphous material, cell debris, and neutrophils. Macrophages are common. Degenerated acinar cells, with irregular pyknotic nuclei, and reactive ductal cells may be seen. In addition, granulation tissue and evidence of fat necrosis, including degenerated or dead adipose tissue, globules of lipid, and lipophages as well as amorphous calcium deposits (basophilic in Papanicolaou stain, colorless in Diff-Quik stain), representing saponification, are common. Sheets of markedly reactive mesothelial cells, mimicking adenocarcinoma, also may be prominent.

Chronic Pancreatitis

Chronic pancreatitis is characterized clinically by chronic recurrent abdominal pain that is not necessarily accompanied by an increased serum amylase level. The classic clinical diagnostic triad of steatorrhea, diabetes mellitus, and weight loss (ie, signs of pancreatic insufficiency) may occur late in the course of the disease.

Chronic pancreatitis can be focal or diffuse. Microscopically, the main features of chronic pancreatitis are chronic inflammation and fibrosis with loss of acini (acinar atrophy), leaving ducts |i17.9|. The ducts are frequently dilated and filled with protein plugs. Preservation of islets of Langerhans is characteristic (until very late). The amount of chronic inflammation and fibrosis is variable but may be marked, resulting in a hard pancreas, grossly mimicking infiltrating carcinoma at surgery. Microscopically, a tissue biopsy may show glands trapped and distorted by fibrosis, mimicking infiltrating carcinoma.

The FNA biopsy of chronic pancreatitis is similar to that of chronic sialadenitis. Ductal cells usually outnumber acinar cells, in contrast with normal pancreatic tissue, although the overall

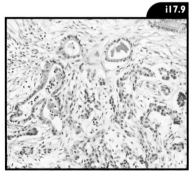

i17.9

Chronic pancreatitis, tissue (H&E)

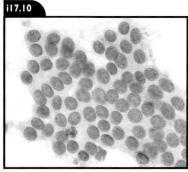

Chronic pancreatitis—ductal cells (P)

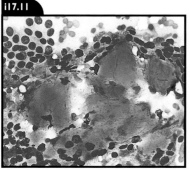

Chronic pancreatitis—duct plugs (DQ)

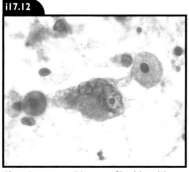

Chronic pancreatitis—myofibroblast (P)

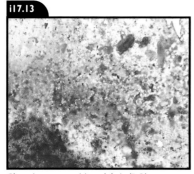

Chronic pancreatitis—debris (DQ)

cellularity usually is low |i17.10|. Fat necrosis consists of dead fat cells (ie, adipocytes sans nuclei) and lipophages, which can be cytologically atypical in appearance. Protein deposits from plugged ducts may be seen |i17.11|. Reactive myofibroblasts, deriving from mesenchymal repair, are spindle or stellate cells that can have large lobulated nuclei and prominent or irregular nucleoli, mimicking malignancy |i17.12|, particularly in Diff-Quik stain. However, in Papanicolaou stain they have pale, bland chromatin, similar to reparative cells. A variable amount of chronic or acute inflammation usually is present.

In summary, in chronic pancreatitis, there is a potpourri of mucus, degenerated cells, debris, macrophages (a few multinucleated), granulation tissue, connective tissue fragments (metachromatic in Diff-Quik stain) containing fibroblasts, and, occasionally, calcification |i17.13|. Atypical (reactive) cells also can be present but usually are few. Be cautious diagnosing malignancy in the presence of significant inflammation. However, pancreatic cancer is frequently surrounded by a zone of pancreatitis; therefore, pancreatitis or inflammation does not exclude malignancy.

Pancreatic Pseudocyst

Pseudocysts of the pancreas are by far the most common, clinically important cysts of the pancreas. Pseudocysts form by destruction and necrosis of pancreatic tissue, usually due to pancreatitis, which is walled off by fibrous tissue. Continued pancreatic secretion leads to accumulation of fluid, which results in formation of a cyst. The cyst lacks an epithelial lining (ergo, pseudocyst). Clinical findings may include jaundice, pain, nausea and vomiting, and weight loss—findings that may suggest pancreatic cancer.

Pseudocysts usually are small but can grow very large and become clinically palpable. Most pseudocysts occur in the tail of the pancreas. They are usually solitary (85%) and unilocular. Multiloculated cysts are more likely to be neoplastic. Drainage of pseudocysts may be therapeutic. Occasionally, pseudocysts become infected (usually coliform bacteria), resulting in a pancreatic abscess (see p 330).

The FNA biopsy obtains turbid fluid that varies from yellow to hemorrhagic to chocolate brown or, occasionally, is milky. The amylase level is characteristically elevated. The cytologic features of pseudocysts are nonspecific, consisting mostly of histiocytes and debris, with few epithelial cells. The histiocytes can be mononucleated or multinucleated and often contain phagocytosed debris or hemosiderin. Necrosis, inflammation, granulation tissue, fibrosis, calcification, cholesterol crystals, and iron or bile pigment also may be present. A few, sometimes strikingly atypical, mesenchymal cells, ie, reactive myofibroblasts, derived from mesenchymal repair, as well as atypical histiocytes, can be seen that could be mistaken for malignancy.

17.4 Ductal Adenocarcinoma

Carcinoma of the pancreas is the fifth most common cause of cancer-related deaths in the United States. The prognosis is grim; most patients (90%) die within a year of diagnosis. Ductal adenocarcinoma accounts for at least 75% of pancreatic malignancies. Most patients are elderly, often in their 70s, although there is a wide age range. Women are slightly more commonly affected than men. The development of pancreatic carcinoma has been associated with cigarette smoking, high fat diet, diabetes mellitus, and industrial pollutants, but it has no proven association with alcohol or coffee consumption. The classic clinical triad of symptoms of pancreatic carcinoma consists of jaundice, weight loss, and pain. This triad, however, is nonspecific, and, unfortunately, by the time symptoms develop, the cancer usually is incurable. Metastases occur to local lymph nodes, liver, and lung, as well as almost any other site in the body.

Most ductal carcinomas (two thirds) arise in the head of the pancreas. Ductal carcinomas range from very well-differentiated to poorly differentiated to anaplastic. Although most pancreatic adenocarcinomas are moderately differentiated, the prognosis does not correlate well with the grade of the tumor. Carcinoma of the pancreas is characterized histologically by irregularly shaped glands surrounded by dense concentric fibrosis. However, benign accessory ducts trapped in fibrous connective tissue can mimic this histologic appearance. Consequently, the cytologic details of the cells are critical in diagnosis, even in tissue studies.

The FNA biopsy usually is cellular, consisting predominantly of ductal-type cells; acinar cells usually are absent or sparse. Malignant ductal cells typically form disorderly clusters and sheets, with an increase in the number of single cells. Malignant cellular features (eg, nuclear enlargement and pleomorphism, irregular nuclear membranes, and abnormal chromatin, as well as nuclear crowding and overlapping, high nuclear/cytoplasmic ratios, prominent nucleoli, mitosis, and necrosis) are usually obvious |i17.14|, |i17.15| but may be subtle in well-differentiated tumors |i17.16|, |i17.17|.

Well-differentiated carcinoma, although fully malignant, may appear deceptively bland and can pose a diagnostic problem. The first clue to the diagnosis is a highly cellular aspirate dominated by ductal cells without acinar cells. The architectural configuration of the cells is abnormal: the cell aggregates are either too crowded or too loosely arranged ("drunken honeycombs"). Nuclear enlargement and increased mitotic figures are suspicious findings. Nuclear membrane irregularity is an important feature of malignancy |i17.18|. Macronucleoli, if present, also suggest malignancy. On diligent search of an adequate specimen, there are often

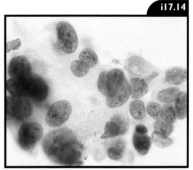
Adenocarcinoma (P)

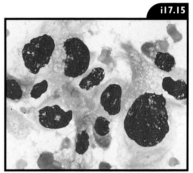
Adenocarcinoma (DQ)

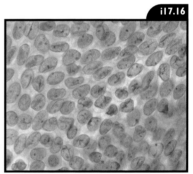
Well-differentiated adenocarcinoma (P)

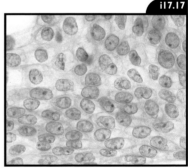
Well-differentiated adenocarcinoma (P)

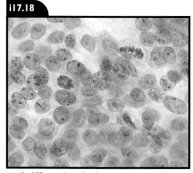

Well-differentiated adenocarcinoma (P)

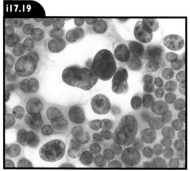

WD AdCA—obvious malignant cell (P)

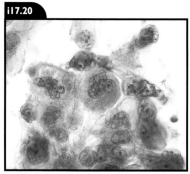

Adenocarcinoma—squamoid cytoplasm (P)

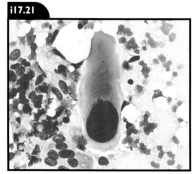

Adenocarcinoma—tombstone cell (DQ)

at least a few scattered, more obviously malignant-appearing cells present, even in well-differentiated adenocarcinoma (WD AdCA), that help make the diagnosis of malignancy |i17.19|. (Conversely, even in poorly differentiated pancreatic carcinomas, there often is a component of well-differentiated carcinoma.)

An abundance of large goblet cells, in large sheets or singly, is suspicious for malignancy. Although adenosquamous carcinoma is traditionally considered rare, squamoid cytoplasm (dense with distinct cell boundaries) is common in all but the best differentiated pancreatic adenocarcinomas |i17.20|. "Tombstone cells" |i17.21|, which are very large, very tall, well-formed columnar cells, also are frequently present in pancreatic carcinoma (except when very well-differentiated). Signet ring cells may be present, and when numerous, they indicate signet ring carcinoma. Rarely, oncocytic or clear cell change is prominent.

The background of the smear often is necrotic, but necrosis is nonspecific and commonly seen in benign diseases of the pancreas, particularly pancreatitis. Also, pancreatic carcinoma often is surrounded by a zone of pancreatitis. Mucin may be seen in the background; when abundant, this can be designated colloid carcinoma. Pseudomyxoma peritonei also can occur.

17.4.1 Anaplastic Carcinoma of the Pancreas

Most anaplastic pancreatic carcinomas are of ductal origin and usually occur in the body or tail of the pancreas. Their morphologic characteristics are distinctive; their behavior, aggressive.

Pleomorphic giant cell carcinoma of the pancreas is characterized by the presence of a significant proportion of bizarre, pleomorphic, multinucleated tumor giant cells |i17.22|. Emperipolesis of inflammatory cells, particularly neutrophils, by giant tumor cells is common. Hyaline cytoplasmic inclusions (eosinophilic in Papanicolaou stain, metachromatic in Diff-Quik stain) may be seen.

Spindle cell, or sarcomatoid, carcinoma of the pancreas is composed predominantly of pleomorphic spindle-shaped tumor cells |i17.23|. The differential diagnosis includes primary spindle cell sarcomas of the pancreas, which are very rare, and spindle cell endocrine neoplasms.

Giant and spindle cell carcinoma is composed of malignant giant and spindle epithelial cells.

Osteoclastic giant cell tumor of the pancreas is characterized by the presence of benign-appearing osteoclastic giant cells that have multiple uniformly small, bland nuclei with conspicuous nucleoli |i17.24|. A second population of mononucleated spindle tumor cells appearing singly or in groups and having similar nuclear features, also is usually present. The background cellularity may include adenocarcinoma.

Small cell carcinoma of the pancreas is morphologically similar to small cell carcinoma of the lung, which is far more common, and a metastasis must be excluded.

17.4.2 Adenosquamous Carcinoma

The diagnosis of adenosquamous carcinoma classically requires the presence of well-formed glands and obvious squamous differentiation, eg, squamous pearls or heavy cytoplasmic keratinization. In surgical and autopsy series, adenosquamous carcinoma is generally considered an unusual variant of pancreatic carcinoma (< 5% of cases). However, on careful search, this variant may be much more common; in fact, some squamoid features (ie, dense cytoplasm, distinct cell borders) are very common in cytologic specimens of ordinary ductal pancreatic carcinoma.

In FNA biopsy specimens, classic adenosquamous carcinoma shows a dual population of glandular and distinctively squamous malignant cells |i17.25|. Rarely, the squamous component is the predominant cell population, sometimes suggesting pure squamous cell carcinoma. Diff-Quik stain can be useful in identifying the squamous component by demonstrating cytoplasmic density and distinct cell boundaries. (See discussions in Chapters 8 and 15.)

17.5 Metastatic Tumors

Metastatic and hematologic neoplasms involving the pancreas may be indistinguishable clinically and radiologically from primary pancreatic carcinoma. Consider metastatic carcinoma if the tumor is not typical of pancreatic adenocarcinoma, particularly if the morphologic findings are small cells or pure squamous cells. The most common sources of secondary deposits are lymphomas; carcinomas of lung, kidney, breast, liver, and gastrointestinal tract; and melanoma.

17.6 Neoplastic Cysts

Neoplastic cysts account for 10% to 15% of all pancreatic cysts and approximately 2% of all pancreatic neoplasms. Although many different kinds of cysts occur in the pancreas, the two major types of neoplastic cysts are mucinous and serous. Solid and papillary epithelial neoplasms also can be cystic. Solid malignant neoplasms of the pancreas can undergo

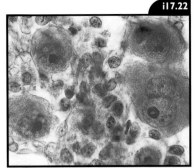

i17.22

Pancreatic carcinoma—giant cells (P)

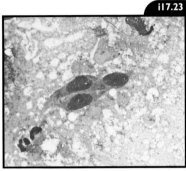

i17.23

Pancreatic carcinoma—spindle cells (DQ)

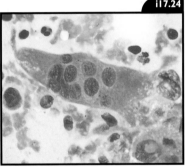

i17.24

Pancreatic carcinoma—osteoclast (DQ)

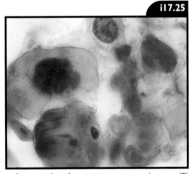

i17.25

Pancreatic adenosquamous carcinoma (P)

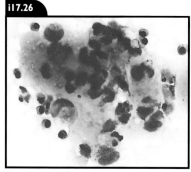

Pseudocyst (DQ)

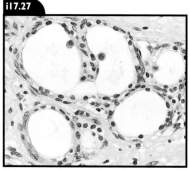

Serous cystadenoma, tissue (H&E)

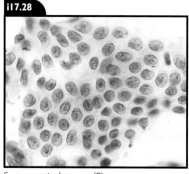

Serous cystadenoma (P)

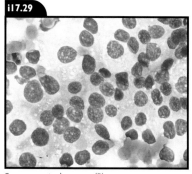

Serous cystadenoma (P)

necrosis with cystic degeneration, but they have the usual dismal prognosis. Cystic endocrine neoplasms and acinar carcinomas also occur, rarely.

A combination of clinical and radiologic features, analysis of the fluid, and FNA biopsy can be useful in differentiating the various types of pancreatic cysts. Pancreatic pseudocysts usually have a high amylase level and a low carcinoembryonic antigen (CEA) level, while the reverse usually is true of pancreatic mucinous cystic neoplasms and cystic carcinomas, although exceptions occur. Slight elevations of amylase and CEA have been reported in serous adenomas. In an abscess, neither amylase nor CEA levels are elevated. To review, pancreatic pseudocysts are characterized by cell debris, macrophages, and few or no epithelial cells in an inflammatory background |i17.26| (see p 326).

17.6.1 Serous Cystadenoma (Microcystic Adenoma)

Serous cystadenoma, also known as microcystic adenoma or glycogen-rich cystadenoma, usually is benign. The tumor is asymptomatic or causes nonspecific symptoms, such as abdominal pain, weight loss, and jaundice; a mass may be palpable. Serous cystadenomas typically occur in elderly patients, women more often than men. In some cases, the tumor destroys the islets of Langerhans, resulting in diabetes mellitus. Although these tumors are benign, death may occur due to biliary tract obstruction or complications of surgery on elderly debilitated patients. Some patients have von Hippel-Lindau disease, an autosomal dominant disorder consisting of hemangioblastomas of the central nervous system and retina, epididymal cystadenomas, renal cysts and renal cell carcinoma, and pheochromocytoma.

Serous cystadenomas can arise anywhere in the pancreas, but they occur more often in the head of the pancreas and can be multiple. The lesions are well circumscribed and may have a central stellate scar. Serous cystadenomas average more than 10 cm in diameter (range, 1-25 cm) and are composed of a myriad of small cysts (< 2 cm in diameter), grossly resembling a sponge. The cysts contain serous fluid that is rich in glycogen. Histologically, the cysts are lined by small cuboidal cells set in a fibrovascular stroma that may be focally calcified and contain cholesterol clefts and hemosiderin |i17.27|.

The aspirate obtains clear, watery, sparsely cellular fluid with only a few clusters of flattened ductal-like cells and no acinar cells |i17.28|, |i17.29|. A potential clue to the diagnosis is that the tumor does not collapse on aspiration. The cells are present singly or in cohesive honeycombed sheets and palisaded strips. Occasional papillae may be present. The nuclei are small, round, and slightly pleomorphic and may be somewhat hyperchromatic, but they do not overlap or have prominent nucleoli. Irregular nuclear membranes, nuclear grooves, and intranuclear cytoplasmic invaginations may be seen, but mitotic figures are absent. The cytoplasm is moderate in amount and clear to finely granular or vacuolar. It contains abundant glycogen, little or no mucin, and no zymogen granules. Foamy or hemosiderin-laden macrophages may be present. However, the background is clean without cell debris or mucus. Islet cells, present in the tissue between the microcysts, may be seen.

17.6.2 Mucinous Cystic Neoplasms

Mucinous cystic neoplasms are rare tumors (~ 1%) of the pancreas, which usually are regarded as at least potentially malignant. Mucinous cystic neoplasms usually occur in middle-aged patients (40s), but there is a wide age range. Women are more commonly affected than men. Clinically, patients may present with abdominal pain and weight loss; belching, nausea, vomiting, and diarrhea also are possible. These clinical findings are nonspecific and could be seen with other pancreatic tumors. Absence of a history of trauma or alcoholism helps exclude pancreatic pseudocyst.

Mucinous cystic neoplasms average about 10 cm (range, 2-20 cm). Larger lesions may be clinically palpable. The neoplasm is composed of cysts, usually 2 cm or more in diameter |i17.30|. The cysts can be unilocular or multilocular and usually are surrounded by a fibrous capsule that eventually becomes focally calcified. Small cysts usually behave in a benign fashion; complicated cysts usually are malignant. Radiologic findings, including size, configuration, and pattern of calcification, can be helpful in diagnosis. Mucinous cystic neoplasms usually occur in the body and tail of the pancreas (in contrast with ordinary pancreatic carcinomas).

The FNA biopsy obtains mucoid material, a key diagnostic feature that usually can be appreciated grossly |i17.31|. The aspirate is variably cellular, depending on the amount of mucus obtained. Sheets of cohesive, orderly, bland cells alternate with disorderly groups of cells that show cytologic atypia |i17.32|. Papillary clusters may be present |i17.33|. The tumor cells are similar to those of mucinous ovarian tumors. They are tall and columnar and characteristically contain mucin. Numerous benign muciphages also may be present, which may closely resemble the mucinous tumor cells |i17.34|. The stroma ranges from acellular and hyalinized to highly cellular, reminiscent of ovarian stroma, to pseudosarcomatous. Hemorrhage, necrosis, and calcification may occur.

Previously described features of well-differentiated pancreatic carcinoma may be seen, eg, crowding and overlapping,

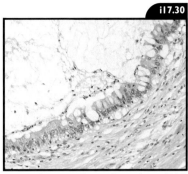
Mucinous cystic neoplasm, tissue (H&E)

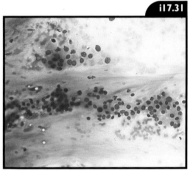
Mucinous cystic neoplasm (DQ)

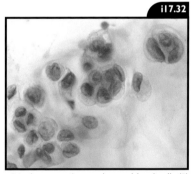
Mucinous cystic neoplasm—bland cells (P)

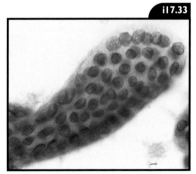
Mucinous cystic neoplasm (P)

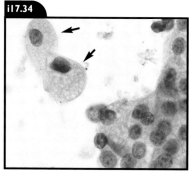

Mucinous cystic neoplasm—muciphages (P)

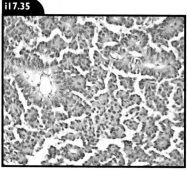

SPEN, tissue (H&E)

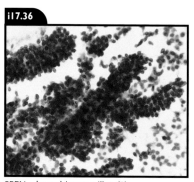

SPEN—branching papillae (P)

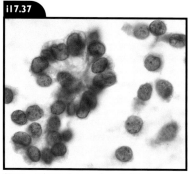

SPEN—microacini, single cells (P)

cellular and nuclear enlargement, increased nuclear/cytoplasmic ratios, irregular nuclear membranes, and nucleoli. Well-differentiated tumor cells resemble benign endocervical cells. Transitions from benign-appearing to malignant-appearing cells are common. Scattered cells may show obvious malignant features (when predominant, diagnose mucinous cystadenocarcinoma). Numerous goblet or signet-ring cells may be present and provide a clue to the diagnosis.

17.6.3 Solid and Papillary Epithelial Neoplasm

Solid and papillary epithelial neoplasm (SPEN), also known as papillary cystic neoplasm, is a rare, low-grade pancreatic malignancy that typically affects young women, often in their twenties, but it can be seen rarely in old age or in men |i17.35|. Clinically, most patients present with vague upper abdominal pain accompanied by an enlarging abdominal mass, but they are not jaundiced nor do they have hormonal abnormalities. This tumor should be suspected in a young woman with a cystic or partially cystic pancreatic mass.

The tumor is an encapsulated or well-circumscribed, multiloculated cystic and solid mass, usually located in the body or tail of the pancreas. It usually is solitary but can be multifocal. Grossly, the tumor has a variegated appearance with solid hemorrhagic and cystic necrotic areas.

The FNA biopsy may obtain only clear fluid or predominantly necrotic debris, precluding diagnosis. However, many cases yield highly cellular smears. A characteristic finding consists of branching fibrovascular papillae lined by one or more layers of neoplastic cells |i17.36|. The cells may be present singly, in loose fragments, or as microacinar structures |i17.37|. Sometimes, the stroma surrounding the vascular cores of the papillae is myxoid and stains metachromatically in Diff-Quik stain.

The cells are relatively uniform, with bland nuclei and a moderate amount of cytoplasm. In some cases, the cells have long, slender, cytoplasmic processes |i17.38|. The nuclei are round to oval, eccentrically located, and have fine chromatin. Nuclear grooves are typical. Nucleoli are not prominent. A few more atypical cells may be present in some cases. Mitotic figures are absent or rare.

Metachromatic hyaline globules (intracellular, extracellular, or in microacinar lumens) may be seen—a very rare finding in other primary pancreatic neoplasms |i17.39|. Macrophages with foamy cytoplasm, multinucleated giant cells (neoplastic and nonneoplastic), cholesterol, and necrotic debris also may be present. Metastases can show more cytologic atypia, including bizarre tumor cells, and an increased mitotic rate.

17.7 Acinar Cell Carcinoma

Acinar cell carcinoma is rare, only about 1% of all pancreatic malignancies |i17.40|. Acinar cell carcinoma occurs over a wide age range, including children, and is slightly more common in males. There is no predilection for head, body, or tail of the pancreas. Although acinar cell carcinomas usually are nonfunctional, a clinical syndrome occurs rarely, consisting of disseminated fat necrosis, polyarthralgia, and eosinophilia, due to release of pancreatic digestive enzymes. The prognosis is poor.

The FNA biopsy specimen is similar to that of acinic cell carcinoma of the salivary gland. The aspirate is cellular, characteristically composed only of acinar cells without ductal cells. Groups of tumor cells exhibit overlapping and crowding and form solid nests, short cords, and acinar structures. There also is an increased number of single cells.

The nuclei are eccentrically located and relatively large with increased nuclear/cytoplasmic ratios. The chromatin varies from dense and granular to open and coarse. Irregular nuclear membranes and prominent nucleoli may be seen. The mitotic rate is variable. The cytoplasm is abundant and may be coarsely granular due to zymogen granule content or clear due to degranulation.

Well-differentiated tumors are composed of cells that closely resemble the normal acinar cells and, therefore, may be difficult to diagnose |i17.41|. However, obtaining small, dissociated acinar cells with increased nuclear/cytoplasmic ratios, in the absence of ductal cells, from a mass in the pancreas suggests this diagnosis, especially if the clinical syndrome is present. (The differential diagnosis with endocrine neoplasms is discussed on p 335.) Trypsin usually is expressed immunocytochemically and favors acinar carcinoma over ductal and endocrine tumors. A minor component of the tumor also may express neuroendocrine markers.

17.8 Endocrine Neoplasms: Islet Cell and Carcinoid Tumors

Pancreatic endocrine neoplasms (PENs), including islet cell tumors and pancreatic carcinoid tumors, are relatively rare pancreatic tumors (< 5%). Pancreatic carcinoid tumors arise from neuroendocrine Kulchitsky cells or their precursors in the pancreatic ducts. Islets of Langerhans probably also develop, embryologically, from the ductal system. Thus, islet cell and carcinoid tumors are closely related developmentally and are essentially identical morphologically.

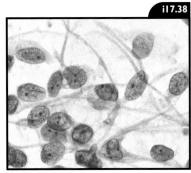

i17.38

SPEN—nuclear grooves, cytoprocesses (P)

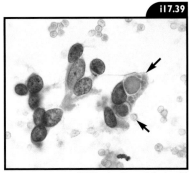

i17.39

SPEN—hyaline globules (P)

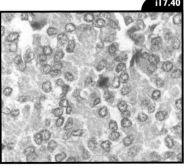

i17.40

Acinar cell carcinoma, tissue (H&E)

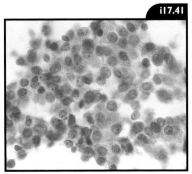

i17.41

Acinar cell carcinoma (P)

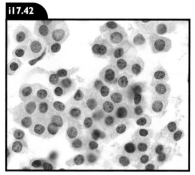

PEN, islet cell tumor, gastrinoma (P)

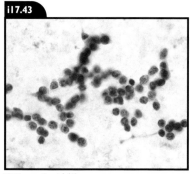

PEN, carcinoid (P)

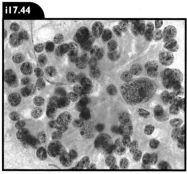

PEN, islet cell tumor, insulinoma (P)

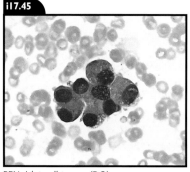

PEN, islet cell tumor (DQ)

Pancreatic endocrine neoplasms occur predominantly in older adults, but no age is spared. Pancreatic endocrine neoplasms are important because many are benign and treatable, whereas ordinary pancreatic carcinoma is usually incurable. On the other hand, pancreatic endocrine neoplasms, even when small and benign, can be life-threatening due to hormone production.

Pancreatic endocrine neoplasms can be associated with a variety of clinical syndromes, which can be helpful in diagnosis. More than one hormone may be produced, and the hormones are not necessarily native to the pancreas (eg, corticotropin, parathormone, serotonin, human chorionic gonadotropin). Tumors producing ectopic hormones, particularly corticotropin or parathormone, are more likely to be malignant. The most common syndromes are hypoglycemia due to insulin secretion; Zollinger-Ellison (ulcerogenic) syndrome due to gastrin secretion; and multiple endocrine neoplasia.

Islet cell tumors are more common in the body and tail than in the head of the pancreas, reflecting the distribution of islets of Langerhans. The tumors vary from one to several centimeters in diameter and can be multiple. They usually are well circumscribed but may have microscopically infiltrating borders. Rarely, the tumors are cystic. Histologically, islet cell tumors grow in a variety of patterns, including glandular, solid, ribbons, and cords.

The FNA biopsy specimen usually is cellular; the cells are found singly, in loosely cohesive irregular sheets |i17.42|, or crowded clusters, ribbons |i17.43|, and, occasionally, rosettes |i17.44|. Perivascular tumor growth, with cells attached to capillaries, is a characteristic feature. The cells are small to medium and, usually, strikingly monotonous. The cells usually have a plasmacytoid appearance with eccentrically located nuclei |i17.45|. The nuclei are usually uniform, round to oval, with smooth membranes, "salt-and-pepper" chromatin, inconspicuous nucleoli, and little or no molding. The cytoplasm may contain fine metachromatic granules, corresponding to neurosecretory granules (NSGs) |i17.46|, |i17.47|. As is common in endocrine tumors, significant pleomorphism can be seen, focally, even in benign neoplasms ("endocrine atypia"). Conversely, malignant tumors can be composed entirely of bland, uniform cells. Mitotic figures or a tumor diathesis are unusual in both benign and malignant pancreatic endocrine neoplasms, but their presence would suggest malignancy. Ultimately, the best indicator of malignancy is metastasis |i17.48|, |i17.49|.

Rarely, pancreatic endocrine neoplasms have oncocytic, clear, or lipid-rich cytoplasm. In some cases, dual glandular and endocrine differentiation may occur (analogous to adenocarcinoids). Fibrosis, calcification, ossification, amyloid deposition, and psammoma bodies also can occur.

Special stains, such as Grimelius argyrophil stain, or electron microscopy can help demonstrate neurosecretory granules. Nowadays, however, immunocytochemistry is used more often to demonstrate synaptophysin, chromogranin, or neuron-specific enolase, as well as specific secretory products (eg, insulin, gastrin). The tumors can then be named accordingly (eg, insulinoma, gastrinoma).

The differential diagnosis includes normal and neoplastic acinar cells. Acinar cells have abundant coarsely granular (zymogen) or foamy cytoplasm and usually present in more cohesive (acinar) groups than do neoplastic islet cells. Islet cell tumors often have characteristic salt-and-pepper chromatin, which helps distinguish this cell type. Note that a minor component of the tumor cells in acinar carcinoma may express neuroendocrine, including islet cell, markers by immunocytochemistry.

Some pancreatic endocrine neoplasms may be more atypical, analogous to atypical carcinoid tumors, with spindle cells, occasional nuclear molding, increased mitoses, and necrosis. Such tumors are likely to be aggressive. Rarely, small cell carcinoma (poorly differentiated neuroendocrine carcinoma) arises in the pancreas (exclude lung metastasis). Islet cell hyperplasia (adenosis) may be difficult or impossible to distinguish from islet cell tumors by cytology alone; the cells are essentially identical.

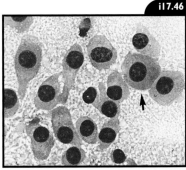

i17.46

Gastrinoma—metachromatic granules (DQ)

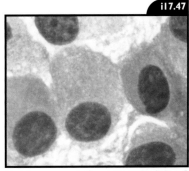

i17.47

Gastrinoma—metachromatic NSGs (DQ, oil)

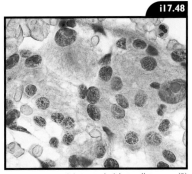

i17.48

Metastatic islet cell tumor (P)

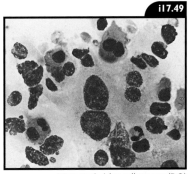

i17.49

Metastatic islet cell tumor (DQ)

Kidney

Hematuria, flank pain, and abdominal mass are the classic findings suggestive of a renal neoplasm. The workup of a suspected renal lesion may begin with an intravenous pyelogram to define the mass. Next, ultrasonography or computed tomography can be used to determine whether the mass is solid or cystic. Solid masses can be studied arteriographically: renal cell carcinoma (RCC) has a characteristic vascular pattern. However, many cases of RCC are hypovascular, and, conversely, vascular lesions, such as angiomyolipoma or inflammation, can be benign. The differential diagnosis of hypovascular renal masses includes benign and malignant diseases such as cysts, abscess, hematoma, oncocytoma, transitional cell carcinoma (TCC), lymphoma, metastatic carcinoma, and cystic RCC. Fine needle aspiration (FNA) biopsy of renal masses can provide the definitive diagnosis, which may obviate surgery.

The sensitivity of FNA biopsy of the kidney (for cancer) averages about 85%, and the specificity averages about 98%, a diagnostic accuracy exceeded only by surgical exploration. False-negative diagnoses are primarily related to problems obtaining sufficient diagnostic material, eg, from large, extensively necrotic, hemorrhagic, or cystic tumors, as well as a geographic miss of the lesion. False-positive diagnoses can occur due to chronic inflammation, infarcts, polycystic kidney disease, cysts, hematoma, angiomyolipomas, and other benign neoplasms.

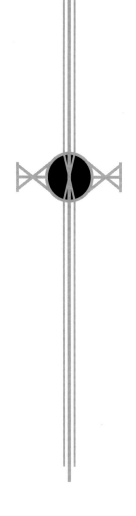

18.1 The Cells

Most benign cells aspirated from normal kidney are tubular in origin, and most of those derive from the proximal renal tubule |i18.1|. Renal tubular cells form cohesive flat sheets of orderly cells, reminiscent of honeycombed sheets of endocervical cells in the Pap smear. Occasional gland-like acinar structures or intact tubules also can be seen.

The nuclei are small, round, and uniform, and the nuclear/cytoplasmic (N/C) ratios are moderately high. The chromatin is finely granular. One or two small inconspicuous nucleoli may be present. The cytoplasm of the proximal renal tubule is moderate in amount and finely granular (owing to numerous mitochondria). The cytoplasm stains pink in Papanicolaou stain, gray-blue in Diff-Quik stain. The cells of the distal tubule and loop of Henle are similar to proximal tubular cells but are smaller and have paler, less granular, and less abundant cytoplasm. The cells may contain lipofuscin pigment (paranuclear bodies), which suggests the cells are benign. Normal tubular cells do not contain

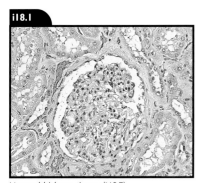

Normal kidney, tissue (H&E)

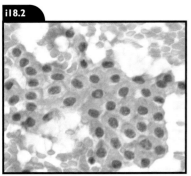

Renal tubular cells (P)

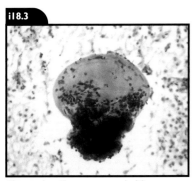

Glomerulus, Bowman capsule (P)

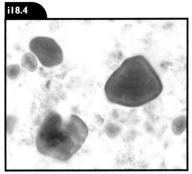

Renal cyst—Liesegang rings

intracytoplasmic vacuoles, and there is no cytoplasmic clearing |i18.2|. In contrast, RCC frequently has cytoplasmic vacuoles or clearing (due to lipid or glycogen content). However, tubular cells may contain lipid vacuoles in benign disease, such as the nephrotic syndrome.

Rarely, intact glomeruli are aspirated |i18.3|. These are lobulated capillary aggregates, sometimes contained in a fibrous capsule (Bowman capsule).

18.2 Benign Diseases

18.2.1 Renal Cysts

Renal cysts can be congenital (single, multiple, poly-cystic) or acquired (including cysts of von Hippel-Lindau disease, tuberous sclerosis, dialysis, and polycystic kidney disease, as well as solitary and multilocular cysts). Virtually any kind of renal cyst could be associated with neoplastic transformation.

Acquired cysts of the kidney are usually asymptomatic and incidentally discovered. Their frequency increases with age, and they must be differentiated from RCC. Aspiration of the fluid may be curative in patients with benign renal cysts.

The fluid from a benign renal cyst usually looks like urine. Blood-tinged or, especially, chocolate-colored fluid is suspicious for malignancy, although rarely RCC is associated with clear fluid. The fluid is poorly cellular; most cells are small bland epithelial cells and macrophages, which may contain hemosiderin pigment. The background commonly contains a small amount of fresh blood and debris. Liesegang rings, similar to corpora amylacea, may be seen |i18.4|. Significant reactive atypia is rare but can occur.

18.2.2 Abscess

Occasionally, an abscess forms in the kidney (renal abscess) or near it (perinephric abscess). Predisposing factors include urinary tract infection with obstruction, renal calculi, diabetes mellitus, skin infections, general debility, and chronic illness. The patients are clinically sick, with fever, chills, costovertebral angle tenderness, and pyuria.

The FNA biopsy shows abundant acute and chronic inflammation and granulation tissue. Organisms, usually gram-negative bacilli, often are present. Epithelial repair may yield atypical cells that could suggest malignancy. FNA biopsy can provide material for culture and may help relieve pain.

18.2.3 Xanthogranulomatous Pyelonephritis

Xanthogranulomatous pyelonephritis is a rare, benign, inflammatory disease of the kidney that can mimic malignancy clinically, radiologically, and microscopically. It occurs in association with urinary tract obstruction, infection, and stones. Clinical findings include flank pain, renal mass, hematuria, and recurrent urinary tract infections (usually *Escherichia coli, Pseudomonas,* or *Proteus*). Similar signs and symptoms can be seen in patients with renal cancer. Radiologic findings may include a hypovascular, nonfunctioning mass, which also can mimic cancer. Renal enlargement and staghorn calculi may be demonstrated with diagnostic imaging techniques.

Grossly, the kidney usually is enlarged and nodular and may be focally necrotic or cystic. The lesion appears yellow to orange ("xantho") owing to the accumulation of lipid in collections of histiocytes ("granuloma").

The FNA biopsy shows histiocytes and giant cells, with foamy vacuolated cytoplasm containing neutral fat and phospholipids (ie, xanthoma cells). The histiocytes may be clustered around capillaries, as in granulation tissue. Necrosis, cholesterol crystals, and inflammation also may be present.

Atypical lipid-laden histiocytes, perivascular growth, and necrosis can mimic RCC. Granulomatous kidney disease, eg, due to tuberculosis, sarcoid |i18.5|, |i18.6|, or bacillus Calmette-Guérin therapy for bladder carcinoma, also can occur and is recognized cytologically by the presence of epithelioid histiocytes and giant cells.

18.2.4 Renal Infarct

Infarcts of the kidney usually are due to emboli, often of cardiac origin. A renal infarct typically results in a wedge-shaped area of parenchymal destruction, with the base of the lesion at the surface of the kidney. The patients can have a variety of nonspecific clinical findings, including flank pain, fever, leukocytosis, hematuria, renal failure, and hypertension.

The FNA biopsy may obtain necrotic glomeruli and tubules, allowing the correct diagnosis to be made. However, regenerating tubular cells with atypia, including nuclear enlargement and pleomorphism, irregular nuclear membranes, prominent nucleoli, and cytoplasmic vacuolization, can mimic RCC. Be cautious diagnosing RCC when the aspirate is scanty and the atypical cells have repair-like features.

18.2.5 Angiomyolipoma

Angiomyolipoma is an uncommon tumor (a choristoma), that occurs most often in the kidney but can arise in the liver, retroperitoneum, and, rarely, elsewhere |i18.7|, |i18.8|. Angiomyolipomas occur in two distinct clinical settings, one inherited

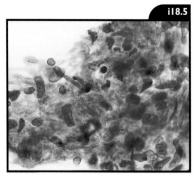
Granuloma, sarcoid (P)

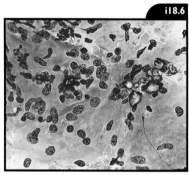
Granuloma, sarcoid (DQ)

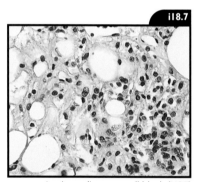
Angiomyolipoma—cell block (H&E)

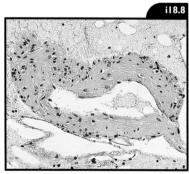
Angiomyolipoma—thick-walled vessel (H&E)

339

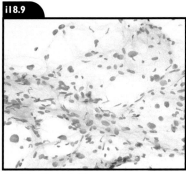

Angiomyolipoma (P)

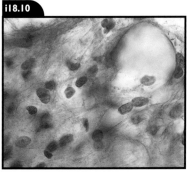

Angiomyolipoma (P)

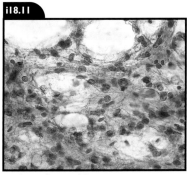

Angiomyolipoma (P)

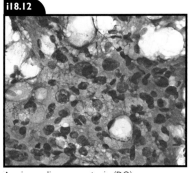

Angiomyolipoma—atypia (DQ)

(usually multiple small tumors associated with tuberous sclerosis), the other sporadic (usually large unilateral tumors, more often occurring in middle-aged women). Usually benign and often asymptomatic, angiomyolipomas can hemorrhage severely, which can be fatal.

The lesions have a variegated appearance, and hemorrhage and necrosis are common, which can grossly mimic RCC. Although angiomyolipomas have characteristic radiologic features, it is not always possible to differentiate them from RCC by using diagnostic imaging techniques.

The FNA biopsy obtains blood vessels ("angio"), smooth muscle ("myo"), and mature fat cells ("lipoma"), in varying proportions |i18.9|, |i18.10|. In cell blocks and tissue, the blood vessels are tortuous and thick-walled, surrounded by hyperplastic smooth muscle, and set in fibroadipose tissue. Fibrous tissue containing spindle cell fibroblasts also may be obtained. However, epithelial cells are not a component of the tumor. Disrupting the vessels may result in a bloody, poorly cellular aspirate.

The presence of mature adipose tissue in an aspirate of a renal tumor is suggestive of this lesion, although fat could be inadvertently sampled from perinephric adipose tissue. Evidence of fat necrosis can be present, including histiocytes, multinucleated giant cells, and pleomorphic nuclei of adipocytes. In some cases, the adipose tissue is scant or absent, making the diagnosis difficult.

Similarly, masses of smooth muscle are not found commonly in other renal tumors or in normal kidney, and, therefore, their presence suggests angiomyolipoma |i18.11|. The smooth muscle can be present as single cells or clusters of spindle-shaped cells with fibrillar or granular cytoplasm and indistinct cell borders. The smooth muscle cells can have an epithelioid appearance, suggesting RCC. The nuclei can vary from round to oval to spindle or cigar-shaped, usually with fine chromatin and small nucleoli. Naked nuclei are common.

Atypia of the smooth muscle cells or the fatty component could suggest malignancy |i18.12|; however, despite a sometimes alarming cytologic appearance, angiomyolipomas usually behave in a benign fashion, although occasionally the tumors are locally aggressive and rarely are fully malignant. Actin and vimentin are positive and cytokeratin is negative in immunocytochemical studies. Unexpectedly, HMB-45 (a marker for melanoma) is usually positive in the perivascular epithelioid cells of the tumor.

18.3 Malignant Diseases

Malignant diseases of the kidney include RCC arising from the renal parenchyma and TCC arising in the transitional epithelium of the renal pelvis. These are usually tumors of adults. Wilms tumor is the most common renal malignancy in children. A variety of other rare tumors, including sarcomas, also occur.

18.3.1 Renal Cell Carcinoma

RCC is, by far, the most common primary malignant tumor of the kidney. It is more common in men than women (3:2), reaching a peak incidence in the late 50s, but can occur rarely in children. The etiology of RCC is unknown, but tobacco smoking is probably the most important risk factor. Also, obesity, dialysis, and genetic defects have been implicated in its development. Most cases of RCC are associated with a genetic abnormality (often involving chromosome 3).

The classic clinical triad of findings in RCC is hematuria, flank pain, and an abdominal mass, but the full triad is seldom present, and when it is, the disease is usually far advanced. Hematuria is a frequent presenting complaint, but hematuria is common and nonspecific. Rarely, malignant cells are found in the urine but usually late in the course of the disease.

RCC is known clinically as the "great imitator" because many patients present with systemic effects or paraneoplastic syndromes, which can be misleading in the diagnosis of RCC. RCC can produce hypercalcemia (with mental confusion and weakness due to release of a parathormone-like substance), hypertension (renin), polycythemia (erythropoietin), or anemia (normochromic, normocytic), as well as gynecomastia, virilization, Cushing syndrome, amyloidosis, masculinization, and leukemoid reactions. Hepatic dysfunction, with hepatomegaly and abnormal serum liver function tests mimicking hepatitis, unrelated to metastatic disease, is the most common paraneoplastic syndrome.

RCCs are usually solitary but can vary greatly in size; most arise in the upper pole of the kidney. Unfortunately, many patients have metastases at diagnosis, in expected sites, such as lung, liver, and bone, as well as in unexpected sites, such as the thyroid, ovary, or salivary gland, which can mimic a primary tumor at the metastatic site. The presence or absence of metastases is the single most important prognostic factor.

In the past, renal cell neoplasms less than 3 cm were considered adenomas; tumors greater than 5 cm, carcinomas. Although the size of the tumor roughly correlates with its propensity to metastasize, small size alone does not exclude malignant behavior. Therefore, most so-called adenomas should be considered at least potentially malignant. However, two subtypes are possibly benign: oncocytomas (when strictly defined, see "Oncocytoma and Oncocytic Neoplasms," p 345) and papillary adenomas (< 1 cm in diameter, composed of small, basophilic

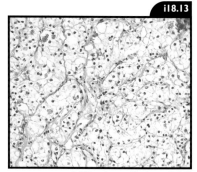

i18.13

RCC—clear cell, tissue (H&E)

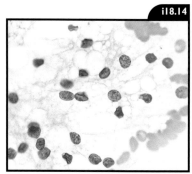

i18.14

RCC—clear cell (P)

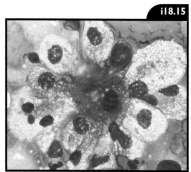

i18.15

RCC—clear cell (DQ)

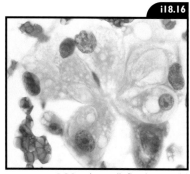

i18.16

RCC—clear cell, floral group (P)

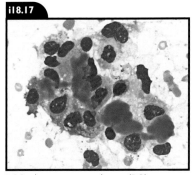

RCC—basement membrane (DQ)

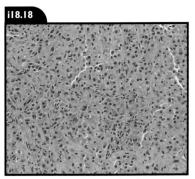

RCC—granular cell, tissue (H&E)

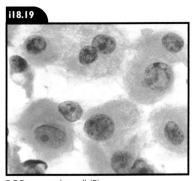

RCC—granular cell (P)

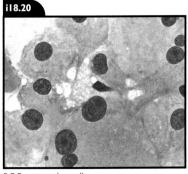

RCC—granular cell

cells). Necrosis, degeneration, or any significant degree of atypia excludes a diagnosis of adenoma.

Microscopically, RCC can have clear, granular, papillary, sarcomatoid, or mixed morphology. Clear cell morphology has the best prognosis, sarcomatoid the worst, but grading is more important than cell type. Well-differentiated tumors are characterized by monomorphous cells with little atypia that may be difficult to distinguish from normal tubular cells. As the grade of the tumor increases, cellular and nuclear atypia increases, while intercellular cohesion decreases. Poorly differentiated RCC may resemble other high-grade malignancies, including sarcomas, cytologically. Coexpression of keratin and vimentin is characteristic of RCC but not specific.

The FNA biopsy specimen is usually bloody but cellular. The cells are found in clusters, sheets, glands, papillae, or singly. Hemorrhage, necrosis, and degeneration are common. Although the various cell types will be discussed individually, mixtures are common.

Clear Cell RCC

The cells of clear cell RCC |i18.13|, |i18.14|, |i18.15| characteristically grow along capillaries and may form short papillary groups. Floral groups of clear cells, radiating from a central point, also may be seen |i18.16|. The presence of cells adherent to metachromatic basement membrane–like material is a characteristic feature |i18.17|.

The tumor cells are usually much larger than benign tubular cells, with low N/C ratios. The cytoplasm is abundant, pale, and multivacuolated. In Papanicolaou stain, it tends to be wispy and delicate or foamy, staining a gossamer blue. In Diff-Quik stain, clear cells are characterized by numerous fine vacuoles that are sharply outlined against the intervening densely stained cytoplasm. The vacuoles in malignant cells contain lipid or glycogen or both, but not mucin. Hyaline globules may be present in the cytoplasm. Phagocytosed RBCs and hemosiderin may be seen, and occasionally hemosiderin accumulation is massive.

The nuclei can range from small, uniform, and bland to large and bizarre, depending on the grade of the tumor. The nuclear membranes can vary from smooth to irregular and the chromatin from fine to coarse, depending on grade. Similarly, nucleoli can range from inconspicuous to enormous. However, the most characteristic nuclei have fine pale chromatin and single cherry-red macronucleoli. Intranuclear cytoplasmic invaginations also can be seen. Naked nuclei may be numerous.

Benign foamy histiocytes often are present and, in some cases, may be difficult to distinguish from tumor cells (obvious nucleoli favors tumor). Necrosis, fibrosis, cartilage, bone, hemosiderin, cholesterol, and fat may be seen in the background. Rarely, psammoma bodies may be present.

Granular Cell RCC

The cells of granular RCC are usually smaller than those of the clear cell variety, but they have more atypical nuclei, higher N/C ratios, and of course, granular cytoplasm |i18.18|, |i18.19|, |i18.20|. The granules correspond primarily to mitochondria; some cases mimic oncocytomas (oncocytic carcinoma). Granular and clear cell types are frequently mixed. Even single cells may show mixed features, usually with a granular center and clear periphery. Finding such cells in a metastasis suggests renal origin. Hemorrhage and necrosis are common, particularly in larger tumors.

The cells of well-differentiated granular RCC resemble benign proximal renal tubular cells. However, tumor cells are usually larger and more numerous than benign tubular cells and have malignant nuclear features. The presence of vacuolated clear cells also helps in the diagnosis of RCC.

Benign hepatocytes may be incidentally sampled and can mimic granular cell RCC, including granular cytoplasm and atypical (reactive) nuclei. Oncocytoma also may be considered in the differential diagnosis; nuclear anaplasia, among other features, excludes oncocytoma (see "Oncocytoma and Oncocytic Neoplasms," p 345).

Sarcomatoid RCC

Sarcomatoid RCC is renal carcinoma with a sarcomatous appearance. It is characterized by aggressive behavior and a poor prognosis. Sarcomatoid RCC is relatively rare, accounting for less than 5% of cases. The tumor cells are epithelial rather than mesenchymal in origin, maintaining epithelial features, ultrastructurally and immunologically.

The FNA biopsy usually shows a dimorphic population of cells, consisting of a high-grade epithelial component (clear or granular RCC) plus a sarcomatoid component, in varying proportions. Pure sarcomatoid RCC is rare. There are three basic morphologic appearances of the sarcomatoid cells: spindle (fibrosarcoma-like) |i18.21|, strap (rhabdomyosarcoma-like) |i18.22|, and pleomorphic (malignant fibrous histiocytoma–like) |i18.23|. Benign-appearing osteoclastic giant cells also can be seen in some cases.

18.3.2 Papillary (Chromophil) Carcinoma

Papillary carcinoma is a malignant renal tumor in which at least half of the lesion grows as well-defined papillae |i18.24|. Papillary RCC accounts for up to 15% of all renal carcinomas. These tumors are characteristically hypovascular on intravenous pyelogram, mimicking a benign lesion. Papillary RCC usually is composed of low-grade cells, and the cytoplasm is characteristically dense and granular (aka chromophil carcinoma). Clear cell papillary carcinomas or tumors composed of high-grade cells

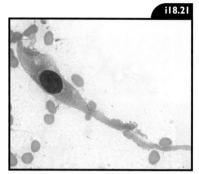

i18.21

RCC—spindle cell

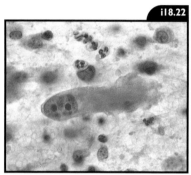

i18.22

RCC—strap cell

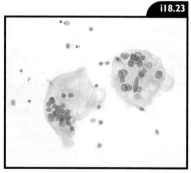

i18.23

RCC—giant cells

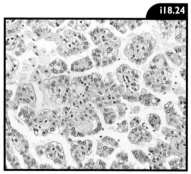

i18.24

Papillary carcinoma, tissue (H&E)

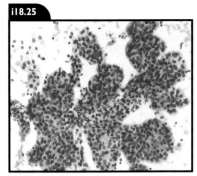

Papillary carcinoma (P)

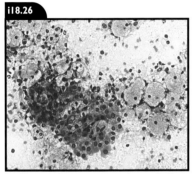

Papillary carcinoma—macrophages (DQ)

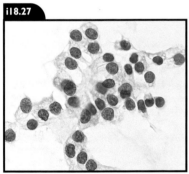

Papillary carcinoma (P)

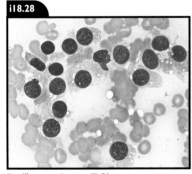

Papillary carcinoma (DQ)

probably should not be included in this diagnosis because their behavior is more aggressive.

The FNA biopsy specimen is usually cellular, obtaining characteristic papillae surrounded by bland uniform tumor cells |i18.25|; single cells are relatively few. The papillae are often distended with macrophages containing lipid (foam cells) or hemosiderin (siderophages), which also are found in the background |i18.26|. The tumor cells are cuboidal to columnar with bland nuclei and high N/C ratios |i18.27|, |i18.28|. The nuclear membranes can vary from smooth to irregular, but the chromatin is usually fine and nucleoli are small, single, and inconspicuous. The cytoplasm is dense and granular in character (chromophil) and scant to moderate in amount. Psammoma bodies are most common in this variant of RCC. Focal areas of necrosis and hemorrhage are frequent.

The differential diagnosis includes well-differentiated papillary TCC of the renal pelvis and ordinary RCC. The lining of the papillae of TCC is more stratified; the cells have more abundant, denser cytoplasm; and there may be a high-grade component or mucin positivity. Ordinary RCC has fewer shorter papillae with more single cells, lower N/C ratios, and more cytologic atypia than papillary RCC. Psammoma bodies and abundant foamy histiocytes favor papillary RCC.

18.3.3 Collecting Duct Carcinoma

The collecting (Bellini) ducts of the kidney and the renal calyces, pelvis, and ureter share a common embryologic origin from the ureteric bud, which is derived from the mesonephric duct. The majority of RCCs are probably derived from the metanephric portion of the kidney.

Collecting duct carcinoma characteristically has a mixed tubular-papillary growth pattern |i18.29|. The cells are present singly and in clusters, tubules, and occasionally papillary groups. They are medium-sized with scant to moderate amounts of finely granular cytoplasm and high N/C ratios. The nuclei are mildly pleomorphic with coarse hyperchromatic chromatin and inconspicuous to prominent nucleoli. Some cases of collecting duct carcinoma are mucin-positive and, thus, an exception to the general rule that RCC is mucin-negative. The cytologic findings are reminiscent of carcinoma of the breast.

18.3.4 Chromophobe Cell RCC

Chromophobe cell RCC accounts for approximately 5% of renal epithelial tumors. Most patients are middle-aged, and the sexes are equally affected. It has a better prognosis than ordinary RCC. The tumor is thought to arise from intercalated cells in the collecting ducts. The gross appearance is similar to onco-cytoma (mahogany brown), although there is no central scar, and hemorrhage and necrosis may occur. Multiple chromosomal monosomies have been reported in this tumor.

The cytology shows polygonal cells with moderate to abundant and pale to granular cytoplasm, some with character-istic perinuclear pale zones |i18.30|. A few cases show more intense cytoplasmic staining, similar to oncocytes |i18.31|. The nuclei vary in size and have irregular outlines; binucleation is common. The chromatin is coarse and granular, and nucleoli are conspicuous. The cells are reminiscent of oncocytes or hepato-cytes. Metachromatic hyaline globules may be seen in some cells |i18.32|. Characteristically, the cells stain positive with Hale colloidal iron and show paranuclear cytoplasmic vesicles by elec-tron microscopy. Keratin, but not vimentin, is expressed, in contrast with ordinary RCC (both are expressed).

18.3.5 Oncocytoma and Oncocytic Neoplasms

Oncocytoma is a controversial renal cortical neoplasm. If strict criteria are followed in diagnosis, ie, a tumor composed exclusively of well-differentiated (nuclear grade 1) oncocytes, malignant behavior is rare. If cytologic atypia is present, there is a risk of malignancy. Because of possible sampling error, the desig-nation *oncocytic neoplasm* is better than oncocytoma for a biopsy diagnosis. Oncocytomas lack the characteristic cytogenetic abnormality (affecting chromosome 3) of ordinary RCC but may have other chromosome alterations, such as loss of chromo-somes 1 and Y. Oncocytomas are usually diploid but can be tetraploid or aneuploid; hence, ploidy cannot help distinguish between benign and malignant oncocytic renal neoplasms.

Oncocytomas account for about 5% of all renal neoplasms. Like RCC, oncocytomas have a propensity to occur in older men. They also occur in women and, rarely, in adoles-cents. Oncocytomas are usually asymptomatic, even when large. Oncocytomas average about 6 cm; many are larger than 10 cm. They are usually solitary, well-circumscribed, and encapsulated. Larger tumors usually have a central stellate fibrous scar, an almost pathognomonic gross appearance, that can be detected on diagnostic imaging studies. Another characteristic gross feature of this tumor is its uniform mahogany (ie, reddish-tan) appearance. There is no necrosis or hemorrhage, and oncocy-toma also lacks the typical variegated appearance of RCC. Some oncocytomas are bilateral, a few are multicentric, and an occa-sional one is cystic. Locally aggressive behavior, such as capsular or renal vein invasion, is evidence of malignant potential.

The FNA biopsy specimen is cellular and contains a monotonous population of oncocytes, isolated and in small loose

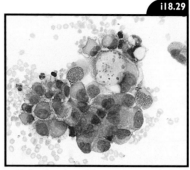
Collecting duct CA—mucin vacuole (DQ)

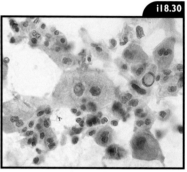
Chromophobe carcinoma (P)

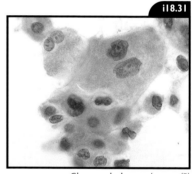
Chromophobe carcinoma (P)

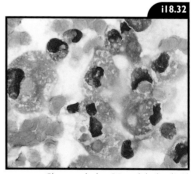
Chromophobe CA—globules (DQ)

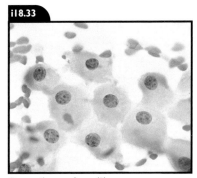

Oncocytic neoplasm (P)

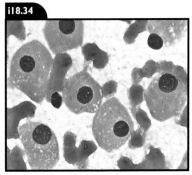

Oncocytic neoplasm (DQ)

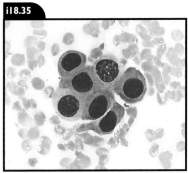

TCC (DQ)

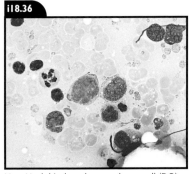

Non-Hodgkin lymphoma—large cell (DQ)

clusters. Oncocytes are large polygonal or rounded cells with abundant finely granular cytoplasm (due to mitochondria) and well-defined cell borders |i18.33|, |i18.34|. By definition, the nuclei are small, uniform, round, and cytologically bland with finely granular chromatin and inconspicuous nucleoli. Mitotic figures are absent.

There is a morphologic spectrum from oncocytoma to oncocytic carcinoma to granular RCC. Although a few cytologically atypical cells can be seen focally in benign tumors (akin to "endocrine atypia"), any significant degree of atypia or pleomorphism carries with it a definite risk of malignant behavior. Benign oncocytoma is never mixed with clear or spindle cells, nor does it exhibit mitosis, necrosis, or more than focal papillary growth. Stains for lipid and glycogen are negative in oncocytoma.

18.3.6 Transitional Cell Carcinoma of the Renal Pelvis

TCC of the renal pelvis accounts for about 5% to 10% of all renal malignancies and about 5% of all urothelial tumors. It usually occurs in an older population, predominantly men. The presenting symptoms of renal pelvic TCC may be similar to those of ordinary RCC. Radiologically, a filling defect of the renal pelvis, with maintenance of the architecture of the rest of the kidney, is characteristic. Stones are found in about 10% of cases. Survival depends on stage and grade of the tumor. Unfortunately, renal TCC is usually infiltrative and high grade when discovered. Metastases occur in lung, liver, lymph node, and bone.

The cytology of TCC is similar to that described in Chapter 5 |i18.35|. Low-grade TCC is characterized by papillary aggregates of minimally abnormal transitional cells with little nuclear atypia, except slight nuclear membrane irregularity. High-grade TCC is characterized by obvious malignant nuclear features, including marked pleomorphism, coarse irregular chromatin, and prominent nucleoli. The cytoplasm is relatively dense with scattered vacuoles. In addition, squamous cells, mucin-positive glandular cells, or mixed adenosquamous features, as well as spindle, clear, or bizarre cells, may be seen. Occasionally, pure squamous cell carcinoma and, rarely, pure adenocarcinoma arise in the renal pelvis.

18.3.7 Lymphoma

Primary malignant lymphoma of the kidney is rare. Most renal lymphomas represent extension from adjacent sites or secondary involvement in generalized disease. Most cases are high-grade non-Hodgkin lymphomas, particularly large cell |i18.36| or Burkitt types. The differential diagnosis includes Wilms tumor and metastatic poorly differentiated carcinoma.

The presence of a single cell pattern and lymphoglandular bodies favors lymphoma.

18.3.8 Sarcoma

Primary sarcomas of the kidney are rare (< 1%). Leiomyosarcoma is, by far, the most common primary renal sarcoma, but virtually any sarcoma could arise in the kidney. Distinction from sarcomatoid RCC, which is more common, may be difficult (look for expression of epithelial antigens). The differential diagnosis also includes renal angiomyolipoma and adrenal cortical spindle cell carcinoma. The prognosis is poor.

18.3.9 Metastasis

Metastases to the kidney are more common than primary renal neoplasms, but they usually are diagnosed only at autopsy. Most cases are asymptomatic, but patients can have features of primary RCC, such as flank pain, hematuria, or mass. Adenocarcinoma of the breast, lung, pancreas, and stomach, as well as lymphoma and melanoma, are common sources |i18.37|. However, the tumor with the greatest propensity to metastasize to a kidney is carcinoma of the other kidney.

18.4 Malignant Renal Tumors in Children

Malignant renal tumors of children are rare. Among these cancers, Wilms tumor is by far the most common, accounting for about 85% of cases. Other pediatric renal tumors include anaplastic Wilms tumor, rhabdoid tumor, mesoblastic nephroma, and clear cell sarcoma.

18.4.1 Wilms Tumor

Wilms tumor, also known as nephroblastoma |i18.38|, is the most common renal malignancy of infancy and childhood; most patients are younger than 3 years old, and 90% are younger than 10 years old. Boys and girls are affected equally. Rarely, Wilms tumor occurs in adults, is bilateral, or arises in extrarenal locations. Some patients have a genetic predisposition (autosomal dominant inheritance) or chromosome abnormality (trisomy E, deletion in the short arm of chromosome 11). Patients usually have an asymptomatic abdominal mass. Symptoms associated with RCC, such as hematuria and flank pain, may occur. Bone metastases are unusual with Wilms tumor, while lung metastases

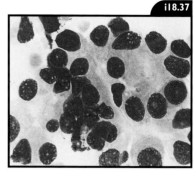
i18.37

Metastatic carcinoma—prostate (DQ)

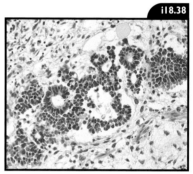
i18.38

Wilms tumor, tissue (H&E)

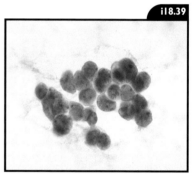
i18.39

Wilms tumor—blastema (P)

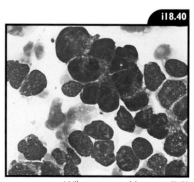
i18.40

Wilms tumor—blastema (DQ)

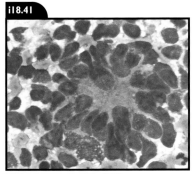

Wilms tumor—rosette (DQ)

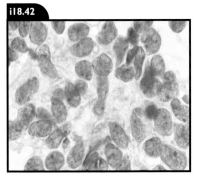

Wilms tumor—tubule formation (P)

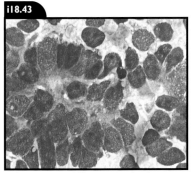

Wilms tumor—differentiation (DQ)

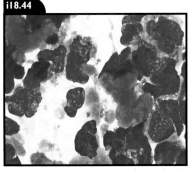

Wilms tumor—basement membrane (DQ)

are frequent, which is the opposite of neuroblastoma, the other common intra-abdominal malignancy of childhood.

The FNA biopsy specimen is usually cellular but may be bloody. Wilms tumor, or nephroblastoma, recapitulates the embryologic development of the kidney, represented by blastema, epithelial cells, and stroma. Any or all of these elements can be seen in Wilms tumor.

Blastema is composed of classic small blue cells about twice the size of a lymphocyte, with dark blue nuclei, fine chromatin, inconspicuous nucleoli, and very scanty cytoplasm |i18.39|, |i18.40|. The cells form dense groups with variable nuclear molding. Occasionally, rosettes are seen |i18.41|. In some cases, the cells are strongly PAS positive.

Epithelial cells are larger than blastema cells, with slightly larger nuclei and more abundant cytoplasm, and they may form nests, glands, and tubules |i18.42| or glomeruloid bodies. Subtle epithelial differentiation may be easier to appreciate in cytologic compared with histologic specimens |i18.43|. The cells may be outlined by or attached to metachromatic basement membrane–like material, as seen in ordinary RCC |i18.44|.

Stromal cells vary morphologically. The most common appearance is spindle cells set in a metachromatic myxoid stroma |i18.45|. The spindle cells (usually fibroblasts) have a small amount of delicate cytoplasm and elongated active nuclei |i18.46|. Well-differentiated muscle, usually smooth muscle but occasionally skeletal muscle (rhabdomyocytes), also can be seen. Rarely, other stromal elements such as bone and cartilage may be present.

The differential diagnosis of Wilms tumor includes a variety of other small blue cell tumors: embryonal rhabdomyosarcoma, Ewing sarcoma, lymphoma, and neuroblastoma. The special features of Wilms tumor are the presence of stroma, epithelium, tubules, or glomeruloid bodies, in addition to small blue cells.

Anaplastic Wilms Tumor

Cellular anaplasia is the major morphologic correlate of unfavorable outcome of Wilms tumor |i18.47|. Anaplasia consists of a triad of cytologic abnormalities: marked nuclear enlargement (≥ 3 diameters), marked hyperchromasia, and markedly abnormal mitotic figures. These changes are obvious even under scanning power in the microscope but can be focal.

18.4.2 Rhabdoid Tumor

Rhabdoid tumor is a rare, highly aggressive renal tumor that occurs predominantly in infants and young children, more often boys (3:2). Similar tumors have been reported in other body sites.

The FNA biopsy obtains rhabdoid cells (formerly thought to be rhabdomyoblasts), which have characteristic, dense, intracytoplasmic inclusions and nuclei with prominent nucleoli |i18.48|. The inclusions are composed of intermediate filaments, mostly vimentin. By definition, there is no tissue-specific differentiation. In addition, spindle cells and, occasionally, multinucleated giant cells may be seen. Naked nuclei and mitotic figures are common. Intracytoplasmic inclusions occur in a wide variety of other tumors and are not specific for rhabdoid tumor.

18.4.3 Clear Cell Sarcoma of the Kidney

Clear cell sarcoma of the kidney is a rare but aggressive tumor of young children, with a propensity to metastasize to bone, particularly the skull.

The FNA biopsy obtains bland, polygonal, stellate, or spindle-shaped cells in small clusters or singly, often loosely arranged in a myxoid background.

18.4.4 Mesoblastic Nephroma

Mesoblastic nephroma is a low-grade malignancy, most commonly seen in newborns (congenital) or infants. The FNA biopsy obtains a scant amount of material in a clean background. The cytology shows clustered and single mildly pleomorphic round or spindle cells with minimal nuclear atypia, coarse chromatin, and scanty cytoplasm. Occasionally, heterologous elements (cartilage) may be present. However, there is no blastema or epithelial, tubular, or glomeruloid differentiation.

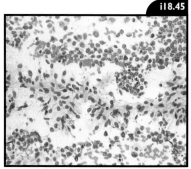

i18.45

Wilms tumor—stroma (P)

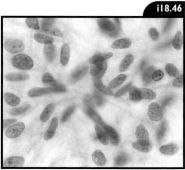

i18.46

Wilms tumor—stromal cells (P)

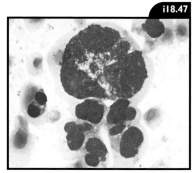

i18.47

Wilms tumor—anaplasia (DQ)

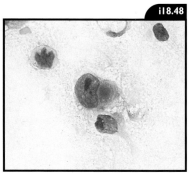

i18.48

Rhabdoid cell (DQ)

CHAPTER NINETEEN

Adrenal Glands

O On top of the kidneys sit the adrenal glands, which are small, paired, retroperitoneal organs. The normal weight of each adrenal gland is about 4 to 5 g. The adrenal gland is composed of an outer rind, the cortex, which makes up about 90% of the gland, and a soft inner core, the medulla. The cortex and medulla are actually separate glands of different embryologic origins (coelomic mesoderm and neural crest, respectively) |i19.1|, |i19.2|.

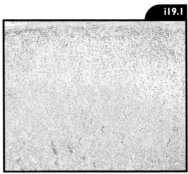

Adrenal cortex, tissue (H&E)

The adrenal cortex manufactures steroid hormones, including mineralocorticoids, primarily aldosterone, and glucocorticoids, eg, hydrocortisone or cortisol. The adrenal gland is also an important extragonadal source of sex hormones—estrogens and androgens. The adrenal medulla is a component of the sympathetic nervous system. It produces catecholamines, particularly norepinephrine and epinephrine, involved in the "fight or flight" reaction.

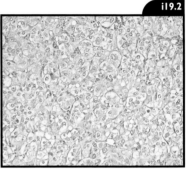

Adrenal medulla, tissue (H&E)

19.1 Evaluation of Patients With Adrenal Masses

Asymptomatic adrenal masses are commonly discovered incidentally during investigation of another disease, raising the spectre of metastatic tumor. In patients without a history of malignancy, most incidental adrenal masses are benign (mostly adenomatous nodules). Even in patients with a known history of malignancy, up to half of newly found adrenal masses are benign. Functioning primary adrenal tumors are rare.

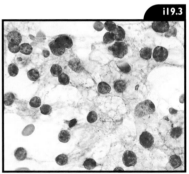

Adrenocortical cells (P)

19.2 Adrenal Cortex

19.2.1 The Cells

Adrenal cortical cells are normally found in fine needle aspiration (FNA) biopsy specimens in cords, small aggregates, or singly. The cells are generally uniform and polygonal; however, cytologic atypia can be seen even in a normal gland ("endocrine atypia") |i19.3|, |i19.4|.

The nuclei are usually round and uniform with granular chromatin and distinct nucleoli. However, focal, marked nuclear abnormalities, including pleomorphism, multiple large nucleoli, and binucleation, can occur in benign cells. Intranuclear cytoplasmic invaginations also can be seen. The cytoplasm ranges from

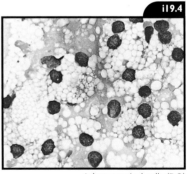

Adrenocortical cells (DQ)

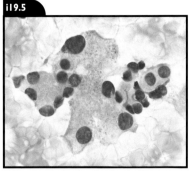

Adrenocortical cells—lipofuscin (P)

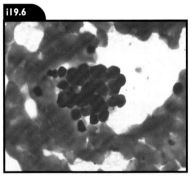

Naked nuclei mimic small cell CA (DQ)

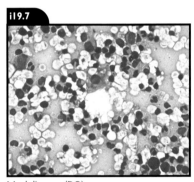

Myelolipoma (DQ)

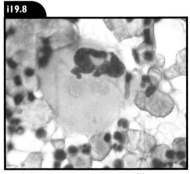

Myelolipoma—megakaryocyte (P)

finely lipid vacuolated to dense. Lipofuscin vacuoles may be seen in dense cytoplasm |i19.5|. Naked nuclei are common and can mimic lymphoma or small cell carcinoma |i19.6|. The background shows microvesicular fat but is otherwise clean.

19.2.2 Adrenal Cysts

Pseudocysts, without an epithelial lining, are the most common clinically recognized type of adrenal cyst. Pseudocysts are thought to result from hemorrhage followed by organization. The causes of adrenal hemorrhage encompass trauma (including birth trauma), burns, sepsis, and shock, as well as bleeding disorders or leukemia.

Epithelial cysts include cystic adenomas and mesothelial cysts. Rarely, small adrenal cysts are associated with hypertension, Cushing syndrome, or virilization. Parasitic cysts, eg, echinococcal cysts, also can occur in the adrenal gland. FNA biopsy is performed primarily to exclude malignancy, but cyst drainage can be curative.

The FNA biopsy obtains turbid or clear yellow fluid, which can be thin or viscous. Turbidity correlates with the presence of cholesterol crystals, other lipids, and proteinaceous debris. The fluid is usually sparsely cellular, consisting predominantly of foamy macrophages and a few leukocytes. A few benign adrenal epithelial cells also may be present. In hemorrhagic cysts, blood and hemosiderin-laden macrophages are seen.

19.2.3 Adrenal Myelolipoma

Adrenal myelolipoma is a rare, hormonally inactive, benign tumor of the adrenal gland or, rarely, other sites. Myelolipomas occur over a wide age range but are usually diagnosed in middle age. Women and men are equally affected. Most are asymptomatic incidental findings that FNA biopsy can help distinguish from more ominous lesions of the adrenal gland. Myelolipomas are usually unilateral and range in size from minute to massive.

The FNA biopsy specimen consists, in essence, of mature adipose tissue and immature hematopoietic cells in variable proportions |i19.7|. The hematopoietic elements can include megakaryocytes, immature granulocytes, erythroid precursors, eosinophils, and lymphocytes, resembling an aspiration of bone marrow (best appreciated in Diff-Quik). The single most helpful cell in the diagnosis of adrenal myelolipoma is the megakaryocyte |i19.8|.

19.2.4 Inflammatory Lesions of the Adrenal Gland

The anti-inflammatory action of adrenal steroid hormones provides a protected environment for certain microorganisms to flourish. Fungus (eg, *Histoplasma* species, *Cryptococcus* species), mycobacteria, and viruses (cytomegalovirus, herpes) are among the most common infectious agents. Cytomegalovirus infection is particularly common in patients with AIDS.

The FNA biopsy of an adrenal abscess consists of an abundance of neutrophils with necrotic debris. A specific infectious agent may be identified. The biopsy is useful in excluding neoplastic disease, and material can be obtained for culture and special stains.

19.2.5 Hyperplasia, Adenoma, and Adenomatous Nodules

Adrenal Hyperplasia

Adrenal cortical hyperplasia can be hormonally functional, eg, producing Cushing syndrome (hypercortisolism) or Conn syndrome (hyperaldosteronism), or nonfunctional, ie, unassociated with clinical symptoms. In adults, an adrenal gland that weighs more than 6 g is considered enlarged. Grossly, adrenal cortical hyperplasia can be diffuse or nodular. Large hyperplastic nodules are commonly referred to as "adenomas," but only very rarely are they true neoplasms (see "Adenomatous Nodules," below).

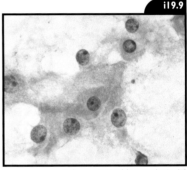

Adrenocortical hyperplasia (P)

Adrenal Cortical Adenoma

True adenomas usually maintain some semblance of normal hormonal function. Therefore, the contralateral gland and the uninvolved portion of the ipsilateral gland usually are suppressed, or at least not hyperplastic, in contrast with nodular hyperplasia. A true adenoma is usually solitary, encapsulated, and clearly demarcated, and it compresses the adjacent gland. Adenomas are usually less than 4 cm in diameter but can grow larger. Grossly, the lesions are usually bright yellow but may be black owing to massive lipofuscin accumulation (black adenoma). Black adenomas have no special clinical significance other than their striking appearance. Hemorrhage is rare, and necrosis is absent.

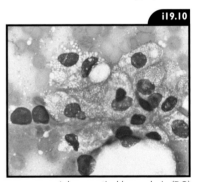

Adrenocortical hyperplasia (DQ)

Adenomatous Nodules

Nodules of the adrenal gland are common, and the incidence increases with age. Adenomatous nodules also can occur in patients with diabetes mellitus, hypertension, and certain malignancies, including renal cell carcinoma (RCC). Nodular adrenal hyperplasia can be associated with normal function, hyperfunction, or hypofunction, including hormonal syndromes such as Cushing or Conn syndromes. Prominent hyperplastic nodules are commonly, though incorrectly, designated adenomas. Diagnostic imaging studies may demonstrate a small nodule, usually less than 3 cm, with the remainder of the gland, as well as the contralateral gland, being relatively unremarkable. The radiologic appearance

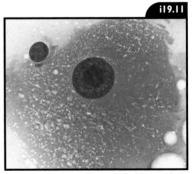

Adrenocortical hyperplasia

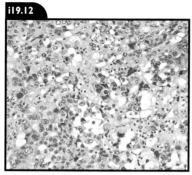

Adrenocortical carcinoma, tissue (H&E)

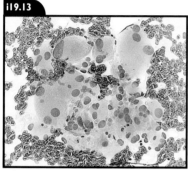

Adrenocortical carcinoma (P)

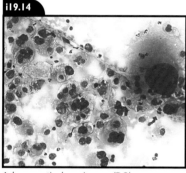

Adrenocortical carcinoma (DQ)

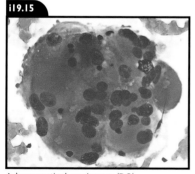

Adrenocortical carcinoma (DQ)

of an adenomatous nodule cannot be distinguished from a metastasis; either lesion can be bilateral.

FNA Biopsy of Adenomas and Adenomatous Nodules

The FNA biopsy of a normal, hyperplastic, or neoplastic adrenal gland can show similar cytologic findings. The needle obtains loose aggregates, fascicles, or whorls of cells with small uniform nuclei and indistinct cell borders. The cytologic studies may show essentially normal-appearing adrenal cortical cells (previously described) in a microvesicular lipid background |i19.9|, |i19.10|. Oncocytic adenomas (due to mitochondria) and black adenomas (due to marked lipofuscin accumulation) occur rarely. Spironolactone bodies, which are laminated cytoplasmic inclusions, may occur in aldosteronomas treated with spironolactone. As is common in benign endocrine tumors, focal cytologic atypia may be present, which has no clinical significance ("endocrine atypia") |i19.11|. However, no necrosis and, at most, rare mitotic figures are present.

The distinction among adrenal cortical hyperplasia, adenoma, and (well-differentiated) carcinoma can be difficult or impossible by cytology alone, because any of these lesions can be composed of essentially normal-appearing cells. Clinical features, including size of the tumor, symptoms, or endocrine function, are important in the differential diagnosis.

19.2.6 Adrenal Cortical Carcinoma

Adrenal cortical carcinoma is a very rare and usually highly aggressive tumor |i19.12|. Men and women are equally affected, but women tend to be younger at diagnosis (mean age, 40 vs 50 years). A few cases are bilateral. Metastases are commonly present in liver, lymph node, or lung and provide definite proof of malignancy. Adrenal cortical carcinomas are usually larger than 6 cm, frequently encapsulated, and often functional.

The FNA biopsy obtains an abundance of poorly cohesive aggregates, disorderly clusters, and single cells. The cytologic appearance ranges from bland adrenal cortical cells to anaplastic malignant tumor cells |i19.13|, |i19.14|, |i19.15|, |i19.16|, |i19.17|. Cytoplasmic lipid content tends to decrease with increasing atypia. Spindle cells or bizarre tumor giant cells may be seen |i19.18|. Some tumor cells surround capillaries or are embedded in metachromatic stroma. Necrosis, hemorrhage, fibrosis, and calcification are common in carcinomas; in some cases, there is a prominent neutrophilic infiltrate. Note that highly atypical cells can occur focally in adenomas, and, conversely, rare cases of cancer are composed of benign-appearing cells. Atypical mitotic figures and, of course, metastases, indicate malignancy.

19.3 Adrenal Medulla

19.3.1 The Cells

Adrenal medullary cells are polygonal to elongated and vary more in size and shape than adrenal cortical cells. The cytoplasm is finely granular and contains neurosecretory granules (epinephrine, norepinephrine) and, frequently, lipofuscin. Intracytoplasmic hyaline globules, probably of lysosomal origin, are common. The nucleus has granular chromatin and a distinct nucleolus.

19.3.2 Pheochromocytoma and Paragangliomas

Paragangliomas, including pheochromocytomas, are neurogenic tumors of neural crest origin showing gangliocytic differentiation. They produce catecholamines and express neuroendocrine cell markers. Pheochromocytomas arise from the sympathetic nervous system and can be adrenal (vast majority) or extra-adrenal in origin; they frequently are associated with clinical symptoms due to overproduction of catecholamines. Paragangliomas arise from parasympathetic-related organs, including chemoreceptors; they usually are associated with symptoms related to neuroendocrine hyperfunction.

Although rare, pheochromocytoma is the most common primary tumor of the adrenal medulla. Intermittent paroxysmal hypertension accompanied by sweating and palpitations constitute the classic clinical triad characteristic of pheochromocytoma, although the full triad is not always present. The signs and symptoms of pheochromocytoma are due to secretion of epinephrine, norepinephrine, or both by the tumor. Plasma levels and urinary excretion of catecholamines or their metabolite, vanillylmandelic acid, are usually (90%) increased in patients with pheochromocytoma, providing a useful diagnostic test.

Pheochromocytoma is known as the "10% tumor." About 10% affect children; about 10% occur in extra-adrenal sites in adults (in children, about half are extra-adrenal, particularly organ of Zuckerkandl); about 10% are bilateral; about 10% are familial (including clinical syndromes, such as multiple endocrine neoplasia, von Recklinghausen neurofibromatosis, von Hippel-Lindau syndrome [renal, hepatic, and pancreatic cysts, RCC, angiomatosis, and cerebellar hemangioblastoma], and Sturge-Weber syndrome [cavernous hemangiomas in fifth cranial nerve distribution]); and about 10% are malignant.

Unfortunately, pheochromocytoma is a rare situation in which FNA biopsy can be dangerous. Biopsy can possibly induce fatal hypertensive crisis or uncontrollable hemorrhage. Complications also have occurred, very rarely, with aspiration of paragangliomas (see Chapter 7) |i19.19|.

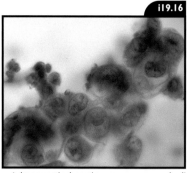
i19.16
Adrenocortical carcinoma—macronucleoli

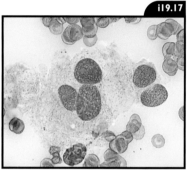
i19.17
Adrenocortical carcinoma (P)

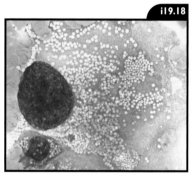
i19.18
Adrenocortical carcinoma—giant cell (DQ)

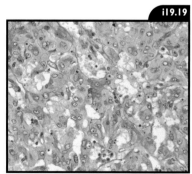
i19.19
Pheochromocytoma, tissue (H&E)

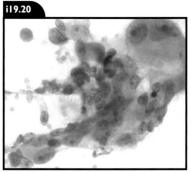

Pheochromocytoma (P)

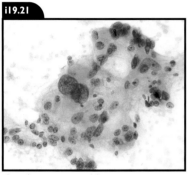

Pheochromocytoma (P)

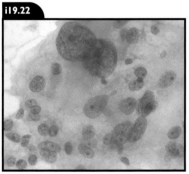

Pheochromocytoma (P)

FNA Biopsy of Pheochromocytoma/Paraganglioma

The FNA biopsy specimen is cellular, obtaining loose aggregates, rosettes, and single cells with ill-defined cell borders. In cell blocks, characteristic "Zellballen" may be seen. The cytologic appearance ranges from relatively bland-appearing, carcinoid-like cells to highly anaplastic tumor cells |i19.20|, |i19.21|, |i19.22|. Generally, however, the cells fall into three categories: epithelioid, spindle, and ganglion. The epithelioid cells can be small and round, essentially identical in appearance to cells derived from carcinoid (neuroendocrine) tumors. Spindle cells are commonly present, and in a few cases, they predominate. The combination of carcinoid-like cells and spindle cells in an adrenal aspirate suggests the diagnosis of pheochromocytoma. The cytoplasm of these cells may have a dusting of fine red (metachromatic) neurosecretory granules in Diff-Quik. Hyaline globules can be seen in some cases. The nuclei range from round or oval and uniform to pleomorphic. The nuclei typically have a "salt-and-pepper" chromatin pattern, but the chromatin texture is variable. Intranuclear cytoplasmic invaginations can be seen. Nuclear atypia does not correlate well with biologic behavior.

Ganglion cells are elongated giant cells with eccentric, sometimes multiple, nuclei, prominent nucleoli, and abundant cytoplasm that may contain Nissl granules (rough endoplasmic reticulum and ribosomes). Sustentacular cells (strongly S-100 positive) also may be present; their absence correlates with malignancy.

Argyrophilic silver stains (eg, Grimelius) are usually positive for neurosecretory granules (epinephrine, norepinephrine), in contrast with adrenal cortical neoplasms. Chromogranin and synaptophysin are typically positive, but keratin is usually negative. Stromal amyloid is present in many cases (Congo red stain and polarization microscopy, showing typical apple green birefringence).

19.3.3 Neuroblastoma, Ganglioneuroblastoma, and Ganglioneuroma

Neuroblastoma is the most common solid (ie, nonlymphoreticular) extracranial malignancy of children. It usually occurs in patients younger than 5 years but occasionally occurs in older children or even adults. Males are slightly more commonly affected than females. Most neuroblastomas arise in the adrenal medulla. Most of the rest occur in sites associated with the sympathetic nervous system, usually in the mediastinum, head and neck, or pelvis. Tumors in adults usually occur peripherally. The differential diagnosis includes metastatic small cell carcinoma of the lung in adults and other small cell tumors, such as Ewing sarcoma, PNET, and Wilms tumor, in children (see Chapter 8).

Neuroblastoma is a classic "small blue cell tumor" |i19.23|, |i19.24|. The cells have hyperchromatic, round, or slightly lobulated nuclei and scanty cytoplasm with an occasional cytoplasmic tag. Primitive neuroblastomas lack features of differentiation and are diffusely composed of these small blue cells. More differentiated tumors are less cellular and have more extracellular matrix (neuropil, ie, tangled neurites). The differentiated cells are larger with more vesicular nuclei containing nucleoli. Homer Wright rosettes, ie, cells arranged around central neuropil, may be seen. Electron microscopy or immunocytochemistry may demonstrate neurosecretory granules. Occasionally, heterologous differentiation, eg, rhabdomyoblasts, may be identified.

Neuroblasts can differentiate into ganglion cells (also Schwann cells), and tumors representing various stages of maturation can be seen. Ganglion cells are larger than neuroblasts with more abundant cytoplasm, finer chromatin, and prominent nucleoli.

Ganglioneuroblastoma is composed of both neuroblasts and ganglion cells. The tumor is of intermediate malignancy |i19.25|.

Ganglioneuroma is a fully differentiated tumor, lacks a neuroblast component, and is benign. Ganglioneuromas usually occur in older patients, more commonly in the posterior mediastinum or retroperitoneum than in the adrenal gland, where they are rare (see Chapter 15).

19.3.4 Metastases

Metastases are far more common than primary malignancies of the adrenal gland. Lung, breast, renal cell, and colorectal carcinomas and melanoma are particularly frequent sources of metastases.

The FNA biopsy obtains cells whose cytomorphology depends on the nature of the patient's primary tumor. If possible, compare the cells in question with those from the primary lesion to see if they "match." Metastatic adenocarcinoma can mimic benign adrenal cortical cells in some cases. RCC is suggested by gland or papillary formation, significant glycogen content, and erythrophagocytosis. Hormonal syndromes related to glucocorticoids, mineralocorticoids, or sex hormones favor a diagnosis of adrenocortical carcinoma but do not completely exclude RCC, the "great imitator" (see Chapter 18). However, the differential diagnosis of adrenal cortical neoplasms and RCC may be impossible with light microscopy alone, and special studies may be needed. Adrenal cortical neoplasms are characterized ultrastructurally by abundant smooth endoplasmic reticulum and mitochondria with characteristic vesicular cristae. RCC is characterized by cells with long microvilli forming glands. Immunocytochemically, epithelial membrane antigen and keratin are usually negative or only focally positive in adrenal cortical neoplasms, but they are usually positive in RCC. Either tumor may be vimentin positive.

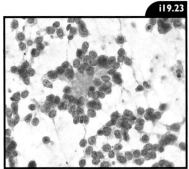

i19.23

Neuroblastoma—rosette (P)

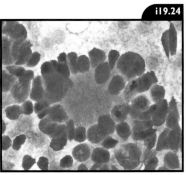

i19.24

Neuroblastoma—rosette (DQ)

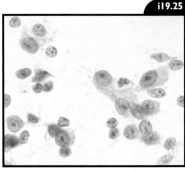

i19.25

Ganglioneuroblastoma (P)

Mucin positivity strongly suggests metastatic carcinoma and at the same time makes both renal and adrenal neoplasms highly unlikely. Note that certain tumors, such as melanoma and RCC, may share ultrastructural features of primary adrenocortical neoplasms, such as melanin and lipid, respectively.

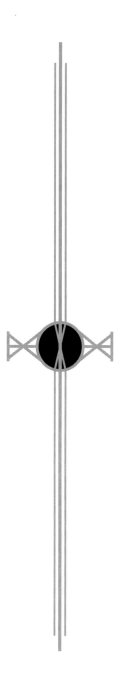

Gonads

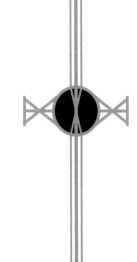

Yin and yang, the gonads include female ovaries and male testes. Some gonadal diseases are similar or identical whether occurring in the testes or the ovaries (eg, sex cord stromal and germ cell tumors [GCTs]); others are unique to the specific organ. Fine needle aspiration (FNA) biopsy of the male genital system (exclusive of prostate) and the female pelvis also are discussed in this chapter.

20.1 Testis and Male Genital System (Exclusive of Prostate)

Incisional (tissue) biopsy of a testicular malignancy carries a significant risk of spread of the tumor. However, the risk is low to nonexistent with FNA biopsy. Still, FNA biopsy of testis is seldom performed because most testicular masses (95%) are malignant, and the dogma is that biopsy is superfluous. FNA biopsy of other scrotal contents is more common, and most scrotal lesions, exclusive of testis, are benign. The most common scrotal lesions are cysts (eg, hydroceles, spermatoceles) and inflammatory lesions, followed by tumors, vascular lesions, and miscellaneous conditions (eg, hernias, lipomas).

20.1.1 The Cells

Seminiferous tubules contain two cell populations: spermatogenic cells and Sertoli cells (supporting cells). The stroma contains androgen-producing Leydig cells, which are necessary for spermatogenesis.

Spermatogonia, spermatocytes, and *spermatids* are primitive cells with round central nuclei, enlarged nucleoli, and homogeneous cytoplasm. Primary and secondary spermatocytes and spermatids are transitional forms to mature spermatozoa.

Sertoli cells are large polygonal cells with finely vacuolated cytoplasm and round to oval vesicular nuclei and prominent nucleoli.

Leydig cells are large with central nuclei and abundant granular cytoplasm. They may contain Reinke crystals.

20.1.2 Cysts, Inflammations, and Neoplasms

Hydrocele: The FNA biopsy obtains clear amber fluid with few cells (macrophages, inflammatory cells, reactive mesothelial cells).

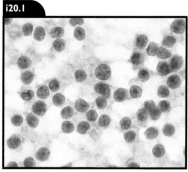

Lymphoma/leukemia—relapse of ALL (P)

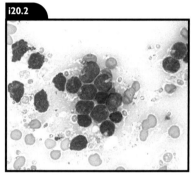

Lymphoma/leukemia—relapse of ALL (DQ)

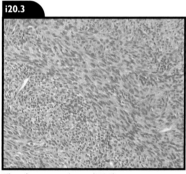

Fibrothecoma, tissue (H&E)

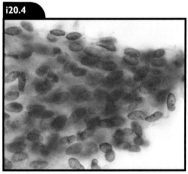

Fibrothecoma (P)

Spermatocele: The FNA biopsy shows sperm, macrophages (characteristically ingesting sperm), and protein precipitate.

Hematocele: Hematocele is usually the result of injury and shows red- to chocolate-colored fluid containing intact or degenerated RBCs and hemosiderin-laden macrophages.

Orchitis, Epididymitis: The FNA biopsy shows acute or chronic inflammation and possibly reparative cells. Various organisms, ranging from acid-fast bacilli to *Filaria*, may be identified.

Adenomatoid Tumor: Adenomatoid tumor is the most common tumor of the paratesticular tissue (epididymis, tunica, spermatic cord) and also occurs in females (uterus, fallopian tube, ovary, and paraovarian tissue). The FNA biopsy obtains sheets and multilayered or branching clusters of bland, monotonous, mesothelial-like cells.

Malignant Lymphoma, Leukemia: Malignant lymphoma is more common in men 50 years of age or older and is rare in younger men or boys. However, testicular involvement by acute lymphoblastic leukemia (ALL) is relatively common in boys |**i20.1**|, |**i20.2**|. Lymphoma also can involve the ovary.

The cytology shows the usual diagnostic features, including dispersed lymphoid cells and lymphoglandular bodies. Many cases of primary testicular lymphoma show lymphoplasmacytoid differentiation. Extramedullary plasmacytoma/myeloma also can be encountered in FNA biopsy of the testis.

Other Malignant Tumors: Rarely, other soft tissue tumors, including embryonal rhabdomyosarcoma, arise in the testis (see Chapter 9).

20.2 Gonadal Tumors

20.2.1 Gonadal Sex Cord Stromal Tumors

In practice, gonadal sex cord tumors, such as Sertoli tumors and granulosa cell tumors, may be difficult to distinguish from one another, as well as from Brenner tumors, by cytology alone.

Ovarian Fibroma/Thecoma

Ovarian fibroma/thecoma |**i20.3**| usually has a low cell yield on FNA biopsy. The tumor is composed of spindle cells |**i20.4**|. Fibroma cells are thin and spindly. Thecoma cells are plumper spindle cells with more irregular nuclei and more abundant, fragile, lipid vacuolated cytoplasm. The cervicovaginal Pap smear may show increased maturation in postmenopausal patients owing to estrogen production by the tumor. The differential diagnosis includes leiomyoma.

Granulosa Cell Tumor

Granulosa cell tumor is a low-grade malignancy; late recurrences are well known, clinically. Call-Exner bodies are particularly characteristic |i20.5|, |i20.6|. These are small spaces containing pale to dense material or degenerated nuclei surrounded by small tumor cells. The tumor cells have pale cytoplasm and uniform round nuclei with characteristic nuclear membrane irregularities (including classic "coffee bean" nuclei) |i20.7|.

Leydig Cell Tumor (Interstitial Cell Tumor)

Leydig cell tumors are rare neoplasms that are usually benign. The FNA biopsy obtains large monomorphic cells with round uniform nuclei and abundant cytoplasm, which may contain characteristic long, rectangular Reinke crystalloids |i20.8|.

Sertoli Cell Tumor

Sertoli cell tumor is a rare tumor composed of cells that resemble normal Sertoli cells. The FNA biopsy shows a glandular pattern composed of columnar cells with cytoplasmic tails and uniform oval nuclei, prominent nucleoli, and irregular chromatin. Large cell and malignant variants also occur.

20.2.2 Germ Cell Tumors

Germ cells are associated with at least five distinct neoplasms: germinoma (seminoma in males, dysgerminoma in females), embryonal carcinoma, yolk sac tumor (endodermal sinus tumor), teratomas (including benign mature teratomas and malignant immature teratomas), and choriocarcinoma. Germinoma is probably the most primitive of the GCTs and acts as a precursor to the other types. Mixtures of cell types are common in GCTs; thus, sampling may be a problem in biopsy diagnosis.

GCTs can occur at any age but are most common in adolescents and young adults, and they usually arise in the gonads. Primary extragonadal GCTs are rare and usually arise in midline structures, eg, sacrococcygeal region, mediastinum, or pineal gland. GCTs often produce β-human chorionic gonadotropin (βHCG) or α-fetoprotein (AFP), which can be detected in the serum or demonstrated immunocytochemically. Rarely, non-GCTs, eg, hepatocellular, lung, pancreas, gastric, or renal cell carcinomas, produce βHCG or AFP. Germinomas are keratin negative, but other GCTs are usually positive.

Germinoma (Seminoma/Dysgerminoma)

Germinoma is an undifferentiated tumor of germ cell origin. It is the most common GCT of the testis (seminoma) and also the most common malignant GCT of the ovary (dysgerminoma). Germinomas are highly radiosensitive.

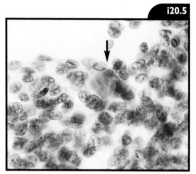

Granulosa cell tumor—Call-Exner body (P)

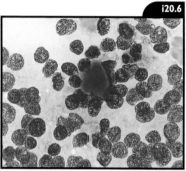

Granulosa cell tumor—Call-Exner body (DQ)

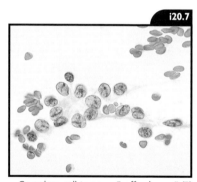

Granulosa cell tumor—"coffee beans" (P)

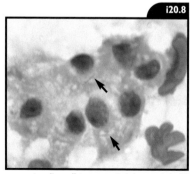

Leydig cell tumor—Reinke crystals (P)

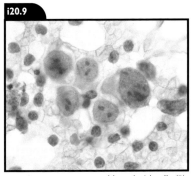

Germinoma—tumor and lymphoid cells (P)

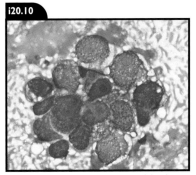

Germinoma—tigroid background (DQ)

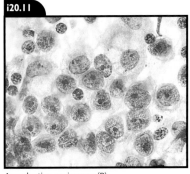

Anaplastic seminoma (P)

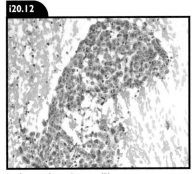

Embryonal carcinoma (P)

The FNA biopsy specimen shows a dual cell population of malignant germinoma cells and reactive chronic inflammation |**i20.9**|. Germinoma cells are large, round, and poorly cohesive. They are obviously malignant appearing, yet rather uniform. The nuclei are large with fine pale chromatin and one or more small to large nucleoli. Naked nuclei are often numerous. The cytoplasm is clear (in Papanicolaou stain) or has sharply punched-out glycogen vacuoles (in Diff-Quik stain).

Chronic inflammation, including lymphoid cells, plasma cells, and eosinophils, is variable. Granulomas are commonly seen and provide a clue to the diagnosis. Isolated syncytiotrophoblast-like multinucleated giant cells also may be seen. These cells may secrete βHCG.

A characteristic feature of germinomas is the presence of a tiger-striped or "tigroid" background |**i20.10**| consisting of interwoven, lacy, PAS-positive material, best appreciated in air-dried slides. Although a tigroid background provides a clue to the diagnosis, it can be seen in other glycogen-rich tumors and may be absent in anaplastic and spermatocytic seminomas. Necrosis is common and may be extensive.

Spermatocytic Seminoma: Spermatocytic seminoma is an unusual, more differentiated variant of seminoma that only occurs in the testis, usually in men 40 years of age or older, and has an excellent prognosis. The FNA biopsy specimen shows round cells that can vary considerably in size, ranging from lymphocyte-like to giant, with high nuclear/cytoplasmic (N/C) ratios. The most characteristic feature is the spireme appearance of the chromatin (similar to meiotic prophase of normal primary spermatocytes). Other characteristic features of seminoma may not be present, such as cytoplasmic glycogen, lymphoid infiltrate, granulomas, and tigroid background.

Anaplastic Seminoma: Compared with classic seminoma, the cells of anaplastic seminoma are larger and more pleomorphic with large pleomorphic nuclei, coarse irregular chromatin, and more prominent, more often multiple, nucleoli |**i20.11**|. There are many naked nuclei as well as nuclear stream artifact. The tigroid background may be absent. The differential diagnosis includes embryonal carcinoma and poorly differentiated adeno-carcinoma or undifferentiated carcinoma.

Embryonal Carcinoma

The FNA biopsy specimen of embryonal carcinoma is cellular and composed of poorly differentiated epithelial-like cells in large cohesive sheets or papillary groups |**i20.12**|. Single cells also may be seen. The cytoplasm is delicate with indistinct cell borders (syncytial growth pattern). The nuclei are large, irregular, and pleomorphic, with coarse chromatin and prominent irregular nucleoli |**i20.13**|, |**i20.14**|. Numerous mitotic figures, including atypical forms, may be seen. Primitive mesenchymal spindle cells also may be present. Necrosis is common.

The differential diagnosis includes germinoma and poorly differentiated adenocarcinoma or undifferentiated carcinoma. In contrast with germinoma, the cells of embryonal carcinoma are more cohesive, the nuclei are more pleomorphic with coarser chromatin and larger nucleoli, and the tigroid background is absent. Embryonal carcinoma cells also tend to be more cohesive and form larger groups than those of ordinary carcinoma. The clinical history can be very helpful. Expression of AFP or βHCG favors a GCT. Keratin expression helps distinguish embryonal carcinoma (+) from germinoma (−) but not from ordinary carcinoma (+).

Yolk Sac Tumor (Endodermal Sinus Tumor)

Yolk sac tumor, also known as endodermal sinus tumor, is composed of irregular, large, cohesive three-dimensional cell balls and papillae with few single cells. The cells are large with abundant, vacuolated, or bubbly cytoplasm. The nuclei are round to irregular with coarse chromatin and prominent nucleoli. Abnormal mitotic figures may be seen.

There are two characteristic features of yolk sac tumor: Schiller-Duval bodies and hyaline globules. Schiller-Duval bodies are glomeruloid structures formed by invagination of a tuft of malignant cells into an empty space |i20.15|. Hyaline globules are relatively large, round, PAS-positive intracytoplasmic inclusions |i20.16|. They also can be seen free in the background. These bodies contain AFP, which also is usually elevated in the blood serum.

Chronic inflammation, including lymphocytes and plasma cells, and epithelioid histiocytes can be seen. Unique to this GCT is intracellular or extracellular mucoid material. Heterologous elements, including embryonal carcinoma and teratoma, are commonly present in yolk sac tumors.

The differential diagnosis includes other GCTs, particularly embryonal carcinoma, and adenocarcinoma. Yolk sac tumor is characterized by more cellular cohesion and more prominent papillary cluster formation than in embryonal carcinoma. Nucleoli are not as prominent as in embryonal carcinoma or germinoma. However, yolk sac tumor and embryonal carcinoma commonly coexist. Mucin can be seen in adenocarcinoma or yolk sac tumor but is absent in other GCTs. PAS-positive hyaline globules, Schiller-Duval bodies, and clinical features help diagnose yolk sac tumor.

Choriocarcinoma

Choriocarcinoma is rare, particularly when pure, but occurs somewhat more often as a component of other GCTs.

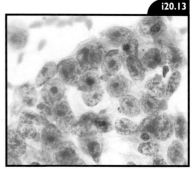

i20.13

Embryonal carcinoma (P)

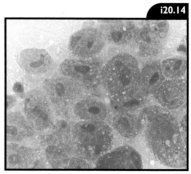

i20.14

Embryonal carcinoma (DQ)

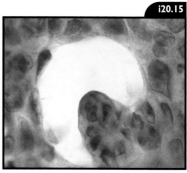

i20.15

Yolk sac tumor—Schiller-Duval body (P)

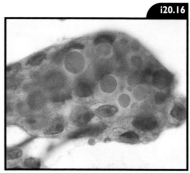

i20.16

Yolk sac tumor—hyaline globules (P)

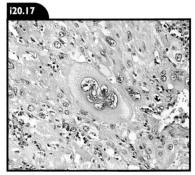

Choriocarcinoma, tissue (H&E)

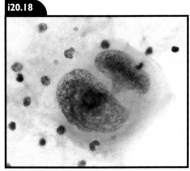

Choriocarcinoma—syncytiotrophoblast (P)

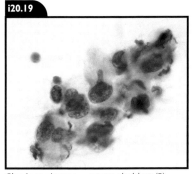

Choriocarcinoma—cytotrophoblast (P)

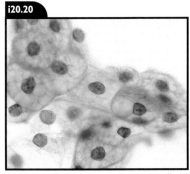

Mature cystic teratoma—sebaceous cells (P)

Also, rarely, it is a component of a poorly differentiated carcinoma. The FNA biopsy specimen shows a characteristic biphasic pattern of cytotrophoblast associated with syncytiotrophoblast; both elements must be present for diagnosis |i20.17|.

Syncytiotrophoblasts are large to giant, pleomorphic, multinucleated, sometimes bizarre-appearing cells |i20.18|. They have pleomorphic hyperchromatic nuclei, prominent irregular nucleoli, and abundant bright blue (in Diff-Quik stain) or eosinophilic (in Papanicolaou stain) cytoplasm that may suggest keratinization.

Cytotrophoblasts are seen in loose clusters and as single smaller cells with indistinct cell borders and pale vacuolated cytoplasm |i20.19|. The nuclei are somewhat pleomorphic, round, and vesicular and have conspicuous nucleoli. Spindle cells also may be present. Hemorrhage and necrosis may be extensive.

Syncytiotrophoblasts are not specific for choriocarcinoma, unless accompanied by cytotrophoblasts. Other pleomorphic malignancies may be considered in the differential diagnosis. Intracytoplasmic βHCG is characteristic of choriocarcinoma but not specific; marked serum elevation of βHCG also is characteristic.

Teratoma

Teratomas are composed of cells from all three germ cell layers (endoderm, mesoderm, and ectoderm).

Mature Cystic Teratoma: Mature cystic teratoma is the most highly differentiated GCT; it is benign. Mature teratomas are predominantly cystic and can grow very large. Calcification is common. The tumor is filled with granular keratinous debris. The FNA biopsy may obtain skin and its appendages (eg, squamous cells, squames, sebaceous cells, hair) |i20.20| and possibly neural, gastrointestinal (including pancreas), cartilage, and ciliated respiratory cells. Granulomas with foreign body giant cells may form in response to keratin. No immature or malignant-appearing cells are present, by definition. In men, the differential diagnosis includes columnar cells and mucus aspirated from a scrotal hernia; in women, it includes squamous contaminants aspirated transvaginally; and in either sex, normal colorectal mucosa, transitional epithelium, mesothelium, or soft tissue is included.

Immature Teratoma: Immature teratoma is usually a solid tumor but can be cystic and is characterized by the presence of immature or malignant cells: epithelial (eg, squamous or adenocarcinoma), mesenchymal (eg, chondrosarcoma or osteosarcoma), or, particularly, neural cells (ie, neuroblasts).

Teratocarcinoma: Teratocarcinoma is the combination of embryonal carcinoma with mature or immature teratoma.

20.3 **Ovary and Female Pelvis**

FNA biopsy of the pelvis can be performed transrectally, transvaginally, transabdominally, or laparoscopically; it is particularly useful in staging or detection of recurrences. Although there is the potential of spillage of malignant cells when aspirating ovarian cysts, the risk is low, particularly for relatively small unilocular cysts.

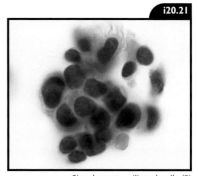
Simple cyst—ciliated cells (P)

20.3.1 Ovarian Cysts

Benign (Simple) Cysts

Benign (simple) cysts include surface germinal epithelial inclusion cysts, paraovarian and paratubal cysts, regressing follicular cysts, and simple serous cysts. These cysts contain clear fluid with a small amount of blood and debris and few cells (mostly macrophages). Psammoma bodies, Curschmann spirals, ciliated cells |i20.21|, and detached ciliary tufts (ciliocytophthoria |i20.22|) sometimes can be seen.

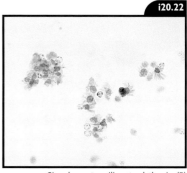
Simple cyst—ciliocytophthoria (P)

Functional Cysts: Follicular Cysts

Follicular cysts are lined by layers of granulosa and theca cells. The FNA biopsy obtains clear, cloudy, or bloody fluid (which has a high estrogen content). The (granulosa) cells can be present singly or in tight clusters and range from small to large |i20.23|. Small cells have a round vesicular nucleus and scant cytoplasm; larger cells have folded, bean-shaped, or grooved nuclei and more abundant granular cytoplasm. Call-Exner bodies may be seen. Some follicular cysts are highly cellular, and the cells may appear atypical (high N/C ratios, hyperchromasia, prominent nucleoli, mitoses), which could result in a false-positive diagnosis.

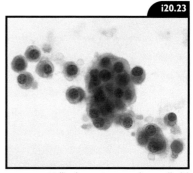
Follicular cyst—granulosa cells (P)

Corpus Luteum Cysts

Corpus luteum cysts are characterized by the presence of luteinized (granulosa) cells. The aspirate may be cellular. Luteinized cells have abundant foamy or granular cytoplasm, sometimes containing fine yellowish pigment and eccentric, small, dark nuclei, sometimes with conspicuous nucleoli or mitotic figures |i20.24|. Single cells resemble macrophages owing to vacuoles and pigment. Fresh and old blood, including hemosiderin-laden macrophages, may be seen in hemorrhagic corpus luteum cysts. Cytoplasmic hyaline globules may occur during pregnancy. In the postpartum period, atypical luteinized cells with increased N/C ratios, irregular nuclei, coarse chromatin, prominent nucleoli, and glandular or papillary formations may be seen.

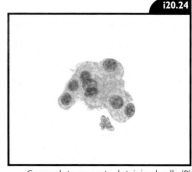
Corpus luteum cyst—luteinized cells (P)

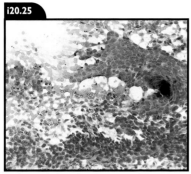

Endometriosis—glands, stroma (P)

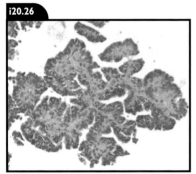

Papillary serous carcinoma, tissue (H&E)

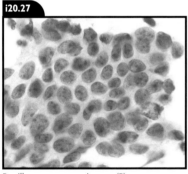

Papillary serous carcinoma (P)

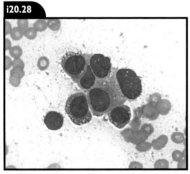

Papillary serous carcinoma (DQ)

Endometriotic Cyst and Endometriosis

The FNA biopsy obtains thick dark brown fluid ("chocolate" cyst). The diagnostic triad consists of hemosiderin-laden macrophages and endometrial epithelial and stromal cells. However, the cellularity is often scant in cysts, consisting only of a few cell balls and macrophages. Degenerated blood may be the only cytologic finding in many cases. The full diagnostic triad is more likely to be found in FNA biopsy of solid endometriosis occurring in diverse sites |**i20.25**|.

20.3.2 Ovarian Epithelial Tumors

The common epithelial tumors of the ovary include serous, mucinous, and endometrioid cell types. Two or more different cell types may be found in a single tumor, although one type usually predominates. It may not be possible to separate low malignant potential, or borderline, tumors from well-differentiated carcinoma based on cytologic studies alone. Moreover, the presence of benign-appearing cells in a biopsy specimen does not exclude the possibility of malignancy in other areas of the tumor.

Brenner Tumor

Brenner tumors are thought to be of transitional cell or urothelial origin. FNA biopsy of a benign Brenner tumor shows clusters and sheets of bland uniform epithelial cells with oval nuclei, irregular, grooved, or coffee bean nuclear membranes, conspicuous nucleoli, and a moderate amount of cytoplasm. Extracellular hyaline globules, which may be fused and multilobated, often are present and usually are surrounded by tumor cells. Borderline and fully malignant varieties of Brenner cell tumors also exist.

Serous Cystadenomas and Carcinomas

Serous cells resemble reactive mesothelial cells, particularly when the tumor is benign or of low-grade malignancy. Some tumor cells may be ciliated; ciliated cells do not completely exclude malignancy in ovarian tumors! Papillary groups and psammoma bodies are characteristic of serous tumors but also can be seen in benign conditions of the ovary and pelvis |**i20.26**|.

FNA biopsy of benign serous tumors typically obtains thin serous fluid with a few, often degenerated, bland cells. Cohesive sheets of uniform mesothelial-like cells with round to oval nuclei, moderate amounts of cytoplasm, well-defined cell borders, and occasional cilia are seen. When well preserved, the nuclei have finely granular chromatin and small nucleoli. Cystadenofibromas may, in addition, yield spindle-shaped stromal cells without atypia.

FNA biopsy of malignant serous tumors obtains thick turbid fluid with increased cellularity, including cell aggregates and single cells |**i20.27**|, |**i20.28**|. Cytologic atypia increases with the grade of the tumor. Malignant atypia includes marked nuclear enlargement, irregular nuclear membranes, hyperchromasia, irregular chromatin, and prominent nucleoli. Psammoma bodies may be present.

FNA biopsy of borderline (low malignant potential) tumors shows sheets and clusters of crowded cells with mild nuclear pleomorphism, irregular nuclear membranes, prominent nucleoli, and increased N/C ratio. Psammoma bodies may be present. The cells appear atypical but not frankly malignant.

The differential diagnosis includes reactive mesothelial cells, papillary mesothelial hyperplasia, endometrioid carcinoma, and metastatic carcinoma.

Mucinous Cystadenomas and Carcinomas

Mucinous tumor cells generally resemble endocervical cells, particularly in benign and low-grade tumors |**i20.29**|.

FNA biopsy of benign lesions characteristically obtains viscous mucus. Tall, uniform, columnar cells with basal bland nuclei, apical mucin vacuolization, and, occasionally, signet ring cells may be seen.

FNA biopsy of malignant lesions obtains highly viscous, sticky mucus with increased cellularity |**i20.30**|. Single cells, irregular clusters, and syncytial fragments with increased cytologic atypia (pleomorphism, multinucleation, coarse chromatin, prominent nucleoli, vacuolated cytoplasm) may be seen, but these findings are often not as prominent as those in serous carcinomas.

Borderline (low malignant potential) lesions show cytologic features intermediate between benign and fully malignant tumors.

The differential diagnosis includes metastatic carcinoma, particularly from the colon or rectum. This differential diagnosis can be very difficult or impossible. However, primary mucinous tumors are rarely bilateral, while metastases commonly are. Colorectal carcinoma often has extensive, "dirty" necrosis. Mucinous ovarian tumors usually have a well-differentiated component. Ovarian carcinoma reacts predominantly with cytokeratin 7 and colonic carcinoma with cytokeratin 20.

Endometrioid Carcinoma

Endometrioid carcinoma resembles serous adenocarcinoma but has scanty, more granular cytoplasm, nuclear crowding, and microacini |**i20.31**|, |**i20.32**|. Squamous differentiation can occur. A mucoid background and hemosiderin-laden macrophages may be seen. The presence of papillae favors a serous tumor. The presence of gross mucoid material favors a mucinous tumor.

Clear Cell Carcinoma

Clear cell carcinoma is characterized by cells with abundant, pale, vacuolated (glycogen) cytoplasm with indistinct cell

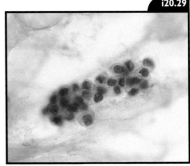

i20.29

Mucinous tumor, low-grade (P)

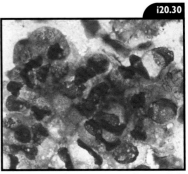

i20.30

Mucinous tumor, malignant (DQ)

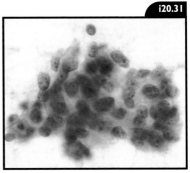

i20.31

Endometrioid carcinoma (P)

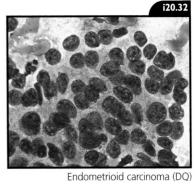

i20.32

Endometrioid carcinoma (DQ)

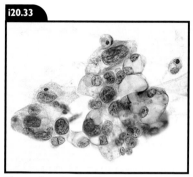

Clear cell carcinoma (P)

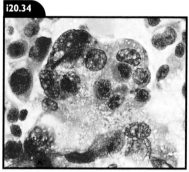

Clear cell carcinoma (DQ)

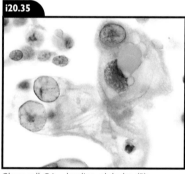

Clear cell CA—hyaline globules (P)

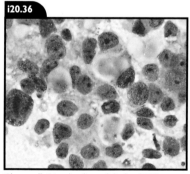

Clear cell CA—hyaline globules (DQ)

borders |i20.33|, |i20.34|. Hyaline cytoplasmic inclusions can be seen |i20.35|, |i20.36|. Although the nuclei can be bland, pleomorphism, binucleation, nuclear irregularities, and macronucleoli commonly are seen. The differential diagnosis includes metastatic renal cell carcinoma.

Miscellaneous Tumors

Undifferentiated carcinoma is characterized by anaplastic malignant tumor cells. Intracytoplasmic hyaline globules may be seen.

Small cell carcinoma is a rare aggressive tumor often associated with hypercalcemia. The tumor may be composed of small cells only, but frequently it has a dimorphic population of small tumor cells and large cells resembling luteinized cells. Hyaline globules may be present.

20.3.3 Metastatic Malignancy

Metastases to the ovary can mimic, clinically and pathologically, a primary ovarian tumor. Common sources include carcinomas of the breast, stomach, pancreas, and colon. Involvement is usually bilateral. Metastatic genital cancers (endometrial, fallopian tube) and pancreatic and colorectal carcinomas are particularly difficult to distinguish from primary ovarian tumors. Metastases can be partially cystic, even though the primary tumor is not cystic. Metastatic signet ring carcinoma, usually from the stomach, is known as Krukenberg tumor. Numerous other tumors can involve the ovary, including lymphomas and leukemias, and may be encountered in FNA biopsy.

20.3.4 Other Female Genital Neoplasms

Endometrial Stromal Sarcoma

The cells generally resemble endometrial stromal cells |i20.37|, |i20.38|. The low-grade tumor is also known as endolymphatic stromal myosis. If benign glands are present, the diagnosis is adenosarcoma; if malignant glands are present, the diagnosis is malignant mixed mesodermal tumor (carcinosarcoma).

The cells are present in loose clusters and singly. The nuclei are plump, oval, and moderately pleomorphic. The chromatin is fine and bland, and one or more small nucleoli may be seen. The cytoplasm is fibrillar to syncytial and stains variably. Mitotic figures are frequent in high-grade tumors.

Malignant Mixed Mesodermal (Müllerian) Tumor

Malignant mixed mesodermal tumor (MMMT) also is known as carcinosarcoma. However, the sarcomatous elements are probably metaplastic, derived from the epithelial component, rather than truly mesenchymal in origin. The specific diagnosis is possible if both components are aspirated. However, poorly differentiated adenocarcinoma may be the only finding in FNA biopsy |i20.39|, |i20.40|. The adenocarcinomatous component also can be papillary, endometrioid, squamous, or clear cell type. The sarcomatous component is usually characterized by the presence of spindle-shaped cells. Heterologous elements, eg, skeletal muscle or cartilage, also could be seen.

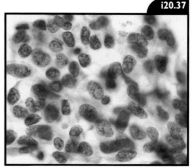

Endometrial stromal sarcoma (P)

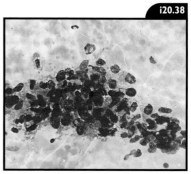

Endometrial stromal sarcoma (DQ)

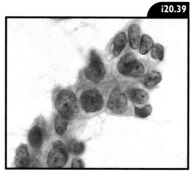

MMMT—carcinomatous component (P)

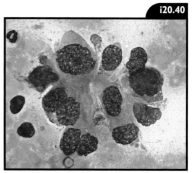

MMMT—carcinomatous component (DQ)

Microbiology

Xenogenous organisms are the subject of this appendix, which is something of a rogues' gallery of microbiologic agents. For more detailed information, please consult a microbiology textbook.

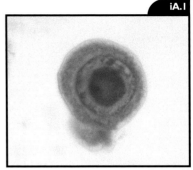
Cytomegalovirus (P)

A.1 Viruses

Cytomegalovirus is characterized by large cells, usually with an enlarged single nucleus (occasionally multinucleated but not molded as in herpes) and large, smooth, amphophilic intranuclear inclusions with a prominent halo in Papanicolaou stain |**iA.1**|. In Diff-Quik stain, the nucleus is enlarged and homogeneous; the halo is not visible. Small satellite nuclear or cytoplasmic inclusions sometimes occur and are better visualized in Diff-Quik stain.

Herpesvirus (simplex or zoster) produces cytologic changes characterized by the three Ms, multinucleation, molding of nuclei, and margination of chromatin, resulting in a diagnostically important ground-glass chromatin pattern. Intranuclear inclusions may be prominent, particularly in secondary infections. |**iA.2**|, |**iA.3**|.

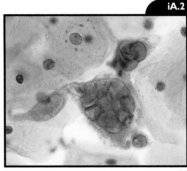
Herpes (P)

Human papillomavirus is characterized by koilocytes, which are pathognomonic. Koilocytes are mature squamous cells with nuclear dysplasia and cytoplasmic halos. The nuclei are enlarged and hyperchromatic; the halos are clear and well-defined with condensation of the peripheral cytoplasm. Binucleation is common (see Chapter 1).

Human polyomavirus is marked by decoy cells, which have large, dark, smudgy nuclear inclusions. They are usually found in transitional cells and, rarely, other cell types (see Chapter 5).

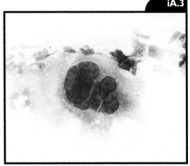
Herpes, air-dried Tzanck prep (DQ)

Molluscum contagiosum is a poxvirus that causes a skin disease (that in the case of sexual transmission can involve vulva and vagina) characterized by large cells filled with dense, red or polychromatic intracytoplasmic inclusions (ie, molluscum bodies) that compress the degenerated or pyknotic nucleus to the periphery of the cell |**iA.4**|.

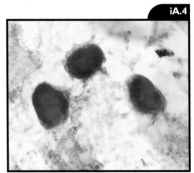
Molluscum contagiosum

A.2 Bacteria

Mycobacteria are not visible with the Papanicolaou or Diff-Quik stain. However, a negative image can sometimes be seen with Diff-Quik when the organisms are abundant (as they

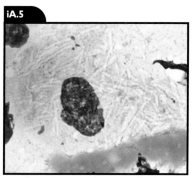

Mycobacteria—negative image (DQ)

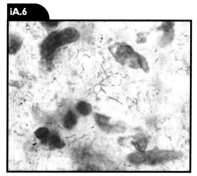

Mycobacteria (acid-fast)

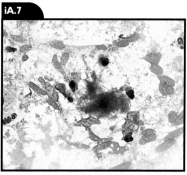

Actinomycosis, cervicofacial (P)

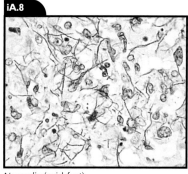

Nocardia (acid-fast)

may be in patients with AIDS) |**iA.5**|; in most of these cases, the organisms are *Mycobacterium avium-intracellulare,* but other types of mycobacteria as well as other entities can produce this finding. The acid-fast stain can confirm the presence of long, red, beaded rods in mycobacterial infection |**iA.6**|. The sensitivity of cytology alone is low; mycobacterial culture is recommended for conclusive diagnosis.

Bacteria can be seen in Papanicolaou- and Diff-Quik–stained smears. Although the shape (eg, coccoid, bacillary) and groupings (eg, clusters, strings) can be identified with these stains, it cannot be determined whether a bacterium is gram-positive or gram-negative without the Gram stain.

Lactobacilli (aka Döderlein bacilli and *Bacillus vaginalis*) are a heterogeneous group of rod-like bacteria that comprise the normal vaginal flora. Enzymes of these bacteria may cause cytolysis, leaving naked nuclei (see Chapter 1).

Gardnerella vaginalis produces a velvety coating of small coccobacilli on random squamous cells, the so-called clue cells, which are clues to the presence of *Gardnerella.* This bacterium can be normal but also may be associated with bacterial vaginosis or "shift in vaginal flora" (see Chapter 1).

Actinomyces organisms may be no more than a saprophyte from tonsils, but occasionally they cause invasive disease with abscess formation and "sulfur granules," followed by scar |**iA.7**|. The organisms are branching filamentous bacilli that tend to stain red in Papanicolaou stain and are frequently associated with other symbiotic bacteria ("dust bunnies"). Clusters may form radiate arrays of bacteria with club-shaped ends, due to the Splendore-Hoeppli phenomenon (antigen-antibody reaction).

Nocardia is a delicately branched, gram-positive, variably acid-fast, filamentous organism associated with respiratory infections but becoming a more frequent finding in central nervous system and subcutaneous infections |**iA.8**|.

Chlamydia trachomatis is a very small intracellular microorganism that is the most common cause of nongonococcal urethritis and cervicitis. Cellular changes include the formation of vacuoles with distinct outlines, which occur with cyanophilic granular inclusions. However, the Pap smear is considered unreliable in its diagnosis. Tissue culture, monoclonal antibodies, or enzyme-linked immunoassays can provide definitive diagnosis.

A.3 Fungi

Alternaria is a pigmented fungus that is usually a stain contaminant and only rarely a pathogen. Its most characteristic feature is a snowshoe-like appearance |**iA.9**|.

Aspergillus (fumigatus, niger) is characterized by a 45° angle branching of true septate hyphae of uniform 3- to 6-μm width |**iA.10**|. Rarely, fruiting heads (conidiophores) are observed. *Aspergillus* (especially *Aspergillus niger*) may be associated with needle-like birefringent calcium oxalate crystals that may form rosettes or wheat sheaf–like clusters. Aspergillosis also can produce cellular atypia mimicking cancer, or it can be associated with actual cancer. Uniform thickness and septa differentiate this organism from *Mucor*; true hyphae and septa differentiate it from *Candida*.

Blastomyces (dermatitidis) organisms are 8 to 15 μm in diameter with refractile cell walls. Broad-based budding (like snowmen) is characteristic. No hyphae are found |**iA.11**|.

Candida (albicans, and other species) is a common inhabitant of the oropharynx and female genital tract. Probably the most commonly encountered fungus, it is often of little or no clinical importance but may be a nuisance and occasionally is life-threatening. Some remember the pattern of pseudohyphae and yeasts as "sticks and stones," respectively. The yeast form is typically 2 to 4 μm in diameter and forms buds. Pseudohyphae (ie, elongated yeasts) occur with additional buds to form what look like "balloon dogs." No true hyphae or septa are found. *Candida* (formerly *Torulopsis) glabrata* is a small yeast-like fungus, without pseudohyphae.

Coccidioides (immitis) is characterized by spherules and endospores. Spherules are nonbudding and thick-walled and measure 20 to 60 μm, and occasionally they are larger than 100 μm. They may be empty or contain round nonbudding endospores measuring 1 to 5 μm. A full spherule resembles a bag of marbles, which when it endosporulates, ruptures; an empty spherule can mimic *Blastomyces*. Arthrospores, similar in appearance to those of *Geotrichum*, or hyphae also may occur.

Cryptococcus (neoformans) organisms measure 5 to 20 μm, but most are on the small end of that range. A very thick, gelatinous capsule (clear zone) may render it almost invisible (ergo, the name "crypto") without special stains such as mucicarmine, alcian blue, or PAS. The mucoid capsule stains red (with variable intensity) with mucicarmine. Single teardrop-shaped budding is characteristic (compare with *Blastomyces*) |**iA.12**|. Infection may elicit little or no inflammatory response or a granulomatous one.

Geotrichum (candidum) produces septate hyphae, spheric cells, and rectangular arthrospores and may branch (at a 90° angle) from the midportion of the hypha without an intervening septum. Because *G candidum* is endogenous and not particularly virulent, its isolation in sputum or feces is not a cause for concern in an asymptomatic person.

Histoplasma (capsulatum) is a small organism, measuring 1 to 5 μm. It is a round to oval budding yeast, which must be identi-

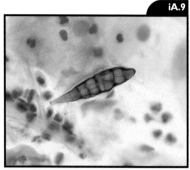

Alternaria—"snow shoe" (P)

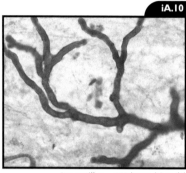

Aspergillus—45° branching (P)

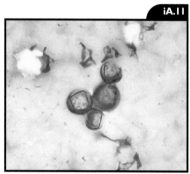

Blastomyces—broad-based budding (P)

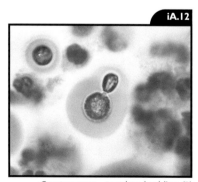

Cryptococcus—teardrop budding (P)

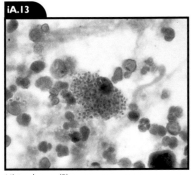

Histoplasma (P)

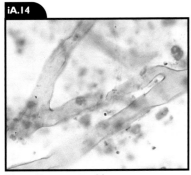

Mucor, Zygomycetes (P)

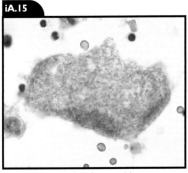

Pneumocystis—alveolar cyst (P)

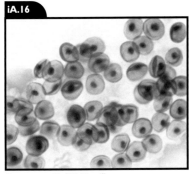

Pneumocystis (GMS, oil)

fied within cytoplasm of a histiocyte or neutrophil to be diagnostic and to differentiate it from similar appearing, but extracellular, contaminants |**iA.13**|. Gomori-methenamine silver (GMS) stain is helpful because the organism is not well visualized with routine stains.

Paracoccidioides (*brasiliensis*) is a round to oval yeast, 4 to 60 μm in diameter (though most are in the 5-30 μm range), with distinctive "ship's wheel" multiple budding. In addition to the unique budding formation, which is often inconspicuous because single and nonbudding cells are more frequent, the marked size variation is highly characteristic.

Zygomycetes (*Mucor, Rhizopus,* etc) exhibit broad (from 5-20 μm), irregular, thin-walled, ribbon-like hyphae with few septations that branch at irregular intervals, often at 90° angles |**iA.14**|. The thin walls often allow for extensive folding, twisting, and wrinkling of the hyphae.

Pneumocystis (*carinii*), though commonly classified as a parasite, is now thought to be a fungus. Formerly rare, the organism has become a common problem with the AIDS epidemic. Organisms often are seen in foamy or flocculent alveolar casts (rounded masses of organisms). Casts stain eosinophilic to basophilic in Papanicolaou stain, but the organisms themselves stain poorly or not at all in Papanicolaou stain, although overlapping ringlets may be seen |**iA.15**|. The alveolar casts are almost diagnostic, but their appearance can be closely mimicked, eg, by aggregates of RBC ghosts; therefore, a special stain may be used to confirm. In GMS, the cell wall of a cyst stains black, often with a central dark dot |**iA.16**|. Cysts are 4 to 8 μm in diameter (slightly smaller than RBCs) and spherical or cup-shaped. The cell wall does not stain in Diff-Quik stain, but a negative image may be seen against a purple background |**iA.17**|. Trophozoites, up to eight per cyst, are about 0.5 to 1.0 μm in diameter. Trophozoites stain in Diff-Quik (tiny purple dots) but not in GMS. Infection is seldom associated with an inflammatory response.

A.4 Parasites

Cryptosporidium is a round, basophilic, protozoal organism normally encountered as oocysts, measuring 2 to 4 μm, that may resemble platelets (which tend to clump) or yeasts (which may bud) |**iA.18**|. The organisms can be visualized with Papanicolaou stain but are better appreciated with an acid-fast or Diff-Quik stain. Oocysts stain vividly red with acid-fast stain. Note the presence of black granules within the oocysts. The organism is associated with the brush border of gastrointestinal tract cells.

Echinococcus granulosus (hydatid disease) often is considered a contraindication to biopsy due to possible anaphylaxis, but has been aspirated with fine needles with no untoward effects (see Chapter 9). Carmine-stained hydatid "sand" aspirated from a hydatid cyst shows scoleces of *Echinococcus* and their hooks |**iA.19**|. Hydatid cysts may form in any tissue but are most common in liver, lung, and the central nervous system.

Entamoeba histolytica is an ameba with trophozoites that characteristically display a prominent vesicular nucleus with a dot-like central karyosome. Cytoplasm is finely granular. A finding of ingested RBCs is considered diagnostic. Trophozoites are encountered most often in the colon and cecum, although invasive forms may be found in a number of organs, including liver, lung, and brain.

Entamoeba gingivalis, like *E histolytica*, produces trophozoites, usually recovered from the oral cavity (it rarely has been reported to occur also in vaginal and cervical smears), that have a small nucleus with a dot-like central karyosome. Unlike *E histolytica*, however, only ingested WBCs will be found, which may sometimes push the nucleus into an eccentric position.

Enterobius vermicularis (pinworm) often is found as eggs (~ 20 × 60 μm), which are ovoid with a double-walled shell that is distinctly flattened on one side. Adult worms also may be encountered occasionally.

Paragonimus (*kellicotti*, *westermani*) eggs are found in fecal matter and in sputum (and occasionally as a vaginal contaminant). They measure approximately 100 μm long, are golden yellow and oval, and have a flattened thick operculum at one end and a rounded thickened shell at the opposite end.

Schistosoma haematobium and *Schistosoma mansoni* ova resemble large uric acid (lemon drop) crystals and are identified by their characteristic lateral and terminal spine, respectively |**iA.20**|.

Strongyloides (*stercoralis*) usually is identified in the form of rhabditoid larvae (180-380 μm long) in human feces. However, filariform (infective-stage) larvae have been recovered from sputum in some cases of hemorrhagic pulmonary infection. Filariform larvae measure 400 to 500 μm and have a closed gullet and an often hard-to-detect notched tail.

Trichomonas (*vaginalis*) is a pear-shaped organism with an elliptical nucleus, red cytoplasmic granules, and flagella. The diagnostic rule of thumb is you must see the nucleus for diagnosis, you may see the red granules in the cytoplasm, but you will never see the flagellum in Pap smears (see Chapter 1). When *Leptothrix* is present, trichomonads also are usually present, but the reverse does not hold (ie, *Trichomonas* often is present without *Leptothrix*).

Trichuris trichiura eggs (~ 25 × 50 μm) are barrel-shaped, thick-shelled, and yellow-brown with unmistakable mucoid polar prominences that are simply called "polar plugs." They rarely are found outside the large intestine, cecum, and appendix.

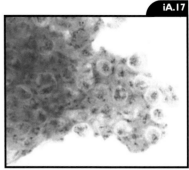

iA.17

Pneumocystis (DQ)

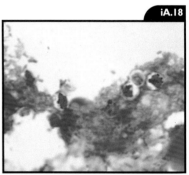

iA.18

Cryptosporidium (acid-fast, oil)

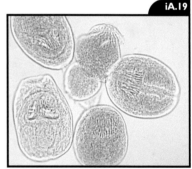

iA.19

Echinococcus—hydatid disease

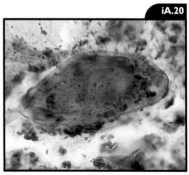

iA.20

Schistosoma, Pap smear (P)

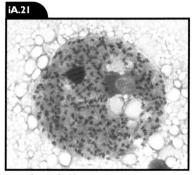

Toxoplasma (DQ)

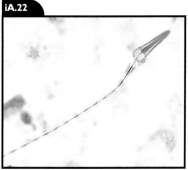

Carpet beetle part (P)

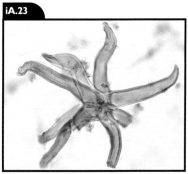

Trichome (P)

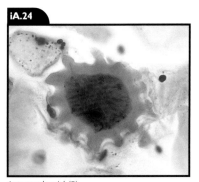

Asterosclereid (P)

Toxoplasma gondii trophozoites are oval to crescent-shaped and measure from 4 to 8 µm long and 2 to 3 µm wide |**iA.21**|. They have relatively large nuclei. Tissue cysts measure between 5 and 50 µm and take different shapes: they are spherical in the brain and more elongated in cardiac and skeletal muscle. Organisms are best visualized by Diff-Quik, PAS, or immunocytochemical stains.

A.5 Arthropods

Arthropods such as the mite, which looks every bit like a tiny crab, sometimes find their way into cytologic samples.

Carpet beetle parts, which can be found in a Pap smear, may be introduced as a contaminant, eg, from a cotton applicator or tampon |**iA.22**|.

A.6 Contaminants

Trichomes are filamentous outgrowths, especially an epidermal hair structure on a plant. Many plants contain trichomes of different size, shape, and color |**iA.23**|.

Asterosclereids are another contaminant derived from higher plants and trees |**iA.24**|.

Pollen appears as colorful bodies with cell walls and spikes. It can be a most attractive contaminant.

Glove powder is now made up of starch crystals (talc is no longer used). This contaminant may obscure cells, when abundant, or may be phagocytosed by cells, producing a signet ring–like appearance. Maltese cross birefringence also is characteristic of starch granules.

Lubricant is a sticky purple-staining material that can interfere with screening by obscuring cells.

INDEX

Numbers in **boldface** refer to pages on which images, figures, and tables appear.

I

M

U